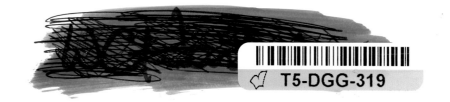

WALTER C. HARTEL, M.D.

Tumors
of the
Eye and Ocular Adnexa

Atlas
of
Tumor Pathology

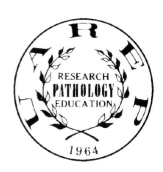

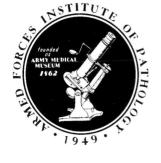

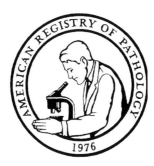

ATLAS OF TUMOR PATHOLOGY

Third Series
Fascicle 12

TUMORS OF THE EYE AND OCULAR ADNEXA

by

IAN W. MCLEAN, M.D.
Chairman, Department of Ophthalmic Pathology
Armed Forces Institute of Pathology
Washington, D.C.

MIGUEL N. BURNIER, M.D., Ph.D.
Professor of Ophthalmology and Pathology
Director, Eye Pathology Laboratory, and
Chairman, Department of Ophthalmology
McGill University
Montreal, Canada

LORENZ E. ZIMMERMAN, M.D.
Chairman Emeritus, Department of Ophthalmic Pathology
Armed Forces Institute of Pathology
Professor of Pathology and Ophthalmology, Georgetown University
Consultant in Ophthalmic Pathology
Washington Hospital Center
Washington, D.C.

FREDERICK A. JAKOBIEC, M.D.
Professor of Ophthalmology and Pathology
Chairman, Department of Ophthalmology, Harvard Medical School
Chief of Ophthalmology, Massachusetts Eye and Ear Infirmary
Boston, Massachusetts

Published by the
ARMED FORCES INSTITUTE OF PATHOLOGY
Washington, D.C.

Under the Auspices of
UNIVERSITIES ASSOCIATED FOR RESEARCH AND EDUCATION IN PATHOLOGY, INC.
Bethesda, Maryland
1994

Accepted for Publication
1993

Available from the American Registry of Pathology
Armed Forces Institute of Pathology
Washington, D.C. 20306-6000
ISSN 0160-6344
ISBN 1-881041-11-5

ATLAS OF TUMOR PATHOLOGY

EDITOR
JUAN ROSAI, M.D.
Department of Pathology
Memorial Sloan-Kettering Cancer Center
New York, New York 10021-6007

ASSOCIATE EDITOR
LESLIE H. SOBIN, M.D.
Armed Forces Institute of Pathology
Washington, D.C. 20306-6000

EDITORS' NOTE

The Atlas of Tumor Pathology has a long and distinguished history. It was first conceived at a Cancer Research Meeting held in St. Louis in September 1947 as an attempt to standardize the nomenclature of neoplastic diseases. The first series was sponsored by the National Academy of Sciences-National Research Council. The organization of this Sisyphean effort was entrusted to the Subcommittee on Oncology of the Committee on Pathology, and Dr. Arthur Purdy Stout was the first editor-in-chief. Many of the illustrations were provided by the Medical Illustration Service of the Armed Forces Institute of Pathology, the type was set by the Government Printing Office, and the final printing was done at the Armed Forces Institute of Pathology (hence the colloquial appellation "AFIP Fascicles"). The American Registry of Pathology purchased the Fascicles from the Government Printing Office and sold them virtually at cost. Over a period of 20 years, approximately 15,000 copies each of nearly 40 Fascicles were produced. The worldwide impact that these publications have had over the years has largely surpassed the original goal. They quickly became among the most influential publications on tumor pathology ever written, primarily because of their overall high quality but also because their low cost made them easily accessible to pathologists and other students of oncology the world over.

Upon completion of the first series, the National Academy of Sciences-National Research Council handed further pursuit of the project over to the newly created Universities Associated for Research and Education in Pathology (UAREP). A second series was started, generously supported by grants from the AFIP, the National Cancer Institute, and the American Cancer Society. Dr. Harlan I. Firminger became the editor-in-chief and was succeeded by Dr. William H. Hartmann. The second series Fascicles were produced as bound volumes instead of loose leaflets. They featured a more comprehensive coverage of the subjects, to the extent that the Fascicles could no longer be regarded as "atlases" but rather as monographs describing and illustrating in detail the tumors and tumor-like conditions of the various organs and systems.

Once the second series was completed, with a success that matched that of the first, UAREP and AFIP decided to embark on a third series. A new editor-in-chief and an associate editor were selected, and a distinguished editorial board was appointed. The mandate for the third series remains the same as for the previous ones, i.e., to oversee the production of an eminently practical publication with surgical pathologists as its primary audience, but also aimed at other workers in oncology. The main purposes of this series are to promote a consistent, unified, and biologically sound nomenclature; to guide the surgical pathologist in the diagnosis of the various tumors and tumor-like lesions; and to provide relevant histogenetic, pathogenetic, and clinicopathologic information on these entities. Just as the second series included data obtained from ultrastructural (and, in the more recent Fascicles, immunohistochemical) examination, the third series will, in addition, incorporate pertinent information obtained with the newer molecular biology techniques. As in the past, a continuous attempt will be made to correlate, whenever possible, the nomenclature used in the Fascicles with that proposed by the World Health Organization's International Histological Classification of Tumors. The format of the third series has been changed in order to incorporate additional items and to ensure a consistency of style throughout. This includes the dropping of the 's possessive in eponymic terms, in accordance with the WHO and the International Nomenclature of Diseases. Close cooperation between the various authors and their respective liaisons from the editorial board will be emphasized to minimize unnecessary repetition and discrepancies in the text and illustrations.

To its everlasting credit, the participation and commitment of the AFIP to this venture is even more substantial and encompassing than in previous series. It now extends to virtually all scientific, technical, and financial aspects of the production.

The task confronting the organizations and individuals involved in the third series is even more daunting than in the preceding efforts because of the ever-increasing complexity of the matter at hand. It is hoped that this combined effort—of which, needless to say, that represented by the authors is first and foremost—will result in a series worthy of its two illustrious predecessors and will be a suitable introduction to the tumor pathology of the twenty-first century.

Juan Rosai, M.D.
Leslie H. Sobin, M.D.

ACKNOWLEDGMENTS

There are a number of individuals whose help and support have contributed to this Fascicle. Our co-workers, particularly Dr. Ahmed A. Hidayat, who has performed much of the consultation for the Department of Ophthalmic Pathology while this Fascicle was in preparation; our colleagues, particularly Dr. Anne Osborne, Salt Lake City, and Dr. James Smirniotopoulos, Washington, who provided figures for this Fascicle; and our wives and families who have given up many evenings and weekends so that we could work on this Fascicle, all deserve special thanks and recognition.

Ian W. McLean, M.D.
Miguel N. Burnier, M.D.
Lorenz E. Zimmerman, M.D.
Frederick A. Jakobiec, M.D.

TUMORS OF THE EYE AND OCULAR ADNEXA

Contents

1. Introduction 1
2. Tumors of the Eyelid 7
   Anatomy and Histology 7
   Classification and Frequency 9
   Tumors of the Epidermis 11
      Squamous Cell Papilloma (Fibroepithelial Papilloma) 11
      Seborrheic Keratosis (Basal Cell Papilloma, Seborrheic Wart, Senile Verruca) 11
      Inverted Follicular Keratosis (Irritated Seborrheic Keratosis) 13
      Pseudocarcinomatous (Pseudoepitheliomatous) Hyperplasia 13
      Keratoacanthoma 14
      Actinic Keratosis (Solar Keratosis, Senile Keratosis) 14
      Bowen Disease 16
      Squamous Cell Carcinoma 17
      Basal Cell Carcinoma 18
   Benign Tumors of Eccrine and Apocrine Gland Origin 22
      Hydrocystoma 22
      Syringoma 22
      Eccrine Acrospiroma (Clear Cell Hidradenoma, Clear Cell Myoepithelioma,
         Eccrine Poroma, Porosyringoma) 22
      Pleomorphic Adenoma (Mixed Tumor of the Sweat Glands, Chondroid
         Syringoma) 24
   Malignant Tumors of Eccrine Sweat Gland Origin (Eccrine
      Adenocarcinoma) 24
   Apocrine Adenocarcinoma 28
   Sebaceous Gland Tumors 28
      Benign Tumors of Sebaceous Origin 28
      Sebaceous Carcinoma (Adenocarcinoma of Sebaceous Gland, Meibomian
         Gland Carcinoma, Zeis Gland Carcinoma) 28
   Tumors of Hair Follicle Origin 35
      Trichoepithelioma (Epithelioma Adenoides Cysticum, Multiple Benign
         Cystic Epithelioma, Brooke Tumor) 35
      Trichofolliculoma 35
      Trichilemmoma 36
      Pilomatrixoma (Calcifying Epithelioma of Malherbe) 36
   Adnexal Carcinoma 38
   Tumors of Melanocytes 38
   Tumors of Hematopoietic and Soft Tissues 38
      Hemangiomas 38
         Capillary Hemangioma (Juvenile Hemangioma, Strawberry Nevus, Nevus
            Vasculosus, Benign Hemangioendothelioma of Childhood) 38
         Nevus Flammeus (Port Wine Stain) 38
         Cavernous Hemangioma 39
   Miscellaneous Tumors 39

Phakomatous Choristoma 39
Merkel Cell Tumor (Trabecular Carcinoma of the Skin, Cutaneous APUDoma,
    Small Cell Neuroepithelial Tumor, Primary Small Cell Cutaneous Carcinoma,
    Neuroendocrine or Merkel Cell Carcinoma) 41
Carcinoma Metastatic to the Eyelid 42

3. Tumors of the Conjunctiva 49
    Anatomy and Histology 49
      Gross Anatomic Features 49
      Microscopic Features 49
    Classification and Frequency 50
    Benign Tumors of Surface Epithelium 52
      Squamous Cell Papilloma 52
      Keratotic Plaque 53
      Pseudocarcinomatous Hyperplasia (Pseudoepitheliomatous Hyperplasia) 53
      Hereditary Benign Intraepithelial Dyskeratosis 53
    Intraepithelial Neoplasia of Surface Epithelium and Related Lesions 55
      Pinguecula, Pterygium, and Actinic Keratosis (Solar Keratosis) 55
      Dysplasia 55
      Carcinoma in Situ 59
    Malignant Tumors of Surface Epithelium 60
      Squamous Cell Carcinoma 60
      Mucoepidermoid Carcinoma 65
    Adnexal Tumors 69
      Oncocytoma (Oncocytic Adenoma, Oxyphilic Adenoma) 69
    Tumors of the Melanocytic System 72
      Nevi 72
      Melanosis 76
        Epithelial Congenital Melanosis 76
        Subepithelial Congenital Melanosis 76
        Secondary Melanosis 77
        Primary Acquired Melanosis (Atypical Melanocytic Hyperplasia,
          Malignant Melanoma in Situ, Benign Acquired Melanosis,
          Precancerous Melanosis) 78
    Malignant Melanoma 82
    Soft Tissue, Lymphoid, Hematopoietic, and Histiocytic Tumors 88
      Kaposi Sarcoma 88
    Choristomas 90
      Limbal Dermoid 91
      Dermolipoma 91

4. Tumors of the Retina 97
    Anatomy and Histology 97
      Retinal Pigment Epithelium 97
      Sensory (Neural) Retina 97
    Classification and Frequency 100
    Retinoblastoma, Retinocytoma, and Pseudoretinoblastoma 101
      Toxocara Canis Endophthalmitis 127
      Persistent Hyperplastic Primary Vitreous 127
      Coats Disease 130

Glial Tumors and Tumor-Like Conditions 135

    Astrocytoma 135

    Massive Gliosis 136

Vascular Tumors and Tumor-Like Conditions 136

    Angiomatosis Retinae (Hemangioblastoma, Capillary Hemangioma,
        von Hippel-Lindau Syndrome) 136

    Cavernous Hemangioma 136

Tumors of Hematopoietic and Lymphoid Tissues 138

    Malignant Lymphoma 138

    Leukemia 138

Neuroepithelial Tumors 142

    Glioneuroma 143

    Medulloepithelioma (Diktyoma, Teratoneuroma) 143

    Acquired Neuroepithelial Tumors of the Ciliary Body 145

    Fuchs Adenoma (Hyperplasia of the Nonpigmented Ciliary Epithelium,
        Pseudoadenomatous Hyperplasia, Coronal Adenoma) 145

    Adenomas of the Nonpigmented Ciliary Epithelium 145

    Carcinomas of the Nonpigmented Ciliary Epithelium 145

    Adenomas and Carcinomas of the Pigmented Ciliary Epithelium 148

    Adenomas and Carcinomas of the Retinal Pigment Epithelium 148

Metastatic Neoplasms 149

5. Tumors of the Uveal Tract 155

Anatomy and Histology 155

    The Iris 155

    The Ciliary Body 157

    The Choroid 157

Classification and Frequency 159

Melanocytic Nevi 159

Malignant Melanoma of the Uveal Tract 161

Hemangioma 195

Choroidal Osteoma 196

Leiomyoma and Mesectodermal Leiomyoma 197

Leukemia 202

Juvenile Xanthogranuloma 202

Well-Differentiated Small Lymphocytic or Lymphoplasmacytic Lymphoma
    and Secondary Lymphomas of the Uvea 204

Metastatic Tumors 207

6. Tumors of the Lacrimal Gland and Sac 215

Anatomy and Histology 215

Classification and Frequency 216

Pleomorphic Adenoma (Benign Mixed Tumor) 217

Pleomorphic Carcinoma (Malignant Mixed Tumor) 220

Adenoid Cystic Carcinoma 222

Adenocarcinoma Arising De Novo 225

Tumors of the Lacrimal Sac 227

    Epithelial Tumors (Papillomas and Carcinomas) 228

7. Tumors of the Orbit 233
    Anatomy and Histology 233
    Classification and Frequency 235
    Capillary Hemangioma 237
    Cavernous Hemangioma 237
    Lymphangioma 238
    Hemangiopericytoma 240
    Fibrous Histiocytoma (Fibroxanthoma) 244
    Fibromatosis (Myofibromatosis, Juvenile Fibromatosis) 249
    Fibrosarcoma (Juvenile Fibrosarcoma) 249
    Leiomyoma 249
    Leiomyosarcoma 250
    Rhabdomyosarcoma 250
    Lipoma 257
    Liposarcoma 258
    Neurofibromas 258
        Plexiform Neurofibroma 258
        Diffuse Neurofibroma 260
        Isolated Neurofibroma 260
    Schwannoma (Neurilemoma) 260
    Malignant Peripheral Nerve Sheath Tumors 262
    Lymphoid Tumors and Inflammation 263
        Inflammatory Pseudotumors 263
        Graves Orbitopathy 263
        Idiopathic Orbital Inflammation (Pseudotumors) 265
        Lymphoid Tumors 270
            Lymphoid Hyperplasia (Benign Lymphoid Tumor) 272
            Malignant Lymphomas 274
            Follicular Lymphomas 274
            Well-Differentiated and Intermediately Differentiated Diffuse
                Lymphomas 274
            Poorly Differentiated Diffuse Lymphomas 280
    Plasma Cell Tumors 282
    Leukemia (Granulocytic Sarcoma) 283
    Histiocytic Disorders 284
        Unifocal and Multifocal Eosinophilic Granuloma (Langerhans Cell
            Histiocytosis) 284
        Sinus Histiocytosis with Massive Lymphadenopathy 285
    Dermoid Cyst 287
    Teratoma 288
    Congenital Melanosis, Cellular Blue Nevus, and Primary Malignant
        Melanoma 289
    Fibrous Dysplasia 291
    Ossifying Fibroma (Juvenile Ossifying Fibroma, Psammomatoid
        Ossifying Fibroma) 291
    Osteogenic Sarcoma 292
    Secondary Tumors of the Orbit 292
    Metastatic Tumors 292

8. Tumors of the Optic Nerve and Optic Nerve Head 299
   Anatomy and Histology 299
   Classification and Frequency 300
   Melanocytoma (Magnocellular Nevus) 301
   Malignant Melanoma 304
   Juvenile Pilocytic Astrocytoma 304
   Malignant Astrocytoma of Optic Nerve and Chiasm 309
   Meningioma 309
   Secondary and Metastatic Optic Nerve Tumors 314

Index 317

TUMORS OF THE EYE AND OCULAR ADNEXA

1

INTRODUCTION

Much has changed regarding our knowledge of ophthalmic tumors since the last Fascicle on ophthalmic pathology was published 37 years ago (7). During this period, investigators documented the behavior of most ophthalmic tumors. Anatomic pathology now extends beyond morphology to molecular pathology. Immunohistochemistry has become a tool routinely used in the differential diagnosis of tumors. Techniques for analyzing alterations in tumor DNA are still experimental but close to practical application. Particularly exciting are the findings concerning the role that the retinoblastoma gene plays in neoplasia. Some of these discoveries are discussed in this Fascicle.

Many general pathologists have only limited experience with intraocular tumors. For this reason, this Fascicle is organized with lengthier discussions of the two most important intraocular tumors, retinoblastoma and uveal melanoma, and shorter discussions of extraocular tumors that have similar counterparts elsewhere in the body. The chapters are arranged anatomically. While having much in common with the skin elsewhere, the eyelid contains unique structures, the meibomian glands and the glands of Zeis and Moll, and is therefore a site of predilection for sebaceous and apocrine tumors. The conjunctiva differs from other mucous membranes because of the high levels of sun exposure it may receive. Actinically related tumors (keratoses, carcinomas, melanomas) are among the most common in the conjunctiva. The tumors of the lacrimal glands are similar to those of the salivary glands except for the Warthin tumor, common in the salivary glands but not seen in the lacrimal glands. Most tumors of the orbit are of lymphoid or soft tissue origin. For unknown reasons, the orbit is a site of predilection for extranodal lymphomas, fibrous histiocytomas, and, in children, rhabdomyosarcomas. The optic nerve has gliomas and

meningiomas in common with the rest of the central nervous system but there is a unique tumor of the optic nerve head, the melanocytoma. These and other features of ophthalmic tumors important to the pathologist are emphasized.

The tumor classification used in this Fascicle is based closely on the scheme proposed by the World Health Organization (WHO) (9). We have added tables with tumor frequencies based on the Armed Forces Institute of Pathology (AFIP) experience and compare them with data from other registries and published series from around the world. Table 1-1 provides comparative frequencies for all ophthalmic neoplasms contained in the AFIP Registry of Ophthalmic Pathology (ROP) and the Brazilian ROP between 1984 and 1989. These tumors are divided on the same anatomic basis as the chapters of this Fascicle. To our knowledge, the Brazilian Registry is the only other data set that provides frequencies of all ophthalmic tumors using the WHO classification.

To better interpret these data, one must be aware of the biases in these data bases. The major bias in both registries is referral. All of the cases in the AFIP Registry are referred by other pathologists who only send selected cases; this registry is weighted with cases that are diagnostically difficult or unusual. This referral bias probably accounts for the lower proportion of eyelid tumors, particularly basal cell carcinoma, in the AFIP Registry (Tables 1-1 and 2-1). Although the Brazilian ROP is hospital based at the Paulista School of Medicine, it also has referral cases. Because this is a teaching hospital, the patients may be selected for unusual diseases. Neither data base represents a random sample of ophthalmic tumors.

We compared the data in the AFIP and Brazilian Registries with data collected by the Surveillance Epidemiology and End Results Study (SEERS) (8). Unfortunately, the SEERS does not

Table 1-1

TUMORS OF THE EYE
AND OCULAR ADNEXA*

Location of Tumor	Number of Cases	
	A-ROP**	B-ROP+
Eyelid	846	869
Conjunctiva	1258	476
Retina	268	150
Uvea	760	148
Lacrimal gland	53	18
Lacrimal sac	33	9
Orbit	396	182
Optic nerve	34	17

*Frequency distribution of 3648 tumors in the AFIP Registry of Ophthalmic Pathology and 1869 tumors in the Brazilian Registry of Ophthalmic Pathology collected between 1984 and 1989.
**AFIP Registry of Ophthalmic Pathology.
+Brazilian Registry of Ophthalmic Pathology.

provide the anatomic site of the eye tumors so that we can only make comparisons of individual tumor types. Because the SEERS data are collected from a defined population in selected areas of the United States, a comparison should provide insight into the population bases of the Brazilian and AFIP Registries. Both registries contain a higher ratio of retinoblastomas to uveal melanomas than does the SEERS. The main reason for this is racial. The incidence of uveal melanoma decreases with increasing racial pigmentation. The Brazilian population and the many cases from Africa and Asia in the AFIP Registry, referred from hospitals without histopathology support, reflect more heavily pigmented individuals than the United States population sampled by the SEERS. A second reason for the excess number of retinoblastomas in the ophthalmic registries is that the patients from Brazil, Africa, and Asia are significantly younger than those from the United States.

Most ophthalmologists in the United States do not use the TNM grading system (5) widely used in Europe and Asia. For this reason, we recommend that pathologists report the tumor measurements and a description of the prognostic features that are present or absent. Because

prognostic factors are often multiple, we and others (3) suggest using multivariate statistical models. Such prognostication can be provided as part of the pathology report or as a separate communication to the clinician.

Cytopathologic diagnosis was not widely used in ophthalmic pathology until recently. The use of modern noninvasive imaging techniques to make a more accurate clinical diagnosis and better localize the tumor is probably the major factor advancing cytopathologic diagnosis in ophthalmic pathology. With experience, pathologists can provide accurate diagnoses on specimens obtained by fine needle aspiration (FNA), conjunctival scrapings, and vitrectomy. Most lesions of the eyelids and orbit can be approached by FNA. Diseases confined to the cornea and the conjunctiva are more often scraped. Vitrectomy is used to obtain an appropriate intraocular cytologic specimen.

Pars plana vitrectomy is used to remove intraocular tissues, such as vitreous, organized fibrovascular membranes, blood, lens fragments, and other types of inflammatory debris. In addition to these therapeutic applications, vitrectomy can also be performed for diagnostic purposes. The large amount of fluid obtained with vitrectomy is processed by the membrane filter technique, cytocentrifugation, and the celloidin-bag technique (4). Techniques that produce a cell block permit histologic processing and preparation of multiple sections used for special stains and immunohistochemistry.

Diagnostic vitrectomy is used to differentiate neoplasms and simulating lesions. In children, retinoblastoma (pl. IA) must be distinguished from inflammatory and developmental lesions. In adults, primary ocular lymphoma (pls. IB, IC, IIA) needs to be differentiated from uveitis (2).

The orbit may contain a wide variety of developmental, inflammatory, and neoplastic lesions. Developmental lesions that can be diagnosed by FNA include dermoid cysts, epithelial inclusion cysts, and ectopic lacrimal gland tissues. Ectopic lacrimal glands have acini with normal cytologic features and should not be misinterpreted as adenocarcinomas, whose nuclei have malignant cytologic features. Precise localization by computerized tomography (CT) or magnetic resonance imaging (MRI) differentiates ectopic from normal lacrimal glands (1).

PLATE I

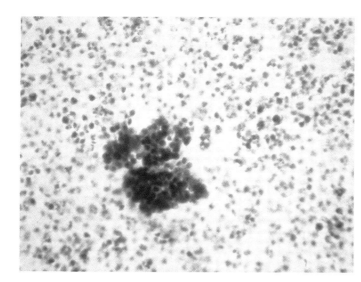

A. RETINOBLASTOMA
Cytologic preparation with both clumps and individual tumor cells.

B. PRIMARY INTRAOCULAR LYMPHOMA
Cytologic preparation of large atypical lymphocytes.

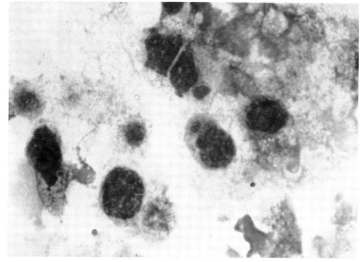

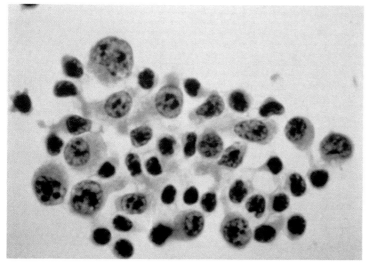

C. PRIMARY INTRAOCULAR LYMPHOMA
Cytologic preparation with marked variation in size of the lymphocytes.

PLATE II

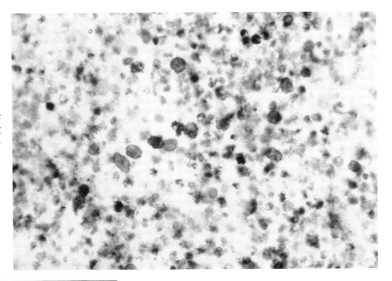

A. PRIMARY INTRAOCULAR LYMPHOMA

Immunohistochemistry of cytologic preparation with B-cell marker staining the plasma membranes of the atypical lymphocytes.

B. ORBITAL LEUKEMIC INFILTRATE OF GRANULOCYTIC SARCOMA

Immunohistochemistry of cytologic preparation for lysozyme.

C. ORBITAL RHABDOMYOSARCOMA

Fine needle aspiration cytologic preparation of cells with long cytoplasmic processes and atypical nuclei. Insert: Immunohistochemistry for muscle-specific actin.

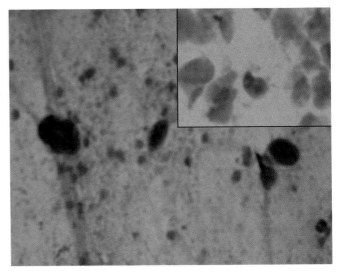

Orbital inflammatory lesions are diagnosed by FNA, including granulomatous inflammation. Special stains are very helpful in determining the nature of these granulomas. Caseous necrosis is usually observed with tuberculosis, noncaseating granulomas with sarcoidosis, and Touton giant cells with juvenile xanthogranuloma.

Benign lymphoproliferative disease may be very difficult to differentiate from malignant lymphoma using FNA. Architectural and cellular details are crucial for distinction. Mixed mononuclear populations favor a benign diagnosis. Leukemic infiltrates (granulocytic sarcoma) can also present as an orbital tumor. Immuno-histochemistry plays a crucial role in establishing the definitive diagnosis (pl. IIB).

Orbital malignant neoplasms, other than lymphoma, include soft tissue sarcomas such as rhabdomyosarcoma (pl. IIC) and primary, secondary, and metastatic melanomas and carcinomas. Because of the broad differential diagnosis, immunohistochemistry may be essential for differentiation (6).

Successful cytologic evaluation of the eye and adnexa depends on wise patient selection, a team of skilled individuals, and particularly, a good interaction between the ophthalmologist, radiologist, and pathologist.

REFERENCES

1. Arora R, Rewari R, Betheria SM. Fine needle aspiration biopsy of eyelid tumors. Acta Cytol 1990;34:227–32.
2. Char DH, Ljung BM, Deschenes J, Miller TR. Intraocular lymphoma: immunological and cytological analysis. Br J Ophthalmol 1988;72:905–11.
3. Fielding LP, Henson DE. Multiple prognostic factors and outcome analysis in patients with cancer. Communication from the American Joint Committee on Cancer. Cancer 1993;71:2426–9.
4. Green WR. Diagnostic cytopathology of ocular fluid specimens. Ophthalmology 1984;91:726-49.
5. Hermanek P, Sobin LH. TNM classification of malignant tumors. 4th ed, 2nd revision. Berlin: Springer-Verlag, 1992:161–88.
6. Kennerdell JS, Slamovits TL, Dekker A, Johnson BL. Orbital fine-needle aspiration biopsy. Am J Ophthalmol 1985;99:547–51.
7. Reese AB. Tumors of the eye and adnexa. Atlas of Tumor Pathology, First Series, Fascicle 38. Washington, D.C.: Armed Forces Institute of Pathology, 1956.
8. Young JL Jr, Percy CL, Asire AJ, et al. Cancer incidence and mortality in the United States, 1973-77. In: Young JL, Percy CL, Asire AJ, eds. National Cancer Institute Monograph 57. Surveillance, epidemiology, and end results: incidence and mortality data, 1973-77. Bethesda, Md.: National Institutes of Health, 1981:157–8.
9. Zimmerman LE, Sobin LH. Histologic typing of tumours of the eye and its adnexa. International Histological Classification of Tumours No. 24. Geneva: World Health Organization, 1984.

2

TUMORS OF THE EYELID

ANATOMY AND HISTOLOGY

The anatomy of eyelids is modified from that of the skin elsewhere to permit greater motility. The eyelids are composed of four layers: skin, muscle, tarsus, and conjunctiva (figs. 2-1, 2-2). The palpebral conjunctiva forms the innermost layer and the epidermis the most external layer. Within the dermis, a circularly oriented striated muscle (orbicularis oculi) closes the lids. Because the orbicularis oculi muscle is superficial, benign lesions of the dermis, such as compound nevi, can involve the muscle without being invasive. There are few places in the body where striated muscle comes as close to the surface epidermis as the orbicularis muscle. The skin of the eyelids has great elasticity and the subcutaneous tissue is loose. These features make the skin of the lids more delicate than skin elsewhere in the body.

The tarsi are semilunar plates of fibroelastic tissue that provide rigidity to the lids. The tarsal plate in the upper lid (fig. 2-1) is about twice as long as the tarsal plate in the lower lid (fig. 2-2). The meibomian sebaceous glands (fig. 2-3) are oriented vertically in the tarsi. There are 30 to 40 meibomian glands in the upper tarsus and 20 to 30 in the lower tarsus. Accessory lacrimal glands (glands of Wolfring) are located at the superior edge of the upper tarsus. The stroma of the palpebral conjunctiva is very thin and adherent to the tarsi. At the mucocutaneous junction, the epithelium of the conjunctiva is stratified squamous; it becomes stratified columnar with goblet cells in the tarsal area.

The orbitopalpebral sulcus (the superior palpebral furrow) subdivides the upper lids into a preorbital portion and a lower pretarsal region. The striated fibers of the levator palpebrae superioris insert anteriorly into a compact fibrous membrane that forms the levator aponeurosis. The levator aponeurosis attaches to the medial and lateral portions of the orbital rim and sends collagenous bands through the orbital septum between bundles of the orbicularis muscle into the dermis. The smooth muscle of Müller originates among the fibers of the levator palpebrae superioris in the upper lid and the inferior rectus in the lower eyelid. The fibers of both the

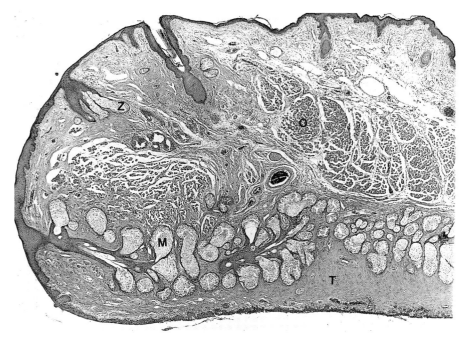

Figure 2-1
NORMAL UPPER EYELID
Structures of the eyelid include cilia, Zeis glands (Z), orbicularis muscle (O), and meibomian glands (M) located within the tarsal plate (T).

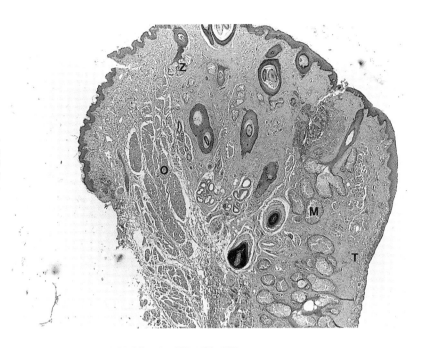

Figure 2-2
NORMAL LOWER EYELID
Structures of the lower eyelid include cilia, Zeis glands (Z), orbicularis muscle (O), and meibomian glands (M) located within the tarsal plate (T). They are similar to those of upper eyelid except that the tarsal plate is smaller.

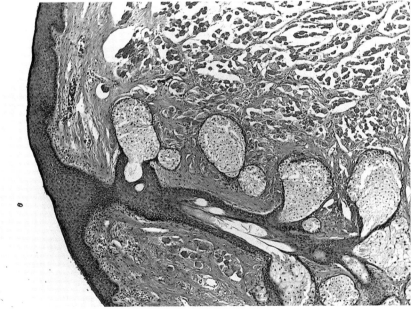

Figure 2-3
NORMAL
MEIBOMIAN GLAND
Sebaceous lobules connect to a sebaceous duct where the ductal epithelium forms valve-like structures.

superior and inferior muscles of Müller insert into the tarsal plates and the dense collagenous tissue attached to the deep fibers of the orbicularis muscle. Modifications of these muscular structures may cause ptosis, ectropion, or entropion. Bundles of orbicularis muscle fibers extend to the margin of the eyelids (muscle of Riolan). At the lid margin are cilia (about 150 cilia in the upper lid and 75 in the lower lid). Associated with the follicles of the eye lashes are large sebaceous glands (glands of Zeis) and large apocrine glands (glands of Moll).

The junction between skin and conjunctiva is located near the posterior edge of the lid margin, just posterior to the openings of the meibomian gland ducts. Anterior to the openings and posterior to the lashes is a pigment sulcus (gray line) extending over most of the length of the eyelid. Surgically, the lids can be split along this landmark into two layers: an anterior layer composed of skin and orbicularis muscle and a posterior layer formed of tarsus and conjunctiva.

The lacrimal puncta, which remove tears from the conjunctiva, are located in the medial aspects of the upper and lower lids; these drain via the canaliculi into the lacrimal sac and then through the nasolacrimal duct into the nose. The pretarsal portion of the orbicularis muscle inserts onto the fascia of the sac and provides a pumping mechanism.

A variety of epidermal appendages are present in the eyelids. The sebaceous glands are of three types: the glands of Zeis are associated with the lashes, the meibomian glands are located in the tarsal plates, and small pilosebaceous units cover the eyelids. In contrast to the apocrine glands of Moll that are related to the lashes, the eccrine sweat glands are located throughout the skin of the eyelids.

The arterial blood supply of the lids is derived mainly from the ophthalmic and lacrimal arteries through their medial and lateral branches. The veins of the eyelids are situated in the upper and lower fornices of the conjunctiva, forming a dense plexus. They are larger and more numerous than the arteries. They drain into the veins of the forehead and the branches of the ophthalmic vein. The lymphatic drainage system is composed of the pretarsal and post-tarsal plexuses that communicate with each other by cross channels. The lymphatics of the outer two thirds of the upper lid and outer one third of the lower lid drain to the preauricular lymph nodes. The lymphatics of the inner two thirds of the lower lid and inner one third of the upper lid drain to the submandibular lymph nodes.

CLASSIFICATION AND FREQUENCY

The many types of tumors that occur in the eyelid reflect the diversity of tissues that are present. Most of these tumors are similar to the same types of tumors observed in other sun-exposed areas of the skin. The most important exceptions to this generalization are the tumors of the specialized sebaceous glands of the eyelid. Sebaceous gland tumors are rarely seen in other parts of the body.

The classification of the World Health Organization (WHO) provides a framework that divides the tumors of the eyelids into groups based on their origin (Tables 2-1–2-8). There is differing opinion on the WHO classification of Bowen

Table 2-1

EPIDERMAL TUMORS OF THE EYELID*

Type of Tumor	Number of Cases
Benign	
Squamous cell papilloma	18
Seborrheic keratosis (basal cell papilloma)	23
Inverted follicular keratosis	28
Pseudocarcinomatous hyperplasia	21
Keratoacanthoma	5
Keratosis, NOS***	13
Premalignant	
Actinic keratosis (senile keratosis)	19
Bowen precancerous dermatosis (in situ carcinoma)	5
Malignant	
Squamous cell carcinoma	50
Basal cell carcinoma	107
Carcinoma, NOS	11

*Frequency distribution of 300 tumors in the AFIP Registry of Ophthalmic Pathology collected between 1984 and 1989.
***NOS = Not otherwise specified.

disease as a premalignant rather than a malignant lesion. There has always been debate as to whether in situ carcinoma is malignant or premalignant, but the more recent tendency is to group dysplasia and carcinoma in situ together as intraepithelial neoplasia, as with the WHO classification of respiratory and uterine cervical neoplasms. In his discussion of eyelid tumors, Font (3) also classifies Bowen disease as a premalignant tumor. One justification for the premalignant designation is that if these lesions are not treated they do not invariably progress to invasive cancer.

The frequency distributions of tumors of the eyelid in the Armed Forces Institute of Pathology (AFIP) Registry of Ophthalmic Pathology (ROP) (Tables 2-1–2-8) reflect the tendency of pathologists to refer difficult and unusual tumors to the AFIP for consultation. In the AFIP ROP, squamous cell carcinoma, sebaceous carcinoma, eccrine and apocrine carcinomas, Merkel cell tumors, and

Table 2-2

TUMORS OF ECCRINE AND APOCRINE GLANDS OF THE EYELID*

Type of Tumor	Number of Cases
Benign	
Hidrocystoma	29
Syringoma	8
Eccrine spiradenoma	0
Eccrine acrospiroma (clear cell hidradenoma)	15
Pleomorphic adenoma (mixed tumor, chondroid syringoma)	15
Papillary syringoadenoma (syringocystadenoma papilliferum)	2
Eccrine dermal cylindroma	1
Apocrine adenoma or cystadenoma	14
Adenoma, NOS**	13
Malignant	
Malignant counterparts of benign tumors	0
Adenocarcinoma, mucous secreting	18
Adenocarcinoma, NOS	15

*Frequency distribution of 130 tumors in the AFIP Registry of Ophthalmic Pathology collected between 1984 and 1989.
**NOS = Not otherwise specified.

Table 2-3

TUMORS OF SEBACEOUS GLANDS OF THE EYELID*

Type of Tumor	Number of Cases
Benign	
Sebaceous hyperplasia	4
Sebaceous adenoma	16
Malignant	
Sebaceous carcinoma	102

*Frequency distribution of 122 tumors in the AFIP Registry of Ophthalmic Pathology collected between 1984 and 1989.

Table 2-4

TUMORS OF PILAR STRUCTURES OF THE EYELID*

Type of Tumor	Number of Cases
Benign	
Trichoepithelioma	6
Trichofolliculoma	1
Trichilemmoma	24
Pilomatrixoma (calcifying epithelioma of Malherbe)	9
Pilar tumor, NOS**	5
Malignant	
Carcinoma	4

*Frequency distribution of 49 tumors in the AFIP Registry of Ophthalmic Pathology collected between 1984 and 1989.
**NOS = Not otherwise specified.

Table 2-5

TUMORS OF MELANOCYTIC ORIGIN OF THE EYELID*

Type of Tumor	Number of Cases
Benign	
Nevi	71
Lentigo simplex	3
Primary acquired melanosis (lentigo maligna)	9
Malignant	
Melanoma	18

*Frequency distribution of 101 tumors in the AFIP Registry of Ophthalmic Pathology collected between 1984 and 1989.

pilar tumors are more prevalent relative to basal cell carcinoma and other benign tumors than in most tumor registries. At the Wills Eye Hospital, 82.4 percent of the malignant tumors were basal cell carcinomas (4) and in the Brazilian ROP, 81.9 percent were basal cell carcinomas (2) compared with 27.8 percent in the AFIP Registry. Malignant tumors were 31.3 percent of the eyelid tumors at the Wills Eye Hospital (4), 38.8 percent in the Brazilian ROP (1,2), and 45.5 percent in the AFIP ROP.

Table 2-6

TUMORS OF LYMPHOCYTIC OR HEMATOPOIETIC ORIGIN OF THE EYELID*

Type of Tumor	Number of Cases
Benign	
Reactive lymphoid hyperplasia	11
Atypical lymphoid hyperplasia	8
Malignant	
Lymphoma	26
Leukemia	1

*Frequency distribution of 46 tumors in the AFIP Registry of Ophthalmic Pathology collected between 1984 and 1989.

Table 2-7

TUMORS OF SOFT TISSUE ORIGIN OF THE EYELID*

Type of Tumor	Number of Cases
Benign	
Lipoma	1
Neurofibroma	14
Schwannoma	3
Fibrous and/or histiocytic	18
Hemangiomas (capillary, nevus flammeus and cavernous)	7
Lymphangioma	1
Malignant	
Liposarcoma	0
Schwannoma	1
Fibrous histiocytoma	5
Rhabdomyosarcoma	4
Juvenile fibrosarcoma	1

*Frequency distribution of 55 tumors in the AFIP Registry of Ophthalmic Pathology collected between 1984 and 1989.

Table 2-8

MISCELLANEOUS TUMORS OF THE EYELID*

Type of Tumor	Number of Cases
Benign	
Phakomatous choristoma	0
Xanthomatous lesions	20
Granular cell tumor	1
Malignant	
Merkel cell tumor	12
Metastatic carcinomas	10

*Frequency distribution of 43 tumors in the AFIP Registry of Ophthalmic Pathology collected between 1984 and 1989.

TUMORS OF THE EPIDERMIS

Squamous Cell Papilloma (Fibroepithelial Papilloma)

Squamous cell papillomas are the most common benign lesions of the eyelid. They can be either sessile or pedunculated and have a color similar to that of the adjacent lid skin. Microscopically, these lesions are composed of finger-like projections of vascularized connective tissue covered by acanthotic epithelium, with focal hyperkeratosis and parakeratosis.

Seborrheic Keratosis (Basal Cell Papilloma, Seborrheic Wart, Senile Verruca)

Seborrheic keratosis is one of the most frequently observed benign skin lesions involving the eyelids of middle-aged and older individuals. The lesions vary from tan to black and are usually darker in heavily pigmented patients. They are well-demarcated, cerebriform excrescences, with a flat, slightly raised, friable surface. They vary in size from a few millimeters to several centimeters.

According to the predominant histologic features, the lesions are classified as three types: hyperkeratotic, acanthotic, and adenoid. Lesions composed of only one of these types are uncommon.

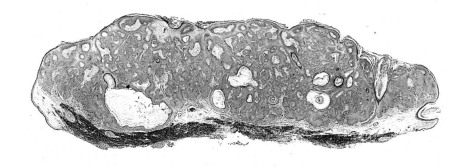

Figure 2-4
SEBORRHEIC KERATOSIS
Plaquoid lesion with anastomosing cords of basaloid cells with numerous horn cysts.

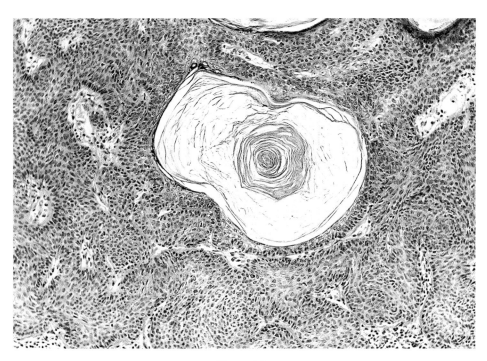

Figure 2-5
SEBORRHEIC KERATOSIS
Higher magnification of the lesion in the previous figure.

Hyperkeratotic lesions have a thickened keratin layer and show the greatest tendency for papillomatosis. In lesions of the acanthotic type, the epidermis is notably thickened and hyperkeratosis is relatively reduced (figs. 2-4, 2-5). Adenoid lesions are even less keratinized and have elongated, branching epithelial strands composed of a double row of basaloid cells. In all three types, the epidermis often contains kera-tin-filled cystic inclusions, referred to as horn cysts (fig. 2-5).

Increased amounts of melanin pigment are almost invariably present within the keratinocytes of a seborrheic keratosis and may be especially observed in the adenoid and acanthotic types. Thus, seborrheic keratosis may be clinically confused with a nevus, a pigmented basal cell carcinoma, or even with a malignant melanoma.

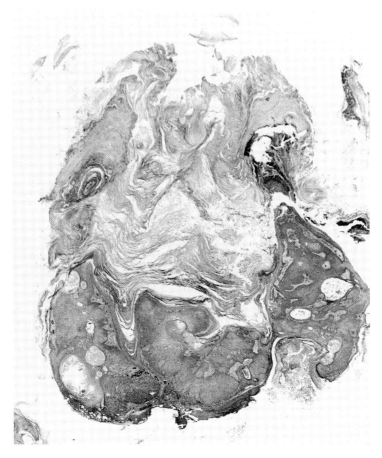

Figure 2-6
INVERTED FOLLICULAR KERATOSIS
Acanthotic epithelium with massive hyperkeratosis forming a cutaneous horn.

Inverted Follicular Keratosis (Irritated Seborrheic Keratosis)

These epithelial lesions have a distinct predilection for the eyelid and usually present as a nodular or wart-like tumor. They often occur at the eyelid margin. They can be pigmented, simulating a melanocytic lesion. There is a tendency to recur if incompletely excised.

Inverted follicular keratosis can be confused by both the clinician and pathologist with squamous cell carcinoma (5,6), especially when severely inflamed and undergoing rapid growth, but there is no evidence that these lesions undergo malignant transformation.

Histopathologically, the overlying epidermis shows lobular acanthosis interspersed with areas of acantholysis (figs. 2-6, 2-7). The acanthosis is due to

the proliferation of both basaloid and squamoid cells. Squamoid eddies, flattened, concentrically oriented epidermal cells found within the areas of acanthosis, are often observed (fig. 2-7).

Pseudocarcinomatous (Pseudoepitheliomatous) Hyperplasia

Pseudocarcinomatous lesions may be confused clinically and histopathologically with either a squamous or basal cell carcinoma. They are usually elevated, with an irregular leukoplakic surface that is often ulcerated. They can occur anywhere in the eyelid and typically are of short duration (a few weeks to several months). Pseudocarcinomatous hyperplasia may be caused by infections (blastomycosis, chromomycosis), insect bites, drugs (bromoderma, iododerma), burns, radiation therapy, and tumors (granular cell tumor), but the cause of many

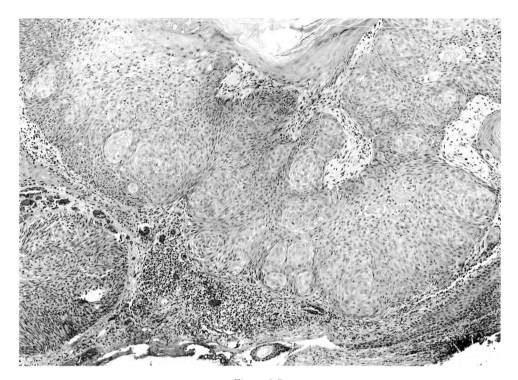

Figure 2-7
INVERTED FOLLICULAR KERATOSIS
Higher magnification of the lesion in figure 2-6 showing numerous squamous eddies within the acanthotic epithelium.

of these lesions cannot be determined. Histologically, there is invasive acanthosis but cytologic features of malignancy are usually absent.

Keratoacanthoma

This is a specialized variant of pseudo-carcinomatous hyperplasia that has a predilection for sun-exposed areas of the skin such as the lower eyelids. In a series of 44 keratoacanthomas of the eyelid, 36 had been present for 2 months or less (7). Clinically and histologically, keratoacanthoma appears as a dome-shaped nodule with a central keratin-filled crater and elevated, rolled margins. Microscopic examination discloses that the squamous epithelium of the cup-shaped lesion is rather uniform and well demarcated from the adjacent dermis by a moderate inflammatory reaction (figs. 2-8, 2-9). Collections of neutrophils forming microabscesses are usually present within some of the islands of squamous epithelium. Proliferating squamous epithelium may invade the orbicularis muscle, which in the eyelid normally lies close to the epidermis.

Actinic Keratosis
(Solar Keratosis, Senile Keratosis)

This is the most common precancerous lesion of the eyelid and results from prolonged exposure to sunlight with inadequate protection. Actinic keratoses usually appear as single or multiple scaly, keratotic, flat-topped erythematous lesions that measure only a few millimeters in diameter. Some lesions have a nodular, horny, or warty configuration.

The natural history of actinic keratosis of the skin has been studied in Australia by Marks et al. (8,9). Of 1040 individuals 40 years and older, 616 (59.2 percent) had one or more actinic keratoses, yielding a total of 4746 tumors. Three patients with 11 actinic lesions received treatment and were excluded from the study. After 1 year of follow-up of the remaining 1037 people, 485 (10.2 percent) of the 4735 actinic keratoses underwent remission and 1535 new tumors developed. Yearly follow-up of 1689 people 40 years and older for 5 years provided 1-year follow-up data on 21,905 actinic keratoses: 10 squamous cell carcinomas

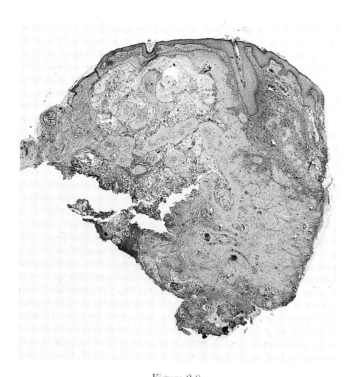

Figure 2-8
KERATOACANTHOMA
Part of a large lesion composed of pale, acanthotic, hyperkeratotic epithelium undermining normal epidermis.

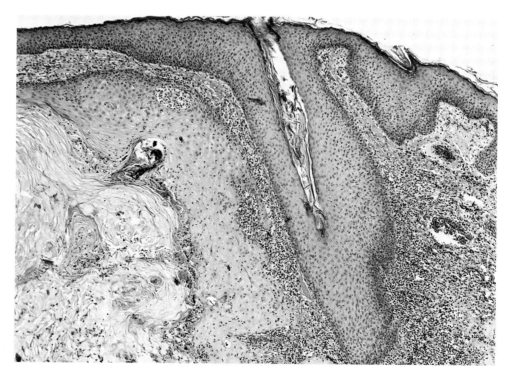

Figure 2-9
KERATOACANTHOMA
Higher power magnification of the lesion in the previous figure.

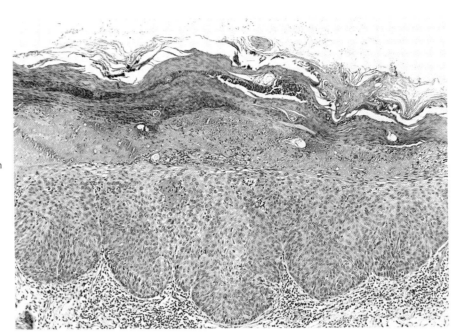

Figure 2-10
ACTINIC KERATOSIS
Irregular acanthosis with atypia and parakeratosis.

definitely arose at the site of a preexistent actinic keratosis, 11 squamous cell carcinomas may have arisen from an actinic keratosis, and 7 carcinomas arose from previously normal skin. From these data we conclude that actinic keratoses rarely (less than 0.1 percent) progress to squamous cell carcinoma; they are at least 100 times more likely to spontaneously regress than to progress to carcinoma.

Histologically, the upper dermis shows moderate to severe basophilic degeneration of collagen (elastotic degeneration) with a moderate lymphoplasmacytic infiltrate. According to the predominant histologic features, two main types of actinic keratosis have been recognized: hypertrophic and atrophic. Whether the epithelium is acanthotic or atrophic, there are always focal areas of parakeratosis. The proliferation of atypical keratinocytes often gives the lesion an irregular papillary structure. The anaplastic keratinocytes may have hyperchromatic nuclei. Multinucleated cells, vacuolated cells, malignant dyskeratotic cells, and abnormal mitotic figures may be present (fig. 2-10). Clefts may form as a result of dysplastic acantholysis with loss of intercellular bridges, giving the lesion an adenoid appearance. When markedly atypical keratinocytes involve the full thickness of the epithelium, mimicking Bowen disease, the lesions are classified as Bowenoid type. These lesions typically spare the

epithelium of the hair follicles, which distinguishes them from Bowen disease.

Bowen Disease

Clinically, the lesions of Bowen disease appear as erythematous, pigmented, crusty, scaly, fissured, keratotic plaques. The plaques are round and sharply demarcated with occasional heaped-up margins. The disease involves both sexes but occurs predominantly in white men with a fair complexion. Although it is ingrained in the pathology literature that Bowen disease is a marker for internal malignancies, particularly of the respiratory, gastrointestinal, and genitourinary systems, newer epidemiologic studies have found no evidence to support this association (10). Chute et al. (10) found that patients with Bowen disease had a relative risk of only 1.1 for internal cancer. Chronic arsenic poisoning is probably one of many causes of Bowen disease (12) and anecdotal reports suggest that Bowen disease due to arsenic poisoning may be associated with internal cancers. Tanimoto et al. (13) described an arsenic miner who at autopsy had primary carcinomas of stomach, lung, pharynx, and prostate in addition to Bowen disease of the skin. Exposure to petroleum byproducts, trauma, or cutaneous injury from ionizing radiation have also been suggested as causes of Bowen disease. Recent studies

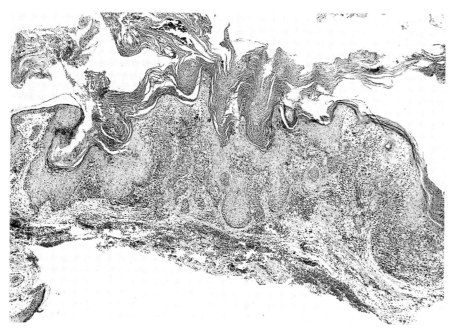

Figure 2-11
ACTINIC KERATOSIS
Actinic keratosis with early invasive squamous cell carcinoma.

employing in situ DNA hybridization have implicated human papilloma virus type 16 or closely related strains in the pathogenesis of some cases of Bowen disease (11). If most cases are not due to arsenic poisoning and if only cases due to arsenic poisoning are associated with internal malignancies, then epidemiologic studies of randomly selected patients with Bowen disease would be unlikely to detect this association.

Microscopically, typical lesions show hyperkeratosis, parakeratosis, and plaque-like acanthosis. The epidermis exhibits a striking loss of normal polarity and abnormal keratinocytic maturation, with markedly atypical keratinocytes present at all levels of the epidermis. Bowen lesions tend to involve the outer sheaths of the hair follicles and may even replace the sebaceous gland cells. Because of the presence of atypical vacuolated cells, frozen sections and lipid stains may be necessary to distinguish between Bowen disease and intraepithelial spread of sebaceous gland carcinoma.

Squamous Cell Carcinoma

Squamous cell carcinoma is not a frequent neoplasm of the eyelid, representing only 2 to 6 percent of malignant neoplasms (14,16). This malignant tumor affects elderly individuals, most commonly involves the margin of the lower lid, and most often arises from a preexisting actinic keratosis (fig. 2-11). Less common precursor lesions are Bowen disease, radiation dermatosis, and xeroderma pigmentosum. Clinically, squamous cell carcinoma presents as a single elevated nodule or plaque with irregular borders. The center portion of these nodules frequently becomes ulcerated. In well-differentiated squamous cell carcinomas, the masses of keratin produced by the neoplastic cells may give the lesion a whitish granular appearance. These tumors have an excellent prognosis: a wide local excision is usually curative. Metastases are rare, which is similar to the behavior of squamous cell carcinoma in other sun-exposed cutaneous sites, where 1.6 percent metastasize (15). This contrasts markedly with the behavior of squamous cell carcinomas of the mucosa in anatomic regions such as bronchus or uterine cervix. When advanced squamous cell carcinomas of the eyelids metastasize, they spread via lymphatics to the preauricular and submandibular lymph nodes.

Microscopically, the neoplastic cells in well-differentiated squamous cell carcinoma are polygonal with abundant eosinophilic cytoplasm. Dyskeratotic cells with keratin pearl formation are often observed. Intercellular bridges may be found. The nuclei of the squamous cells are prominent and hyperchromatic. The histologic

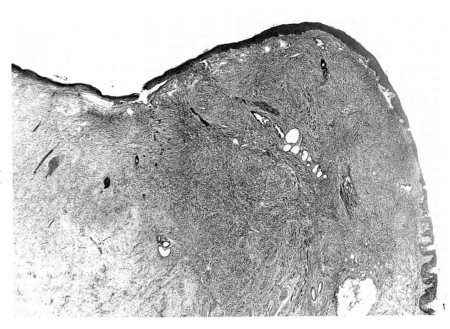

Figure 2-12
SQUAMOUS CELL
CARCINOMA,
SPINDLE CELL TYPE
Atrophic epidermis overlying a highly infiltrative neoplasm.

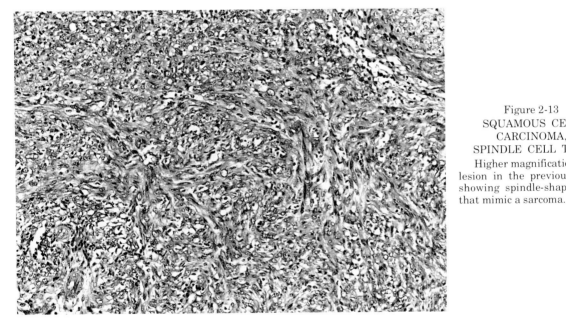

Figure 2-13
SQUAMOUS CELL
CARCINOMA,
SPINDLE CELL TYPE
Higher magnification of the lesion in the previous figure showing spindle-shaped cells that mimic a sarcoma.

findings vary depending on the degree of differentiation of these neoplasms.

A spindle cell variant of squamous cell carcinoma may involve the skin of the eyelids (figs. 2-12, 2-13). Histopathologically, this variant may be confused with undifferentiated sarcomas, fibrosarcomas, and fibrous histiocytomas (fig. 2-13). Multiple sections, however, usually show dysplastic keratinocytes, focal areas of intraepithelial carcinoma of the overlying epider-

mis, and small foci of keratinization. Electron microscopy to demonstrate epithelial features or immunohistochemistry for cytokeratins helps establish the correct diagnosis.

Basal Cell Carcinoma

Basal cell carcinoma is the most common malignant tumor of the eyelid (19,28): it accounts for 80 to 90 percent of all malignant epithelial eyelid neoplasms. Frequently, basal cell carcinoma

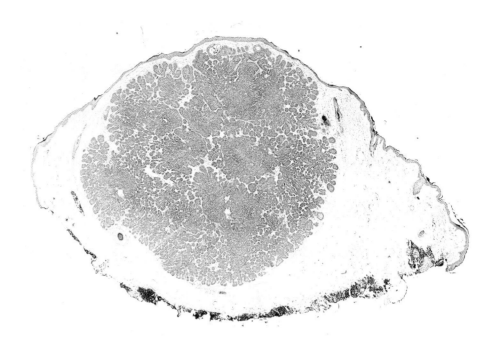

Figure 2-14
BASAL CELL CARCINOMA, NODULAR TYPE
This most common presentation consists of a proliferation of solid lobules of neoplastic basaloid cells.

involves the lower eyelid and the inner canthus in elderly individuals. Prolonged sunlight exposure is an important predisposing factor. Patients with basal cell carcinoma should be closely checked and have follow-up examinations for the development of other actinically related tumors. Wesley and Collins (29) found that 60 percent of patients with basal cell carcinoma of the eyelids had other basal cell carcinoma foci.

Solitary basal cell carcinoma in children and young adults is rare and must be considered a forme fruste of the nevoid basal cell carcinoma syndrome (18). Basal cell carcinoma may be associated with several other lesions, such as nevus sebaceous of Jadassohn and dermatofibromas (22), or as a secondary tumor in adults with heritable retinoblastoma.

Most basal cell carcinomas of the eyelid are of three clinical types: nodular, ulcerative, and sclerosing (morphea form). The nodular type usually presents clinically as a firm pearly nodule, with small telangiectatic vessels on its surface. Quite often, as the nodule slowly increases in size, it undergoes central ulceration becoming an ulcerative type. The sclerosing or morphea type appears as a pale, well-defined, indurated plaque.

Basal cell carcinomas, particularly the nodular type, may become pigmented either due to the presence of melanin (secondary melanosis) or hemorrhage with deposition of hemosiderin. These pigmented lesions may be misinterpreted as malignant melanomas (24). Basal cell carcinomas can also become cystic, and may be confused with inclusion cysts of the eyelid.

Depending on the growth pattern, basal cell carcinomas are classified histologically as multicentric, nodular (fig. 2-14), ulcerative, infiltrative, and mixed types. These types can be subclassified as solid (fig. 2-14), adenoid (fig. 2-15), and metatypical (fig. 2-16). The histologic types differ from the clinical types in three ways. First, some basal cell carcinomas arise as multiple separate foci rather than as a single tumor. Second, some basal cell carcinomas have a mixed nodular and infiltrative pattern or a mixed ulcerative and infiltrative pattern. These tumors appear to be nodular or ulcerative clinically because the infiltrative growth usually occurs at the deep margin and is clinically undetectable. Third, not all infiltrative basal cell carcinomas produce a sclerotic stroma (morphea type) (figs. 2-17, 2-18). This is particularly true with the infiltrative growth that occurs

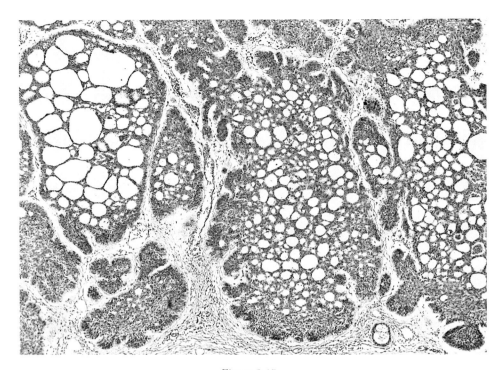

Figure 2-15
BASAL CELL CARCINOMA, ADENOID TYPE
The lobules of basaloid cells have marginal palisading and within the lobules there is a cribriform pattern.

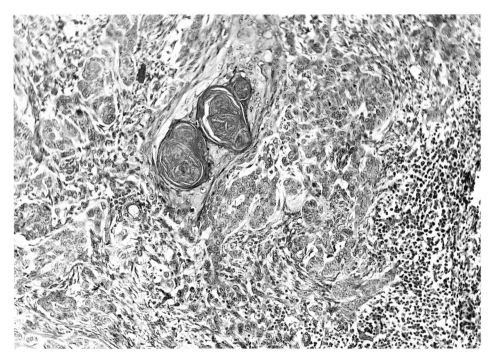

Figure 2-16
BASAL CELL CARCINOMA, METATYPICAL TYPE
Island of squamous cell differentiation within basaloid tumor.

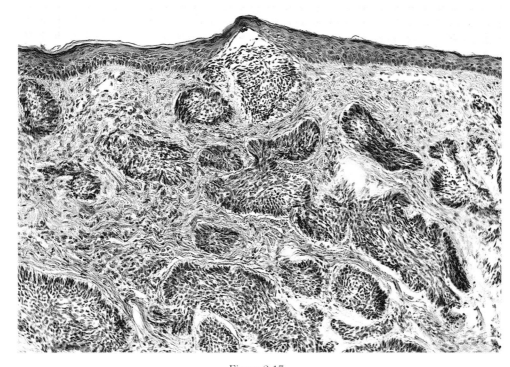

Figure 2-17
BASAL CELL CARCINOMA, MORPHEA TYPE IN A PATIENT WITH HERITABLE RETINOBLASTOMA
Atrophic epidermis overlies small irregularly shaped clusters of basaloid cells.

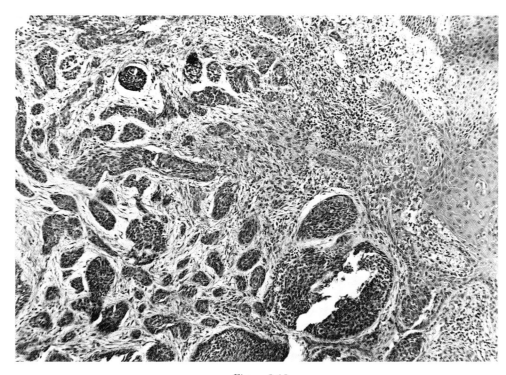

Figure 2-18
BASAL CELL CARCINOMA, MORPHEA TYPE IN A PATIENT WITH HERITABLE RETINOBLASTOMA
Another area composed of highly infiltrative cords of basaloid cells from the tumor illustrated in figure 2-17.

in a mixed type of basal cell carcinoma. Because tumors of multicentric, mixed, and infiltrative types often extend beyond the apparent margins of clinical involvement, these tumors may be incompletely excised. For this reason frozen section control is recommended. Doxanas et al. (20) found that when basal cell carcinomas were excised from the eyelid without frozen section control there was a 5.5 percent recurrence rate. When frozen section control or Mohs microsurgical technique was used, the recurrence rate was reduced to 2 percent or less (20,23,25).

Histologic differential diagnosis of basal cell carcinoma involves two groups of tumors. In our experience, the major problem is confusion between basal cell and sebaceous carcinoma. Pathologists unfamiliar with eyelid tumors may diagnose poorly differentiated sebaceous carcinoma as basal cell carcinoma. This may lead to undertreatment because of the more aggressive behavior of sebaceous carcinoma. The second, less common area of diagnostic confusion is between basal cell carcinoma and benign pilar tumors (26). Because we have seen tumors with features of both basal cell carcinoma and trichoepithelioma, we believe that there is a spectrum of tumors between benign pilar tumors and basal cell carcinoma.

Neglected basal cell carcinomas may invade the paranasal sinuses, orbital and intraocular structures, and meninges of the brain (17,27). They rarely metastasize and death is unlikely (21).

BENIGN TUMORS OF ECCRINE AND APOCRINE GLAND ORIGIN

The eyelid is richly endowed with eccrine and apocrine glands and the entire spectrum of tumors of these glands occur here. Because of the presence of the glands of Moll, the eyelid is a site of predilection for apocrine tumors: the apocrine hidradenoma papilliferum, which is most often a tumor of the labia majora and perianal region, has been described in the eyelid (30,31).

Hydrocystoma

Hydrocystomas of either eccrine or apocrine origin in the eyelid are small bluish, translucent, cystic nodules measuring 1 to 3 mm in diameter. Eccrine hydrocystomas tend to be unilocular and lined by a double layer of small cuboidal cells without papillary projections into the lumen. Apocrine hydrocystomas are usually multiloculated with papillary projections that extend into the lumen. The cyst wall and papillary projections are lined by a double layer of epithelium. The inner layer consists of tall columnar cells showing decapitation secretion and the outer layer is of myoepithelial cells. Apocrine hydrocystoma with numerous papillary projections into the lumen may be diagnosed as apocrine cystadenoma.

Syringoma

Syringoma is a common benign eccrine tumor of the eyelid. It occurs predominantly in young women near puberty or in early adulthood. The lesions are usually multiple, yellowish, waxy nodules averaging 1 to 2 mm in size (32). Microscopically, each nodule is composed of small ducts embedded in a dense fibrous stroma. The ducts are lined by two or more rows of epithelial cells. The inner cells are flat and may be vacuolated or keratinized. Some of the ducts are comma shaped, resembling tadpoles. The lumina of the ducts may contain either mucoid material or keratin.

Eccrine Acrospiroma (Clear Cell Hidradenoma, Clear Cell Myoepithelioma, Eccrine Poroma, Porosyringoma)

Clinically, eccrine acrospiroma is a single, nodular, solid or cystic dermal mass. The skin overlying the nodule varies from flesh color to reddish blue (33). Microscopically, the lesion is a well-circumscribed dermal nodule composed of lobulated masses of epithelial cells (figs. 2-19, 2-20). Two types of epithelial cells are usually present within the epithelial lobules: one type with eosinophilic cytoplasm and another with clear cytoplasm due to the accumulation of glycogen. In many areas there is a transition from eosinophilic cells to clear cells. Some tumors are almost entirely composed of clear cells, hence the name clear cell hidradenoma. Within the lobules of epithelium are branching tubular lumina lined by a single layer of cuboidal or columnar cells. Some lesions contain cysts filled with serous or hemorrhagic fluid. Scattered mitotic figures may be present. Immunohistochemical stains are positive for cytokeratins, carcinoembryonic antigen, and muscle-specific actin (33).

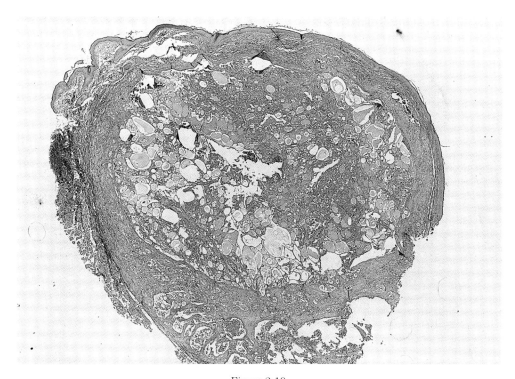

Figure 2-19
ECCRINE ACROSPIROMA
Multinodular tumor within the dermis containing numerous mucin-filled cysts.

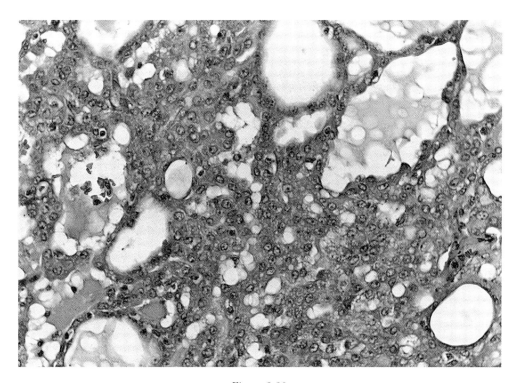

Figure 2-20
ECCRINE ACROSPIROMA
Higher magnification of the tumor in the previous figure showing cuboidal epithelial cells lining the cystic spaces.

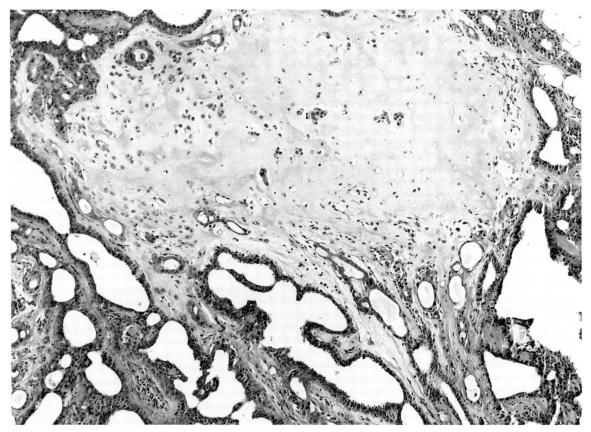

Figure 2-21
PLEOMORPHIC ADENOMA (CHONDROID SYRINGOMA)
Nodular tumor composed of dilated ducts lined by a double layer of epithelium with a chondroid appearance of the stroma.

Pleomorphic Adenoma (Mixed Tumor of the Sweat Glands, Chondroid Syringoma)

Pleomorphic adenoma in the eyelid may be of eccrine (35), apocrine (34), or lacrimal gland origin (36). Clinically, there is an intradermal, multilobulated mass usually ranging from 0.5 to 2 cm in diameter. Histologically, pleomorphic adenomas of eccrine and apocrine origin are similar to pleomorphic adenomas that arise in the lacrimal glands; clinical data are needed to differentiate the former from tumors arising in the palpebral lobe of the lacrimal gland or in the accessory lacrimal glands of Wolfring. Pleomorphic adenomas are composed of tubular structures lined by a double layer of epithelial cells embedded in a stroma that varies from mucoid to chondroid. The inner cells lining the ducts are secretory and the outer cells are myoepithelial (fig. 2-21).

MALIGNANT TUMORS OF ECCRINE SWEAT GLAND ORIGIN (ECCRINE ADENOCARCINOMA)

Clinically, eccrine adenocarcinoma is a nodular, indurated mass with diffuse infiltrating margins. Extension to involve both upper and lower lids may occur. The tumor may invade the orbit and spread to regional lymph nodes. Erythema of the overlying skin may be present. The tumors range in size from 0.4 to 2.5 cm and occur predominantly in middle-aged adults.

Histologically, several different types are recognized including malignant variants of benign types (38,40,43). The eccrine carcinomas are divided into two broad groups dependent on whether mucin production is demonstrated within the tumor cells using Alcian blue or mucicarmine stain. Most eccrine adenocarcinomas are histologically and immunohistochemically

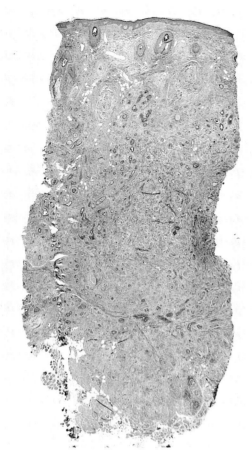

Figure 2-22
ECCRINE CARCINOMA, DUCTAL TYPE
Tumor mimics a syringoma but invades deeply into the eyelid.

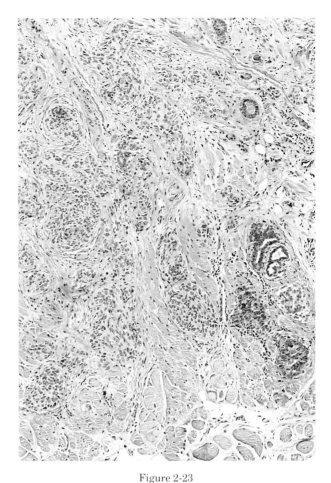

Figure 2-23
ECCRINE CARCINOMA, DUCTAL TYPE
Higher magnification of deep margin of the same tumor in figure 2-22 showing bland cells arranged in ducts and cords infiltrating the orbicularis muscle.

similar to breast carcinoma and include an infiltrating ductal carcinoma (classic type) (figs. 2-22, 2-23) (37), a mucinous type (colloid or gelatinous carcinoma) (fig. 2-24) (46,49), and a poorly differentiated type (histiocytoid or signet ring carcinoma) (figs. 2-25, 2-27) (39,42,44). Some of the infiltrating ductal eccrine adenocarcinomas have a desmoplastic stroma and some of the ducts have a comma shape similar to those of a syringoma (figs. 2-22, 2-23) (38). These tumors are termed *syringoid adenocarcinomas*. The mucinous adenocarcinoma is a variant of mucus secreting adenocarcinoma in which elongated cords and lobules of epithelial cells float in large pools of mucin separated by thin, fibrovascular septa (fig. 2-24). In the undifferentiated type, individual and

small clusters of cells infiltrate the soft tissues of the eyelid, a pattern that has been termed histiocytoid in metastatic carcinoma of the breast to the eyelid (fig. 2-26) (41). The epithelial character of the cells in histiocytoid tumors can be suspected from the atypia of the cells, the tendency for some of the cells to form short chains (single file pattern), and the presence of vacuoles in signet ring cells (figs. 2-25–2-27) and established with immunohistochemical detection of cytokeratin (38). The presence of mucin in the vacuoles can be confirmed with Alcian blue and mucicarmine stains. In all types of eccrine adenocarcinoma, mitotic figures are uncommon. Like breast carcinoma, eccrine carcinoma is frequently estrogen receptor positive (47).

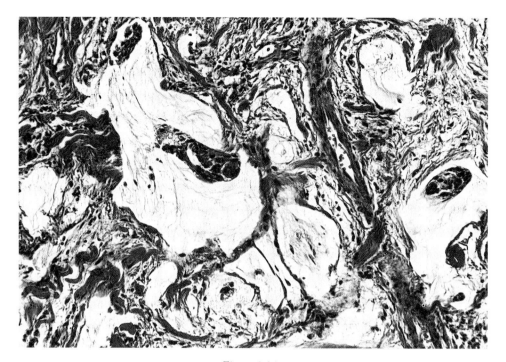

Figure 2-24
ECCRINE CARCINOMA, MUCINOUS TYPE
Small islands of epithelial cells float in large pools of mucin.

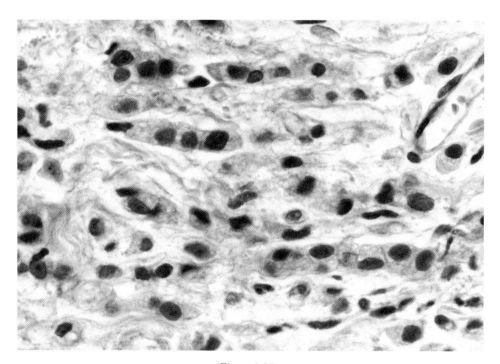

Figure 2-25
ECCRINE CARCINOMA, HISTIOCYTOID TYPE
Anaplastic cuboidal epithelial cells with intracytoplasmic vacuoles are arranged in a single file pattern.

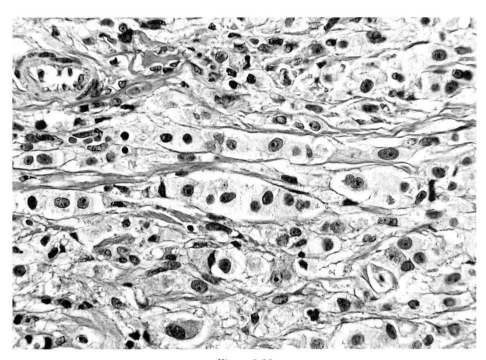

Figure 2-26
METASTATIC BREAST CARCINOMA, HISTIOCYTOID PATTERN
This tumor is very similar to the histiocytoid eccrine carcinoma illustrated in figure 2-25.

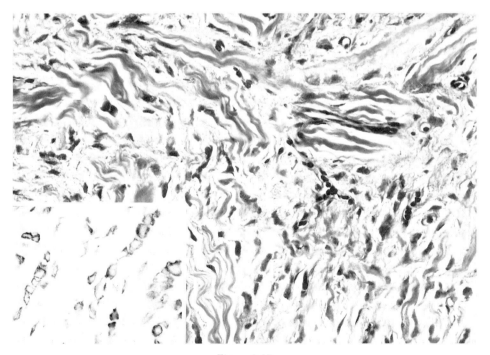

Figure 2-27
ECCRINE CARCINOMA, HISTIOCYTOID TYPE
Intense desmoplastic reaction makes visualization of neoplastic cells difficult. Insert: Immunohistochemistry for cyto-keratin highlights the neoplastic cells arranged in a single file pattern.

The mucinous variant (fig. 2-24) has a better prognosis than the other types. Wright and Font (49) followed 20 patients with mucinous tumors of the eyelid for a median of 8 years. Twelve patients were alive without evidence of recurrence; 8 patients (40 percent) had one or more local recurrences, one of whom died from direct local invasion; and only 1 patient developed metastasis to the submandibular nodes. Of 63 patients with classic and poorly differentiated eccrine adenocarcinomas of skin followed for 5 years or longer, 43 percent developed metastases to regional lymph nodes and 38 percent developed widespread metastatic disease (37). The low metastatic potential of the mucinous variant of sweat gland adenocarcinoma is similar to that observed in patients with the mucinous (gelatinous) variant of adenocarcinoma of the breast.

APOCRINE ADENOCARCINOMA

Apocrine carcinoma of the eyelid is rare. A primary adenocarcinoma of the eyelid is usually of sebaceous or eccrine origin. Apocrine carcinoma arises from the glands of Moll and usually presents as a nodular mass. The most common pattern is that of a cystadenocarcinoma. These tumors are believed to be of low malignant potential with a behavior similar to that of a basal cell carcinoma; however, they may be more likely to metastasize to regional lymph nodes (45,48).

SEBACEOUS GLAND TUMORS

Benign Tumors of Sebaceous Origin

Sebaceous hyperplasia (senile sebaceous nevus) occurs predominantly on the skin of the face and scalp of older individuals. The skin of the lids, the meibomian glands, and the sebaceous glands of the caruncle may be affected. Clinically, there are often multiple lesions that appear as small (2 to 3 mm), elevated, soft, yellowish nodules, some of which are umbilicated. Histologically, each tumor consists of a single enlarged sebaceous gland, with fully mature lobules grouped around a centrally located, dilated sebaceous duct.

Sebaceous adenomas are more likely to be solitary lesions than sebaceous hyperplasias. They may be as large as 1 cm in diameter. Histologically, the tumor is composed of sebaceous lobules that vary in size, shape, and maturity. Within the lobules, germinative cells surround small clusters of sebaceous cells. Mitotic figures may be common in the germinative cells (fig. 2-28).

The *Muir-Torre syndrome* is an association of multiple sebaceous gland neoplasms, other cutaneous lesions, and multiple visceral carcinomas, especially of the colon (50,52). This syndrome is inherited as an autosomal dominant trait and is a cause of familial cancer. Histologically, the sebaceous lesions are usually adenomas, but some are sebaceous hyperplasias, sebaceous epitheliomas (basal cell carcinomas with foci of sebaceous differentiation), or sebaceous carcinomas. Other lesions of the skin associated with this syndrome include epidermal hyperplasias, keratoacanthomas, and squamous cell carcinomas. The visceral internal carcinomas predominantly involve the gastrointestinal tract (colon, stomach, rectum, duodenum), but other organs (urinary bladder, ovary, uterus, and kidney) may also be affected. Rarely, a solitary sebaceous adenoma of the eyelid may be associated with internal carcinoma; this may be a manifestation of the Muir-Torre syndrome (51).

Sebaceous Carcinoma (Adenocarcinoma of Sebaceous Gland, Meibomian Gland Carcinoma, Zeis Gland Carcinoma)

Sites of Origin. Sebaceous carcinoma is the most important malignant neoplasm of the eyelid. It arises almost exclusively in the skin of the eyelid and is extremely rare in the skin elsewhere. Most sebaceous carcinomas of the eyelid arise in the meibomian (tarsal) glands, followed by the sebaceous glands of the lashes (glands of Zeis), and, less frequently, sebaceous glands in the caruncle or the skin of the eyebrow. The upper eyelid is involved in about two thirds of the cases, probably because the meibomian glands are more numerous there. Some tumors appear to originate from both the meibomian glands and the glands of Zeis; in other tumors the exact site of origin cannot be determined. In advanced cases both the upper and lower eyelids may be involved (60).

Clinical Features. Sebaceous gland carcinomas affect elderly patients: the median age at diagnosis is 64 years. Except for one study of 40 cases (55), all large series have disclosed a female preponderance. In a series of 104 patients from

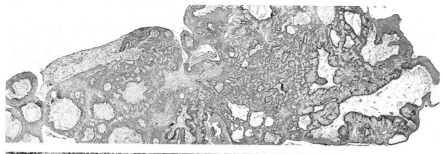

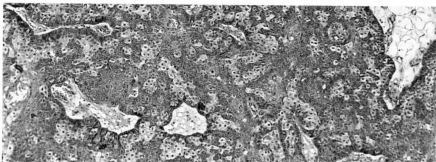

Figure 2-28
SEBACEOUS ADENOMA
Multilobular tumor composed of sebaceous cells with orderly maturation.

the American ROP, 60 percent were female (60) and about two thirds of 156 cases reported from Shanghai were female (58). Sebaceous gland carcinoma is usually a small firm nodule resembling a chalazion. It frequently appears as an atypical or recurring chalazion, with a rubbery consistency. Some patients with meibomian gland carcinoma have a diffuse plaque-like thickening of the tarsus (fig. 2-29) or a fungating or papillomatous growth. Lesions originating from the glands of Zeis are small yellowish nodules located at the lid margin just in front of the gray line. A characteristic finding with sebaceous lesions arising in either meibomian or Zeis glands is loss of lashes caused by intraepithelial neoplastic invasion of the follicles (fig. 2-29). Carcinomas of the sebaceous glands of the caruncle are usually grayish yellow masses covered by an intact epithelium.

A distinctive clinical feature of many sebaceous gland carcinomas is a persistent unilateral conjunctivitis, blepharitis, meibomitis, or blepharoconjunctivitis (fig. 2-29). This clinical picture is referred to as the "masquerade syndrome" (53) and is the inflammatory response caused by invasion of sebaceous carcinoma cells into the conjunctival epithelium. It is often necessary to obtain multiple biopsy specimens from the lid margin as well as the palpebral and bulbar conjunctivas to determine the extent of intraepithelial involvement. Many patients with diffuse pagetoid invasion or

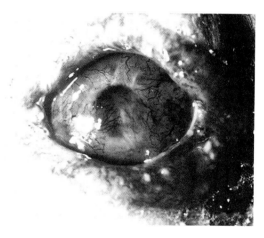

Figure 2-29
SEBACEOUS CARCINOMA PRESENTING
AS CHRONIC BLEPHAROCONJUNCTIVITIS
The tumor involves both upper and lower eyelids with loss of lashes and invades the conjunctival and corneal epithelia with scarring and vascularization.

carcinoma in situ–like changes involving the skin of the lid, the conjunctiva, and the cornea require orbital exenteration.

Sebaceous gland carcinoma should be considered if a patient presents with a lid tumor several years following radiation therapy to the eye or ocular adnexa, or if an orbital mass develops after resection of a histologically unverified tumor of the caruncle or tarsus.

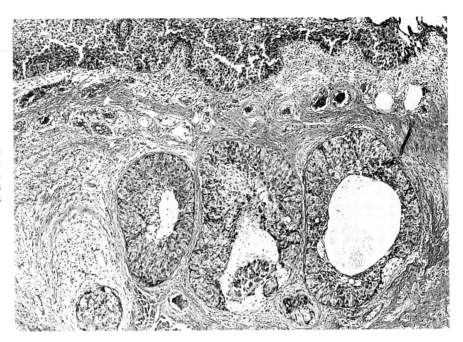

Figure 2-30
SEBACEOUS CARCINOMA
Meibomian glands are replaced by lobules of tumor with a comedocarcinoma pattern and conjunctival epithelium is replaced by neoplastic cells (upper surface).

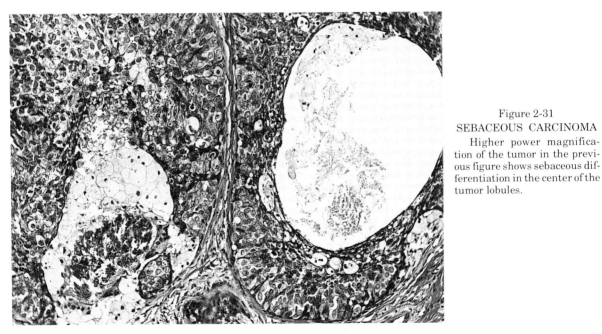

Figure 2-31
SEBACEOUS CARCINOMA
Higher power magnification of the tumor in the previous figure shows sebaceous differentiation in the center of the tumor lobules.

Histologic Findings. Sebaceous carcinoma can be classified by degree of differentiation into three groups. Well-differentiated tumors have a lobular pattern with cells in the center of the lobules exhibiting sebaceous differentiation (figs. 2-30, 2-31). These cells have an abundant, finely vacuolated cytoplasm that appears foamy or frothy. The nuclei are centrally placed. Moderately differentiated tumors show only a few areas of highly differentiated sebaceous cells. The majority of the tumor is composed of anaplastic cells with hyperchromatic nuclei, prominent nucleoli, and abundant amphophilic cytoplasm. In poorly differentiated tumors, most cells exhibit pleomorphic nuclei, with prominent nucleoli and amphophilic cytoplasm. These tumors often show moderate mitotic activity, and the mitotic figures may be atypical or bizarre. Frozen

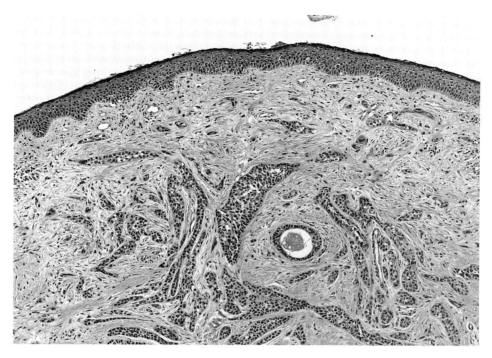

Figure 2-32
SEBACEOUS CARCINOMA
Cords of poorly differentiated neoplastic cells infiltrating the connective tissue of the eyelid mimic a morphea form basal cell carcinoma.

section and oil red 0 stains for lipid may be necessary to establish an unequivocal diagnosis.

Sebaceous carcinoma can have a variety of histologic patterns (60). The most common pattern is lobular, in which the neoplastic cells form well-demarcated lobules of variable size (figs. 2-30, 2-31). The lobules exhibit basaloid features but lack the peripheral palisading that is characteristic of a basal cell carcinoma. In the better differentiated tumors, the cells in the center of the lobules undergo sebaceous differentiation. Sebaceous tumors with a comedocarcinoma pattern have larger lobules with prominent central foci of necrosis. The central necrotic tumor cells usually stain intensely for lipid. Tumors that erode from the tarsus to involve the conjunctival surface or, less commonly, the cutaneous surface may have a papillary pattern. These tumors resemble a squamous cell papilloma or carcinoma but careful histologic examination usually reveals foci of sebaceous differentiation. Poorly differentiated tumors can have an infiltrative pattern that may be confused with basal cell carcinoma (fig. 2-32). Tumors often have mixed patterns; most common is the mixture

of lobular and comedocarcinoma-like areas, but any combination of patterns may be seen.

Modes of Spread. Intraepithelial spread to the conjunctiva, cornea, or skin of the eyelids is frequently observed in sebaceous gland carcinoma (figs. 2-33–2-37). There are two patterns of intraepithelial spread: pagetoid (figs. 2-33, 2-36, 2-37) and carcinoma in situ–like (62,63). The term pagetoid is used because it resembles the invasion of a ductal breast carcinoma into the epidermis of the nipple and surrounding areola in Paget disease of the breast. The neoplastic cells in pagetoid spread invade the overlying epithelium as single cells or as small nests of cells that typically do not form intercellular bridges with the surrounding normal squamous epithelial cells. Pagetoid cells have hyperchromatic nuclei and abundant vacuolated cytoplasm that contains variable amounts of lipid.

The carcinoma in situ–like spread by sebaceous gland carcinoma cells can be a diffuse process, with full thickness replacement of surface epithelium by neoplastic cells (figs. 2-34, 2-35). The changes resemble those observed in

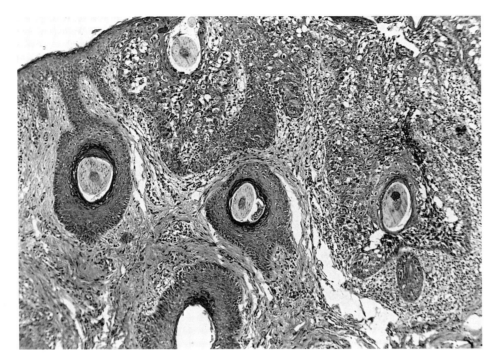

Figure 2-33
SEBACEOUS CARCINOMA
Tumor of Zeis gland involves the epithelium of the cilia and epidermis in a pagetoid fashion.

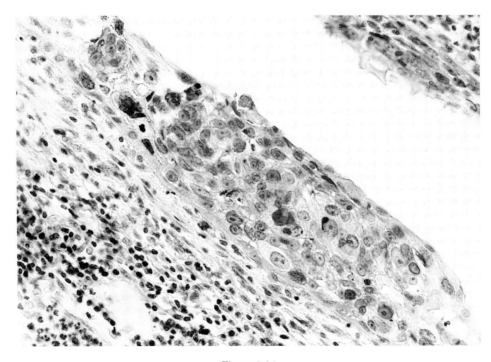

Figure 2-34
SEBACEOUS CARCINOMA
Neoplastic cells have replaced the conjunctival epithelium in a bowenoid pattern.

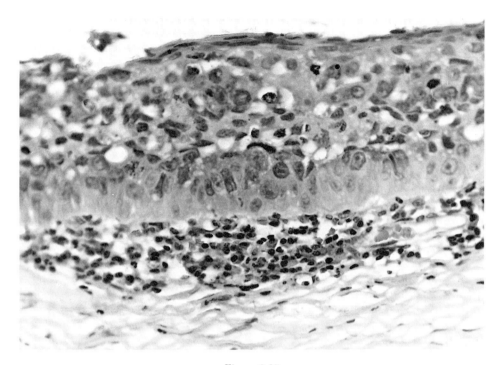

Figure 2-35
SEBACEOUS CARCINOMA
Neoplastic cells have invaded into the corneal epithelium.

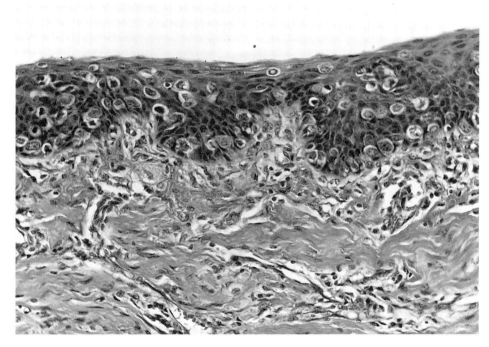

Figure 2-36
SEBACEOUS CARCINOMA
Pagetoid invasion of the epidermis of the eyelid.

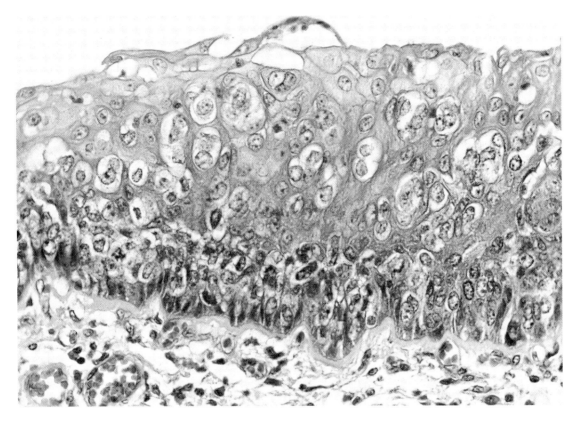

Figure 2-37
SEBACEOUS CARCINOMA
Pagetoid invasion of conjunctival epithelium by neoplastic cells with foamy cytoplasm.

intraepithelial (in situ) squamous cell carcinoma or Bowen disease of the skin. The epithelium of the conjunctiva, cornea, or epidermis of the lids often displays multifocal involvement, with skip areas of unaffected epithelium. The large, pleomorphic, neoplastic cells have increased mitotic activity and are poorly cohesive. The involved epithelium is very friable and if the biopsy specimen is not carefully handled all of the abnormal cells may be lost. Primary intraepithelial carcinoma of the palpebral conjunctiva is exceedingly rare and in situ tumors should be considered secondary spread of sebaceous carcinoma from the eyelid until proved otherwise (57).

Sebaceous carcinoma may spread by direct extension into adjacent structures (lacrimal gland, orbit, paranasal sinuses, intracranial cavity) (fig. 2-38) (54,58,60). Moderate to poorly differentiated tumors with infiltrative growth have perineural infiltration and invade lymphatics. Among the 95 patients studied by Rao et al. (61),

22 developed metastases to the preauricular and cervical lymph nodes (fig. 2-39). Some patients present with a large preauricular mass and a relatively small primary eyelid tumor. In the Rao study, the recurrence rate was 33 percent. Direct orbital invasion occurred in 19 percent of cases and metastases to preauricular or cervical lymph nodes, or both in 23 percent of cases; 22 patients died as a result of the tumor. Distant metastases involving the lungs, liver, brain, and skull often were associated with previous or simultaneous regional lymph node metastases.

Treatment and Prognosis. Rao and colleagues (60) analyzed the prognostic significance of the location and size of the sebaceous gland tumor, its site of origin, the duration of symptoms prior to excision, and the histologic pattern and degree of cellular differentiation. They concluded that a worse prognosis is indicated by origin of the tumor in the upper eyelid; size of 10 mm or more in maximal diameter; origin from

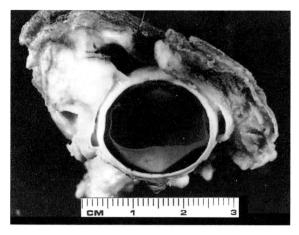

Figure 2-38
SEBACEOUS CARCINOMA
Exenteration specimen with tumor invading from the upper eyelid into the orbit.

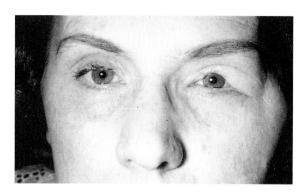

Figure 2-39
SEBACEOUS CARCINOMA
Postoperative reconstruction of upper eyelid with metastasis to the preauricular lymph nodes.

the meibomian glands; duration of symptoms for more than 6 months; an infiltrative growth pattern; moderate to poor sebaceous differentiation; and invasion of lymphatic channels, vascular structures, and the orbit.

It appears that early diagnosis and adequate treatment with primary, wide surgical excision can significantly improve the prognosis. Because of the relatively high recurrence rate of incompletely excised sebaceous gland carcinoma, frozen section control is recommended to insure complete excision. Because of pagetoid invasion, the Mohs surgical technique has been less successful in the management of sebaceous carcinoma than basal cell carcinoma (56). Sebaceous carcinoma is relatively radioresistant and radiotherapy is unlikely to control the disease (59). Radiation may be used for palliation in elderly patients with large tumors who are unable to tolerate extensive radical surgery (59,61). Removal of involved regional lymph nodes has resulted in long-term survival of some patients (60).

TUMORS OF HAIR FOLLICLE ORIGIN

Four benign tumors may arise from hair follicles of the eyelids: trichoepithelioma (solitary and multiple), trichofolliculoma, trichilemmoma, and pilomatrixoma (calcifying epithelioma of Malherbe).

Trichoepithelioma (Epithelioma Adenoides Cysticum, Multiple Benign Cystic Epithelioma, Brooke Tumor)

The eyelids may be involved by both solitary and multiple trichoepitheliomas. Solitary trichoepithelioma is a firm, elevated, skin-colored nodule. It is not inherited and usually appears late in life. Multiple trichoepitheliomas are inherited as an autosomal dominant trait with incomplete penetrance (64). The lesions develop during adolescence and increase thereafter in size and number. Clinically, they appear as multiple, round, firm nodules ranging from 2 to 8 mm in diameter, mainly involving the face and eyelids, and occasionally involving the scalp, neck, and upper trunk.

Histologically, trichoepitheliomas consist of multiple horn cysts with a keratinized center surrounded by a cuff of basaloid cells (fig. 2-40). The cellular stroma of the tumor is well demarcated from the surrounding dermis. Keratinization is typically abrupt and complete, which differs from the gradual and incomplete keratinization observed in the keratin pearls of squamous cell carcinoma.

Trichofolliculoma

This hamartomatous lesion represents the most differentiated form of a pilar tumor. Clinically, the lesion appears as a slightly elevated, small nodule with a central area of umbilication. Small white hairs may protrude from the umbilicated central pore. In a study of 32 cases, all of the patients had solitary lesions, and 26 (81 percent) were located on the face (65).

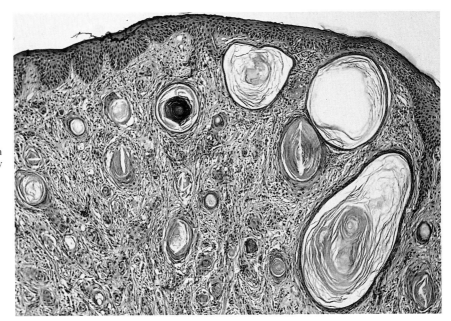

Figure 2-40
TRICHOEPITHELIOMA
Numerous horn cysts within the dermis are surrounded by several layers of basaloid cells.

Microscopically, the tumor is composed of a markedly dilated hair follicle. The cystic structure is lined by keratinized stratified squamous epithelium that is continuous with the epidermis. It is filled with keratin and small hair shafts. Budding from the large cystic follicle are several branching strands of basaloid epithelial cells, which represent secondary hair follicles in which immature hairs can be identified.

Trichilemmoma

This benign tumor of the hair follicles arises from the outer hair sheath (trichilemma), which is mostly composed of glycogen-rich clear cells. In a study of trichilemmomas at the AFIP, 31 of 107 tumors involved the ophthalmic region (28 in the eyelid and 3 in the eyebrow) (67). All 31 were solitary, small, and asymptomatic. Multiple trichilemmomas can occur on the eyelids and face of patients with Cowden disease (66). This syndrome is inherited as an autosomal dominant trait; patients with multiple trichilemmomas are at high risk of developing internal malignancies, particularly breast and thyroid carcinomas.

Histologically, trichilemmomas are composed of lobules of glycogen-rich clear cells. At the periphery of the lobules are columnar cells with a thick basement membrane. Hair follicles may be observed within the lesion (fig. 2-41). Frequently, the center of the lesion has areas of hyalinized collagen that surround epithelial islands of squamoid differentiation. The tumor is frequently misinterpreted histologically as basal cell carcinoma, squamous cell carcinoma, sebaceous neoplasm, or seborrheic keratosis.

Pilomatrixoma
(Calcifying Epithelioma of Malherbe)

Pilomatrixoma is a solid or cystic, freely movable subcutaneous nodule covered by normal skin. The lesion is usually solitary, with a pink or purple discoloration. This tumor tends to occur in children: 40 percent of the lesions are in patients 10 years of age or younger, and 20 percent occur in patients between ages 11 and 20 years (68). The upper lid and the eyebrow are sites of predilection.

Histopathologically, the tumor is a well-demarcated nodule involving the dermis and subcutaneous tissues. It is composed of irregular epithelial islands containing basophilic and shadow cells (fig. 2-42). The basophilic cells are located at the periphery of the epithelial islands and the shadow cells are in the center. The transition from basophilic to shadow cells is abrupt. The tumor contains varying amounts of calcium, which initially appears as basophilic granules within the cytoplasm of shadow cells. Areas of ossification are observed in approximately 15 percent of tumors. The tumor often invokes a foreign body giant cell reaction.

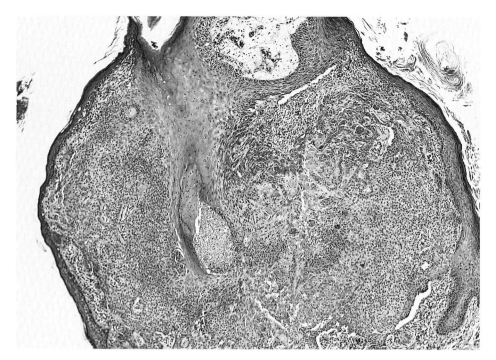

Figure 2-41
TRICHILEMMOMA
A small nodule involving a hair follicle is composed of polyhedral clear cells.

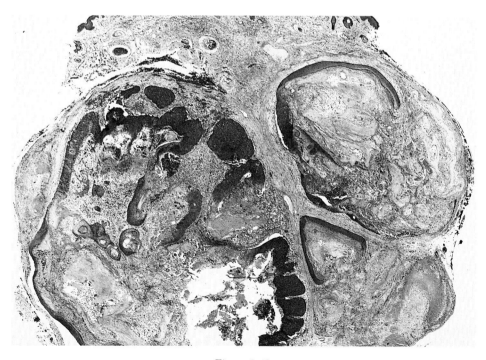

Figure 2-42
PILOMATRIXOMA
Multinodular tumor composed of peripheral basaloid cells and central ghost cells with foci of calcification.

ADNEXAL CARCINOMA

Adnexal carcinoma is a "wastebasket" term that should be restricted to lesions that histologically resemble basal cell carcinoma and exhibit a similar biologic behavior but for which the exact site of origin (from the epidermis or adnexal structures) cannot be determined with certainty.

TUMORS OF MELANOCYTES

Melanocytic tumors of the eyelid (see Table 2-5) are similar to, although less common than, those located in the conjunctiva. The discussion of these lesions in the next chapter is applicable to the eyelid.

TUMORS OF HEMATOPOIETIC AND SOFT TISSUES

Hematopoietic, lymphocytic (see Table 2-6), and soft tissue tumors (see Table 2-7) rarely affect the eyelid and, except for hemangiomas, are similar to their more common orbital counterparts. Only hemangiomas will be discussed in this chapter.

Hemangiomas

Primary angiomatous lesions of the eyelid are hamartomas that may be present at birth or become clinically apparent 1 to 2 weeks after birth (congenital lesions), appear later in childhood or in early adulthood (developmental lesions), or arise at any age as a secondary angiomatous lesion (acquired lesions). The capillary hemangioma of infancy and the nevus flammeus (port wine stain) are the most important congenital lesions, cavernous hemangiomas are developmental lesions, and pyogenic granulomas and varices are acquired angiomatous lesions.

Capillary Hemangioma (Juvenile Hemangioma, Strawberry Nevus, Nevus Vasculosus, Benign Hemangioendothelioma of Childhood). Capillary hemangioma is the most common form of hemangioma. It occurs in approximately one of every 200 live births. The lesion usually appears at birth or in the first or second week of life. Typically, it has a reddish purple color, is elevated, and is soft with small surface invaginations, hence the term strawberry nevus. Involvement of the eyelid is common. Capillary hemangiomas of the eyelid may extend into the conjunctiva or orbit.

The natural history and evolution of capillary hemangiomas are characteristic. They usually appear within the first 2 weeks after birth and rapidly enlarge in the first 6 months of life. Regression occurs over a period of several years and usually is accompanied by fading of the color of the lesion from reddish to a dull grayish red, with concomitant wrinkling of the overlying skin (crepe paper change). About 30 percent of the lesions completely regress by age 3 years and 75 to 90 percent by age 7 years (71).

Histologically, the lesion is composed of lobules of capillaries separated by fibrous septa (72). The capillaries may infiltrate the underlying skeletal muscle and subcutaneous tissues. Frequently, a moderate number of mitotic figures are observed. Early immature lesions have plump endothelial cells that tend to obliterate the vascular lumina. Reticulin stains are extremely helpful in establishing that the proliferation of endothelial cells lies inside the capillary basement membrane. Regression of the capillary hemangioma is accompanied by progressive interstitial fibrosis and peripheral replacement of the tumor lobules by adipose tissue.

The management of these lesions varies with the rate of growth as well as the location. The general approach is to observe and do nothing for smaller lesions that do not produce functional compromise. Rapidly enlarging lesions that cause functional impairment with the threat of amblyopia should be treated. Stigmar et al. (73) found that 22 of 51 children with untreated capillary hemangiomas of the eyelid developed amblyopia. Treatment of choice is intralesional injection of corticosteroids and surgery in older children when the hemangioma fails to regress adequately (69). Unfortunately, there is only anecdotal evidence that corticosteroids increase the rate of tumor shrinkage and adverse effects ranging from depigmentation to eyelid necrosis have been reported (70,74).

Nevus Flammeus (Port Wine Stain). Nevus flammeus is often associated with Sturge-Weber syndrome. Nevus flammeus is always present at birth, and may become darker and more prominent with time. The skin lesion is flat and has a deeper, more purple hue than the cherry red of capillary hemangioma. Additionally, unlike capillary hemangioma, nevus flammeus does not blanch on pressure or enlarge. Histopathologic

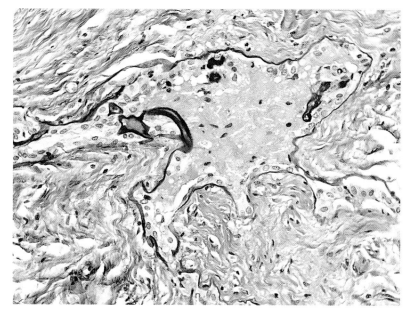

Figure 2-43
PHAKOMATOUS
CHORISTOMA
Island of lens epithelial tissue with a prominent PAS-positive basement membrane surrounded by desmoplastic stroma. (Figures 2-43–2-46 are from the same lesion.)

examination shows large, dilated cavernous spaces in the dermis and not the small blood vessels observed in capillary hemangiomas.

Cavernous Hemangioma. This tumor occurs less frequently in the eyelid than capillary hemangioma. The lesions arise in the second to fourth decades of life, occasionally becoming clinically evident late in the first decade. They differ from capillary hemangiomas in several important respects: a slowly progressive enlargement and no tendency for spontaneous regression. Superficial lesions are often dark blue; deeply located lesions may display little or no change in the color of the overlying skin. The relatively superficial eyelid cavernous hemangiomas are usually well circumscribed but not encapsulated, in contrast to the orbital lesions.

On microscopic examination, cavernous hemangioma is composed of large, dilated, blood-filled vascular spaces that are lined by a flat layer of endothelium (72). The tumor usually has an ill-defined lobular arrangement. The intervascular stroma is fibrotic and contains scattered chronic inflammatory cells. Secondary changes include foci of calcification, fibrosis, and hemosiderin deposits. Phlebolith formation is a frequent finding. The phlebolith represents an organized thrombus which has undergone dystrophic calcification.

In contrast to capillary hemangiomas, most cavernous hemangiomas require surgery. Malignant transformation does not occur.

MISCELLANEOUS TUMORS

Most of the tumors listed in Table 2-8 are adequately described elsewhere in this Fascicle or in other Fascicles. Three requiring additional comment are phakomatous choristoma, Merkel cell tumor, and metastatic carcinoma.

Phakomatous Choristoma

Zimmerman (76) first described three infants who had an unusual choristoma of the lower eyelid. Rare additional cases have been reported (75). All phakomatous choristomas were present at birth or in the first 6 months of life, and all involved the nasal aspect of lower eyelid. The masses ranged from 6 to 20 mm in maximal diameter, and all shared common histopathologic features.

Microscopically, phakomatous choristomas are composed of dense, collagenous tissue containing small epithelial nests and islands that are surrounded by a thick, periodic acid–Schiff (PAS)-positive basement membrane (figs. 2-43–2-46). Inside the basement membrane there is a single layer of large cuboidal cells. Swollen cells resembling the "bladder" cells of human cataractous lenses and amorphous, degenerative eosinophilic material are present within the centers of the epithelial structures. Small foci of dystrophic calcification and psammoma bodies may be present.

Electron microscopic data support the lenticular origin of phakomatous choristomas (75).

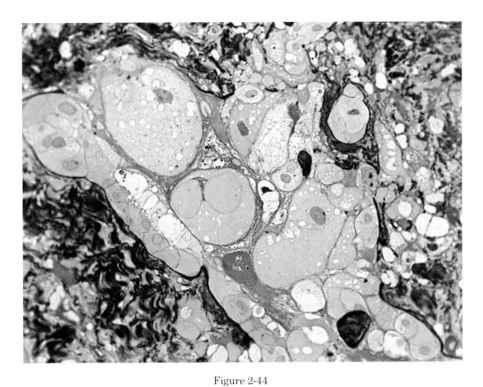

Figure 2-44
PHAKOMATOUS CHORISTOMA
There is proliferation of swollen epithelial cells similar to that seen in a posterior subcapsular cataract.

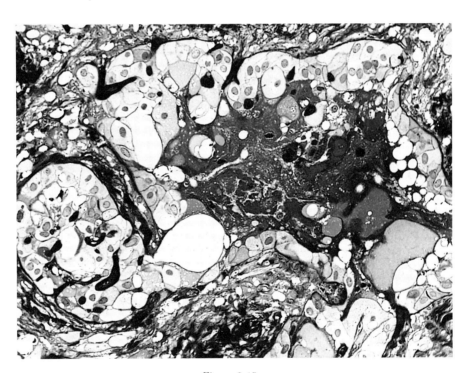

Figure 2-45
PHAKOMATOUS CHORISTOMA
PAS stained island of lenticular tissue with degeneration of the cells in the central area.

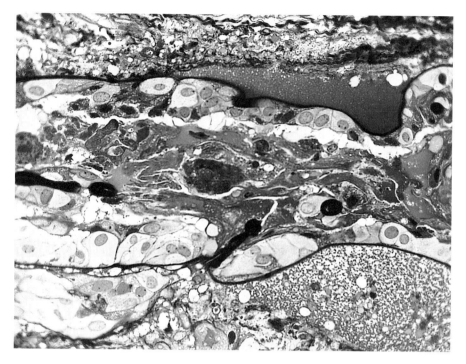

Figure 2-46
PHAKOMATOUS CHORISTOMA
PAS stained thick basement membrane surrounds an island of lenticular epithelial cells.

There is a thick, homogeneous type of basement membrane surrounding the epithelial islands. The degenerated material in the center of the epithelial islands resembles that seen in cataractous lenses. The cuboidal epithelial cells display conspicuous interdigitation of their plasmalemmas (ball and socket configurations), occasional desmosomes, and macula occludens. Some cells have a paucity of cytoplasmic organelles whereas others contain numerous cytoplasmic filaments. Immunohistochemical stains for vimentin are positive in the cells with abundant cytoplasmic filaments.

All these features are characteristic of the cells of the human lens. It has been suggested that the lesion is a choristoma of lenticular anlage that probably results from lens placode cells being left in the mesodermal tissues of the lower eyelid when the lens vesicle forms. The nasal location of the lesion in the lower eyelid probably represents the site where the lens placode is induced in the surface ectoderm. This localization may result from the inferonasal location of the embryonic fissure in the optic cup.

Merkel Cell Tumor (Trabecular Carcinoma of the Skin, Cutaneous APUDoma, Small Cell Neuroepithelial Tumor, Primary Small Cell Cutaneous Carcinoma, Neuroendocrine or Merkel Cell Carcinoma)

In 1875, Friedrich Merkel described clear, nondendritic, oval cells oriented parallel to the skin surface and located in the deeper layers of the epidermis adjacent to hair follicles where they formed complexes with nerve endings. They are best identified with the electron microscope. Although Merkel cell tumors of the skin are uncommon, they have been recognized with increasing frequency in recent years. A common site for Merkel cell tumors is the face, and there have been a number of cases involving the eyelids or eyebrows. Twelve cases were referred to the ROP (see Table 2-8).

Kivelä and Tarkkanen (77) reviewed published reports of Merkel cell tumors. The patients were usually elderly; women were affected in about two thirds of the cases. The tumors,

41

including those involving the eyelid, were painless, cutaneous nodules with violet or reddish blue overlying skin, resembling an angiomatous lesion. Telangiectatic vessels were frequently observed on the surface of the nodules (fig. 2-47). Approximately 10 percent of Merkel cell tumors involved the eyelids and periocular area. Upper eyelid lesions were more common than those of the lower eyelid.

By light microscopy, the tumor cells have a high nuclear-cytoplasmic ratio. The round to oval uniform nuclei contain finely dispersed chromatin and one to three small nucleoli (figs. 2-48–2-50). Mitotic figures may be numerous. The tumor cells that infiltrate the dermis are arranged in diffuse sheets or in a trabecular pattern. Merkel cell tumor in the eyelid is a poorly differentiated round cell neoplasm, and the differential diagnosis includes malignant lymphoma, metastatic oat cell carcinoma, amelanotic melanoma, and sebaceous gland carcinoma.

Ultrastructural examination of Merkel cell tumors confirms their neuroepithelial derivation. The cells contain 80- to 200-nm membrane-bound dense core granules, perinuclear microfilaments (7 to 9 nm in diameter), desmosomes, hemidesmosomes, and focal basal lamina. Another ultrastructural feature observed in normal Merkel cells, as well as in some Merkel cell tumors, is the presence of intranuclear rodlets. Polyribosomes are usually numerous and the Golgi apparatus prominent, whereas mitochondria and rough-surfaced endoplasmic reticulum are scanty.

Immunohistochemical studies are helpful in the diagnosis of Merkel cell tumor. Immunoperoxidase stains for neuron-specific enolase (NSE) show a dark cytoplasmic rim encircling large, round, unstained nuclei. Merkel cells are also cytokeratin positive and typically have a small dot of immunoreactivity within the cytoplasm. Negative reactions for HMB-45 and leukocyte common antigen help to differentiate Merkel cell tumors from melanomas and lymphomas. Other peptides occasionally found in Merkel cell tumors include calcitonin, somatostatin, and corticotropin (ACTH) (67).

Merkel cell carcinomas arising in the eyelid usually grow rapidly and have a diffuse infiltrative pattern. Spread to regional lymph nodes, distant metastases, and death occur in approximately 50 percent of the patients (77). The treat-

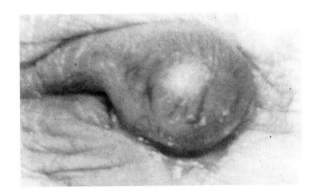

Figure 2-47
MERKEL CELL TUMOR
Tumor of the superficial dermis of the upper eyelid with thinning of the epidermis and prominent blood vessels.

ment of choice is wide surgical excision of the mass with frozen section control of the margins. Because of few cases with lid involvement and incomplete follow-up data, general guidelines regarding tumor response to radiotherapy and chemotherapy are not available.

Carcinoma Metastatic to the Eyelid

Metastatic tumors to the eyelid are uncommon in series based on surgical pathologic material. Only 10 examples were found in a 5-year period in the AFIP ROP (see Table 2-8). Mansour and Hidayat (79) reported on 31 cases in which 35 percent of the metastases were from breast, 17 percent from skin, 10 percent from the gastrointestinal tract, and 10 percent from the urogenital system. Aside from breast carcinoma there was no sex predilection. Only 32 percent were correctly diagnosed clinically. The most common misdiagnoses were chalazion, cyst, and xanthoma. In 45 percent of the cases the eyelid lesion was detected prior to the primary tumor. Morgan et al. (80) reviewed the literature regarding eyelid involvement as the initial manifestation of nonocular cancer. In women the most common primary site was the breast and in men the most common site was the lung.

Hood et al. (78) studied 13 mammary carcinomas metastatic to the eyelids. In 5, metastasis to the eyelid preceded recognition of the primary mammary carcinoma by 1 to 6 months. All 13 of the metastatic tumors were painless. Eight patients had diffuse unilateral swelling of the

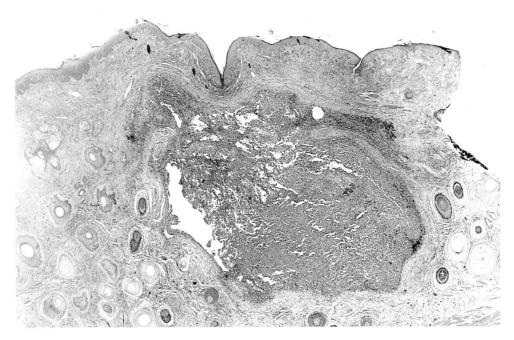

Figure 2-48
MERKEL CELL TUMOR
Well-circumscribed nodule in the superficial dermis.

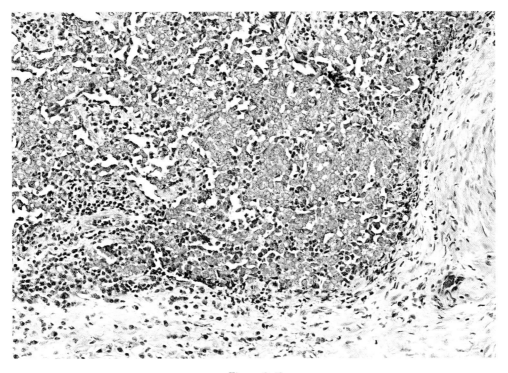

Figure 2-49
MERKEL CELL TUMOR
The neoplastic cells of the tumor seen in figure 2-48 have pale round nuclei with a high nuclear-cytoplasmic ratio.

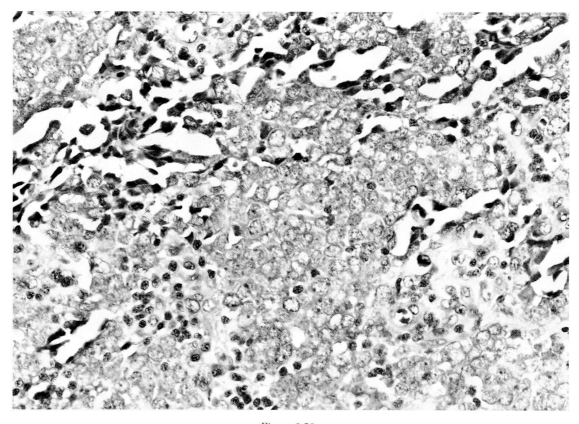

Figure 2-50
MERKEL CELL TUMOR
Higher magnification of the previously illustrated tumor showing the fine nuclear details of the neoplastic cells and reactive lymphocytic infiltration.

upper, lower, or both lids, whereas 5 had mobile nodules. Five of the tumors exhibited the typical morphologic features of metastatic breast carcinoma, whereas 8 had a histiocytoid histologic appearance (see fig. 2-26). Histiocytoid tumor cells have a uniform appearance, with bland, round to oval nuclei containing uniform chromatin and inconspicuous nucleoli. Within the abundant eosinophilic cytoplasm of some of the histiocytoid cells are vacuoles. Signet ring cells may be present. The cells are arranged singly or in small groups with occasional rows of single cells (single file pattern) embedded in a dense collagenous stroma. Mitotic figures are gener-

ally absent or very sparse. These histiocytoid features have led to misinterpretations, resulting in initial diagnoses of xanthelasma, xanthoma, histiocytoma, granular cell myoblastoma, and blastomycosis.

Histochemical stains of metastatic breast carcinoma for mucopolysaccharides often disclose cytoplasmic vacuoles that contain variable amounts of hyaluronidase-resistant Alcian blue–positive material that also stains vividly with the PAS and mucicarmine techniques. Histologically and immunohistochemically, the lesion may be indistinguishable from primary sweat gland carcinoma of the eyelid.

REFERENCES

General References

Jakobiec FA, Iwamoto T. The ocular adnexa: lids, conjunctiva and orbit. In: Fine BS, Yanoff M, eds. Ocular histology: a text and atlas. 2nd ed. Hagerstown, Md.: Harper & Row, 1979:289–342.

Font RL. Eyelids and lacrimal drainage system. In: Spencer WH, ed. Ophthalmic pathology. An atlas and textbook. 3rd ed. Philadelphia: WB Saunders, 1985:2141–312.

Classification and Frequency

1. Burnier MN Jr, Belfort R Jr, Rigueiro MP, et al. Benign tumors of the conjunctiva and eyelids. Arch I P B 1988; 30:17–20.
2. _____, Belfort R Jr, Rigueiro MP, et al. Malignant tumors of the eyelids. Arch I P B 1988;30:58–65.
3. Font RL. Eyelids and lacrimal drainage system. In: Spencer WH, ed. Ophthalmic pathology. An atlas and textbook. 3rd ed. Philadelphia: WB Saunders, 1985:2141–312.
4. Tesluk GC. Eyelid lesions: incidence and comparison of benign and malignant lesions. Ann Ophthalmol 1985; 17:704–7.

Inverted Follicular Keratosis

5. Ni C, Merriam J, Abert DM. Irritated seborrheic keratosis of eyelid and its differential diagnosis. An electron microscopic and light microscopic study. Chin Med J (Engl) 1988;101:555–8.
6. Sassani JW, Yanoff M. Inverted follicular keratosis. Am J Ophthalmol 1979;87:810–3.

Keratoacanthoma

7. Boniuk M, Zimmerman LE. Eyelid tumors with reference to lesions confused with squamous cell carcinoma. III. Keratoacanthoma. Arch Ophthalmol 1967;77:29–40.

Actinic Keratosis

8. Marks R, Foley P, Goodman G, et al. Spontaneous remission of solar keratoses: the case for conservative management. Br J Dermatol 1986;115:649–55.
9. _____, Rennie G, Selwood TS. Malignant transformation of solar keratoses to squamous cell carcinoma. Lancet 1988;1:795–7.

Bowen Disease

10. Chute CG, Chuang TY, Bergstralh EJ, Su WP. The subsequent risk of internal cancer with Bowen's disease. A population-based study. JAMA 1991;266:816–9.
11. Kettler AH, Rutledge M, Tschen JA, Buffone G. Detection of human papillomavirus in nongenital Bowen's disease by in situ DNA hybridization. Arch Dermatol 1990;126:777–81.
12. Ratnam KV, Espy MJ, Muller SA, Smith TF, Su WP. Clinicopathologic study of arsenic-induced skin lesions: no definite association with human papillomavirus. J Am Acad Dermatol 1992;27:120–2.
13. Tanimoto A, Hamada T, Kanesaki H, Matsuno K, Koide O. Multiple primary cancers in a case of chronic arsenic poisoning—an autopsy report. Sangyo Ika Daigaku Zasshi 1990;12:89–99.

Squamous Cell Carcinoma

14. Burnier MN Jr, Belfort R Jr, Rigueiro MP, et al. Malignant tumors of the eyelids. Arch I P B 1988;30:58–65.
15. Nixon RL, Dorevitch AP, Marks R. Squamous cell carcinoma of the skin: accuracy of clinical diagnosis and outcome of follow-up in Australia. Med J Aust 1986;144:235–9.
16. Tesluk GC. Eyelid lesions: incidence and comparison of benign and malignant lesions. Ann Ophthalmol 1985; 17:704–7.

Basal Cell Carcinoma

17. Aldred WV, Ramirez VG, Nicholson DH. Intraocular invasion of basal cell carcinoma of the lid. Arch Ophthalmol 1980;98:1821–2.
18. Anderson DE, Taylor WB, Falls HF, Davidson RT. The nevoid basal cell carcinoma syndrome. Am J Hum Genet 1967;19:12–22.
19. Burnier MN Jr, Belfort R Jr, Rigueiro MP, et al. Malignant tumors of the eyelids. Arch I P B 1988;30:58–65.
20. Doxanas MT, Green WR, Iliff CE. Factors in the successful surgical management of basal cell carcinoma of the eyelids. Am J Ophthalmol 1981;91:726–36.
21. Farmer ER, Helwig EB. Metastatic basal cell carcinoma: a clinicopathologic study of seventeen cases. Cancer 1980;46:748–57.
22. Font RL. Eyelids and lacrimal drainage system. In: Spencer WH, ed. Ophthalmic pathology. An atlas and textbook. 3rd ed. Philadelphia: WB Saunders, 1985:2141–312.
23. Frank HJ. Frozen section control of excision of eyelid basal cell carcinomas: 8½ years' experience. Br J Ophthalmol 1989;73:328–32.
24. Hornblass A, Stefano JA. Pigmented basal cell carcinoma of the eyelids. Am J Ophthalmol 1981;92:193–7.
25. Mohs FE. Micrographic surgery for the microscopically controlled excision of eyelid cancer: history and development. Adv Ophthalmic Plast Reconstr Surg 1986;5:381–408.
26. Simpson W, Garner A, Collin JR. Benign hair-follicle derived tumours in the differential diagnosis of basal-cell carcinoma of the eyelids: a clinicopathological comparison. Br J Ophthalmol 1989;73:347–53.
27. Soffer D, Kaplan H, Weshler Z. Meningeal carcinomatosis due to basal cell carcinoma. Hum Pathol 1985;16:530–2.
28. Tesluk GC. Eyelid lesions: incidence and comparison of benign and malignant lesions. Ann Ophthalmol 1985; 17:704–7.
29. Wesley RE, Collins JW. Basal cell carcinoma of the eyelid as an indicator of multifocal malignancy. Am J Ophthalmol 1982;94:591–3.

Apocrine Adenoma

30. Burnier MN Jr, Belfort R Jr, Rigueiro MP, et al. Benign tumors of the conjunctiva and eyelids. Arch I P B 1988; 30:17–20.
31. Netland PA, Townsend DJ, Albert DM, Jakobiec FA. Hidradenoma papilliferum of the upper eyelid arising from the apocrine gland of Moll. Ophthalmology 1990;97:1593–8.

Syringoma

32. Levine MR, Grossniklaus H. Sclerosing syringoma. Ann Ophthalmol 1990;22:110–11.

Eccrine Acrospiroma

33. Grossniklaus HE, Knight SH. Eccrine acrospiroma (clear cell hidradenoma) of the eyelid. Immunohistochemical and ultrastructural features. Ophthalmology 1991;98:347–52.

Pleomorphic Adenoma

34. Daicker B, Gafner E. Apocrine mixed tumour of the lid. Ophthalmologica 1975;170:548–53.
35. Jordan DR, Nerad JA, Patrinely JR. Chondroid syringoma of the eyelid. Can J Ophthalmol 1989;24:24–7.
36. Parks SL, Glover AT. Benign mixed tumors arising in the palpebral lobe of the lacrimal gland. Ophthalmology 1990;97:526–30.

Eccrine and Apocrine Carcinomas

37. el-Domeiri AA, Brasfield RD, Huvos AG, Strong EW. Sweat gland carcinoma: a clinico-pathologic study of 83 patients. Ann Surg 1971;173:270–4.
38. Glatt HJ, Proia AD, Tsoy EA, et al. Malignant syringoma of the eyelid. Ophthalmology 1984;91:987–90.
39. Grizzard WS, Torezynski E, Edwards WC. Adenocarcinoma of eccrine sweat glands. Arch Ophthalmol 1976;94:2119–23.
40. Headington JT, Niederhuber JE, Beals TF. Malignant clear cell acrospiroma. Cancer 1978;41:641–7.
41. Hood CI, Font RL, Zimmerman LE. Metastatic mammary carcinoma in the eyelid with histiocytoid appearance. Cancer 1973;31:793–800.
42. Jakobiec FA, Austin P, Iwamoto T, Trokel SL, Marquardt MD, Harrison W. Primary infiltrating signet ring carcinoma of the eyelids. Ophthalmology 1983;90:291–9.
43. Jordan DR, Nerad JA, Patrinely JR. Chondroid syringoma of the eyelid. Can J Ophthalmol 1989;24:24–7.
44. Khalil M, Brownstein S, Codere F, Nicolle D. Eccrine sweat gland carcinoma of the eyelid with orbital involvement. Arch Ophthalmol 1980;98:2210–4.
45. Ni C, Wagoner M, Kieval S, Albert DM. Tumours of the Moll's Glands. Br J Ophthalmol 1984;68:502–6.
46. Snow SN, Reizner GT. Mucinous eccrine carcinoma of the eyelid. Cancer 1992;70:2099–104.
47. Swanson PE, Mazoujian G, Mills SE, Campbell RJ, Wick MR. Immunoreactivity for estrogen receptor protein in sweat gland tumors. Am J Surg Pathol 1991;15:835–41.
48. Thomson SJ, Tanner NS. Carcinoma of the apocrine glands at the base of eyelashes: a case report and discussion of histological diagnostic criteria. Br J Plast Surg 1989;42:598–602.
49. Wright JD, Font RL. Mucinous sweat gland adenocarcinoma of eyelid. A clinicopathologic study of 21 cases with histochemical and electron microscopic observations. Cancer 1979;44:1757–68.

Sebaceous Adenoma

50. Jakobiec FA, Zimmerman LE, La Piana F, Hornblass A, Breffeilh RA, Lackey JK. Unusual eyelid tumors with sebaceous differentiation in the Muir-Torre syndrome. Rapid clinical regrowth and frank squamous transformation after biopsy. Ophthalmology 1988;95:1543–8.

51. Tillawi I, Katz R, Pellettiere EV. Solitary tumors of meibomian gland origin and Torre's syndrome. Am J Ophthalmol 1987;104:179–82.
52. Torre D. Multiple sebaceous tumors. Arch Dermatol 1968;98:549–51.

Sebaceous Carcinoma

53. Brownstein S, Codere F, Jackson WB. Masquerade syndrome. Ophthalmology 1980;87:259–62.
54. Bryant J. Meibomian gland carcinoma seeding intracranial soft tissues. Hum Pathol 1977;8:455–7.
55. Doxanas MT, Green WR. Sebaceous gland carcinoma. Review of 40 cases. Arch Ophthalmol 1984;102:245–9.
56. Folberg R, Whitaker DC, Tse DT, Nerad JA. Recurrent and residual sebaceous carcinoma after Mohs' excision of the primary lesion. Am J Ophthalmol 1987;103:817–23.
57. Margo CE, Lessner A, Stern GA. Intraepithelial sebaceous carcinoma of the conjunctiva and skin of the eyelid. Ophthalmology 1992;99:227–31.
58. Ni C, Guo PK. Meibomian gland carcinoma. A clinicopathological study of 156 cases with long-period follow-up of 100 cases. Jpn J Ophthalmol 1979;23:388–401.
59. Nunery WR, Welsh MG, McCord CD Jr. Recurrence of sebaceous carcinoma of the eyelid after radiation therapy. Am J Ophthalmol 1983;96:10–5.
60. Rao NA, Hidayat AA, McLean IW, Zimmerman LE. Sebaceous carcinomas of the ocular adnexa: a clinico-pathologic study of 104 cases, with five-year follow-up data. Hum Pathol 1982;13:113–22.
61. _____, McLean IW, Zimmerman LE. Sebaceous carcinoma of the eyelid and caruncle. Correlation of clinical pathologic features with prognosis. In: Jakobiec FA, ed. Ocular and adnexal tumors. Birmingham: Aesculapius Publishers, 1978:289–342.
62. Swanson PE, Mazoujian G, Mills SE, Campbell RJ, Wick MR. Immunoreactivity for estrogen receptor protein in sweat gland tumors. Am J Surg Pathol 1991;15:835–41.
63. Thomson SJ, Tanner NS. Carcinoma of the apocrine glands at the base of eyelashes: a case report and discussion of histological diagnostic criteria. Br J Plast Surg 1989;42:598–602.

Trichoepithelioma

64. Wolken SH, Spivey BE, Blodi F. Hereditary adenoid cystic epithelioma (Brooke's tumor). Am J Ophthalmol 1968;68:26–34.

Trichofolliculoma

65. Carreras B Jr, Lopez-Marin I Jr, Mellado VG, Gutierrez MT. Trichofolliculoma of the eyelid. Br J Ophthalmol 1981;65:214–5.

Trichilemmoma

66. Bardenstein DS, McLean IW, Nerney J, Boatwright RS. Cowden's disease. Ophthalmology 1988;95:1038–41.
67. Hidayat AA, Font RL. Trichilemmoma of eyelid and eyebrow. A clinicopathologic study of 31 cases. Arch Ophthalmol 1980;98:844–7.

Pilomatrixoma

68. Ni C, Kimball GP, Craft JL, Wang WJ, Chong CS, Albert DM. Calcifying epithelioma: a clinicopathological analysis of 67 cases with ultrastructural study of 2 cases. Int Ophthalmol Clin 1982;22:63–86.

Hemangiomas

69. Boyd MJ, Collin JR. Capillary haemangiomas: an approach to their management. Br J Ophthalmol 1991; 75:298–300.
70. Cogen MS, Elsas FJ. Eyelid depigmentation following corticosteroid injection for infantile ocular adnexal hemangioma. J Pediatr Ophthalmol Strabismus 1989; 26:35–8.
71. Font RL. Eyelids and lacrimal drainage system. In: Spencer WH, ed. Ophthalmic pathology. An atlas and textbook. 3rd ed. Philadelphia: WB Saunders, 1985: 2141–312.
72. Iwamoto T, Jakobiec FA. Ultrastructural comparison of capillary and cavernous hemangiomas of the orbit. Arch Ophthalmol 1979;97:1144–53.
73. Stigmar G, Crawford JS, Ward CM, Thomson HG. Ophthalmic sequelae of infantile hemangiomas of the eyelids and orbit. Am J Ophthalmol 1978;85:806–13.
74. Sutula FC, Glover AT. Eyelid necrosis following intralesional corticosteroid injection for capillary hemangioma. Ophthalmic Surg 1987;18:103–5.

Phakomatous Choristoma

75. Eustis HS, Karcioglu ZA, Dharma S, Hoda S. Phakomatous choristoma: clinical, histopathologic, and ultrastructural findings in a 4-month-old boy. J Pediatr Ophthalmol Strabismus 1990;27:208–11.
76. Zimmerman LE. Phakomatous choristoma of the eyelid. A tumor of lenticular anlage. Am J Ophthalmol 1971;71:169–77.

Merkel Cell Tumor

77. Kivelä T, Tarkkanen A. The Merkel cell and associated neoplasms in the eyelids and periocular region. Surv Ophthalmol 1990;35:171–87.

Metastatic Tumors

78. Hood CI, Font RL, Zimmerman LE. Metastatic mammary carcinoma in the eyelid with histiocytoid appearance. Cancer 1973;31:793–800.
79. Mansour AM, Hidayat AA. Metastatic eyelid disease. Ophthalmology 1987;94:667–70.
80. Morgan LW, Linberg JV, Anderson RL. Metastatic disease first presenting as eyelid tumors: a report of two cases and review of the literature. Ann Ophthalmol 1987;19:13–8.

✧ ✧ ✧

3
TUMORS OF THE CONJUNCTIVA

ANATOMY AND HISTOLOGY

Gross Anatomic Features

The conjunctiva is a mucous membrane that covers the posterior surface of the lids and the anterior surface of the globe, with the exception of the cornea. It is subdivided into the palpebral, fornical, and bulbar regions. The palpebral conjunctiva extends from the mucocutaneous junction at the margins of the upper and lower lids to the superior and inferior fornices. It is firmly adherent to the tarsal plates. Its surface is smooth and contains several crypt-like infoldings of the epithelium (pseudoglands of Henle).

In the fornices, the conjunctiva is loosely attached to the orbital septum. The fornical conjunctiva extends temporally behind the lateral canthus and nasally to the semilunar fold. Ducts of the lacrimal gland open into the temporal portion of the upper fornix, and ducts of the accessory glands of Krause and Wolfring open into the upper and lower fornices.

The bulbar conjunctiva is loosely adherent to the sclera and extends from the limbus to the fornical area. The caruncle lies at the inner canthus. It is composed of a round to ovoid head and a tail blending with the skin at the canthus. Its surface is somewhat irregular. It contains several hairs, sebaceous glands, sweat glands, lobules of lacrimal gland, and striated muscle.

The palpebral conjunctiva and the eyelids share a common arterial blood supply derived from the branches of the ophthalmic artery and supplemented by branches of the facial artery. The bulbar conjunctiva is supplied by branches of the anterior ciliary arteries, which also supply the anterior episclera and form the superficial marginal plexus at the limbus. The palpebral conjunctival veins join the post-tarsal veins of the eyelid and communicate with the orbital veins and the deep facial branches of the anterior facial vein and pterygoid plexus. The bulbar conjunctival veins drain into the episcleral venous plexuses, which also drain the intrascleral plexuses.

Lymphatic channels are present in the conjunctival stroma, and extend much closer to the epithelium than do the lymphatics of the dermis. The lymphatics of the conjunctiva join the lymphatics of the eyelid and drain medially to the submandibular lymph nodes and laterally to the preauricular (intraparotid) lymph nodes. The fifth cranial nerve supplies a network of sensory branches to all portions of the conjunctiva.

Microscopic Features

Epithelium. Two to five layers of stratified columnar epithelium cover most of the conjunctiva except at the limbus, the palpebral margins, and the caruncle where stratified squamous epithelium is present. At the mucocutaneous junction of the lid margin, there is an abrupt transition from keratinized stratified squamous epithelium characteristic of skin to nonkeratinized mucosal epithelium of the palpebral conjunctiva. At the limbus, the epithelium changes gradually from stratified squamous epithelium characteristic of the cornea to stratified columnar epithelium (fig. 3-1). The epithelium of the head of the caruncle is thick and of the nonkeratinized stratified squamous type. There is a gradual transition to keratinized squamous epithelium in the tail of the caruncle.

Melanocytes are present in the basal layer of the conjunctival epithelium and melanin granules may be transferred to adjacent epithelial cells. This is a constant finding in black individuals and is common in heavily pigmented white patients. Langerhans cells are also found within the conjunctival epithelium. Goblet cells normally are present in the middle and superficial epithelial layers. They are most numerous in the semilunar fold and fornices, usually absent at the limbus, and scarce in the remainder of bulbar conjunctiva.

Ultrastructurally, the conjunctival basal cells have a thin basement membrane similar to that of the basal cells of the corneal epithelium. The midepithelial and superficial cells are polygonal and flatten as they approach the surface, where there are microvilli similar to those of surface cells of the cornea. The cell membranes have deep interdigitations, with intercellular desmosomal

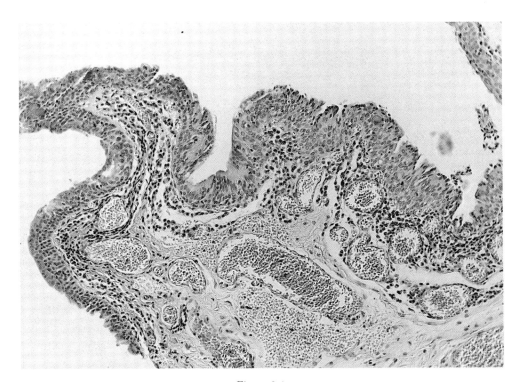

Figure 3-1
NORMAL BULBAR CONJUNCTIVA
Stratified nonkeratinizing squamous epithelium with goblet cells covers a highly vascularized lamina propria.

attachments. The cytoplasm contains bundles of tonofilaments.

Substantia Propria. This layer is composed of fibrovascular connective tissue of varying density and thickness. In the palpebral region it is thin and compact, creating a firm connection between the epithelium and the tarsus. In the fornices and over the globe it is thick and loose, but at the limbus it again thins and becomes more compact as it attaches to the episclera. At the corneal margin the stroma and epithelium form radially oriented rete pegs and papillae (the palisades of Vogt). The substantia propria of the semilunar fold is similar to that of the bulbar conjunctiva; however, occasionally it contains cartilage.

Fibroblasts and inflammatory cells are normally present in the conjunctival stroma. Inflammatory cells are not found in the fetal conjunctiva; however, shortly after birth collections of subepithelial lymphocytes appear, especially in the tarsal region. Lymphocytes also aggregate within subepithelial tissues in the fornices and form follicle-like structures, some of which contain germinal centers.

CLASSIFICATION AND FREQUENCY

The conjunctiva is the most frequent anatomic site for tumors according to the Armed Forces Institute of Pathology (AFIP) Registry of Ophthalmic Pathology (ROP); in the Brazilian ROP only eyelid tumors are more common (see Table 1-1). This difference is mainly because general pathologists do not frequently refer cases of basal cell carcinoma of the eyelid to the AFIP. The schema proposed by the World Health Organization (WHO) provides the basis for classifying conjunctival tumors (Tables 3-1–3-6) with the exception of carcinoma in situ, which is classified with dysplasias and actinic keratoses as an intraepithelial neoplasm rather than as a malignant neoplasm. Data from the Institute of Ophthalmology in England (3), the Brazilian Registry (1,2), and the AFIP Registry (Tables 3-1–3-6) indicate that epithelial tumors account for one third to half of conjunctival neoplasms. The prevalence is highest in Brazil (48.9 percent) and lowest in England (33.8 percent), which probably relates to differences in actinic exposure. Rare

Table 3-1

TUMORS OF SURFACE EPITHELIUM OF THE CONJUNCTIVA*

Type of Tumor	Number of Cases
Benign	
Squamous cell papilloma	74
Keratotic plaque	9
Pseudocarcinomatous hyperplasia	9
Benign hereditary intraepithelial dyskeratosis	5
Intraepithelial neoplasia	
Actinic keratosis (solar keratosis)	149
Dysplasia	76
Carcinoma in situ	26
Malignant	
Squamous cell carcinoma	151
Basal cell carcinoma	1
Mucoepidermoid carcinoma	4
Adenocarcinoma	5

*Frequency distribution of 509 tumors in the AFIP Registry of Ophthalmic Pathology collected between 1984 and 1989.

Table 3-2

TUMORS OF ADNEXAL GLANDS AND SECONDARY ADNEXAL TUMORS OF THE CONJUNCTIVA*

Type of Tumor	Number of Cases
Benign	
Oncocytoma (oxyphilic cell adenoma)	13
Pleomorphic adenoma (mixed tumor, chondroid syringoma)	1
Apocrine adenoma	1
Sebaceous adenoma	1
Malignant	
Sebaceous adenocarcinoma	8

*Frequency distribution of 24 tumors in the AFIP Registry of Ophthalmic Pathology collected between 1984 and 1989.

tumors arise from the accessory glands located in the caruncle (Table 3-2). Regarding melanocytic tumors, two thirds are benign nevi in both the British (3) and AFIP (Table 3-3) Registries and three fourths are benign nevi in the Brazilian Registry (1,2). This probably reflects differences in racial make-up and population age.

Table 3-3

TUMORS OF MELANOCYTIC ORIGIN OF THE CONJUNCTIVA*

Type of Tumor	Number of Cases
Benign	
Nevus	355
Congenital epithelial melanosis (ephelis)	3
Secondary acquired melanosis	3
Primary acquired melanosis	54
Malignant	
Melanoma	127

*Frequency distribution of 542 tumors in the AFIP Registry of Ophthalmic Pathology collected between 1984 and 1989.

Table 3-4

TUMORS OF LYMPHOCYTIC OR HEMATOPOIETIC ORIGIN OF THE CONJUNCTIVA*

Type of Tumor	Number of Cases
Benign	
Reactive lymphoid hyperplasia	54
Atypical lymphoid hyperplasia	33
Malignant	
Lymphoma	29
Leukemia	0
Plasmacytoma	1

*Frequency distribution of 117 tumors in the AFIP Registry of Ophthalmic Pathology collected between 1984 and 1989.

Most lymphoid, hematopoietic, and soft tissue tumors (Tables 3-4, 3-5) are similar to their counterparts in the orbit and these will be discussed in the chapter, Tumors of the Orbit. The major exception is Kaposi sarcoma, which occurs almost always in the conjunctiva or eyelid and has become much more common because of the acquired immunodeficiency syndrome (AIDS). Dermoids and lipodermoids are uncommon choristomatous malformations of the conjunctiva and underlying sclera (Table 3-6) but represented 10 percent of the tumors in the British Registry (3).

Table 3-5

Table 3-5
TUMORS OF SOFT TISSUE ORIGIN OF THE CONJUNCTIVA*

Type of Tumor	Number of Cases
Benign	
Lipoma	1
Neurofibroma	1
Fibrous histiocytoma	7
Myxoma	6
Hemangioma	6
Lymphangioma	2
Malignant	
Fibrous histiocytoma	1
Rhabdomyosarcoma	1
Kaposi sarcoma	4

*Frequency distribution of 29 tumors in the AFIP Registry of Ophthalmic Pathology collected between 1984 and 1989.

Table 3-6
CHORISTOMATOUS TUMORS OF THE CONJUNCTIVA*

Type of Tumor	Number of Cases
Dermoid	16
Dermolipoma	7
Complex choristoma	14

*Frequency distribution of 37 tumors in the AFIP Registry of Ophthalmic Pathology collected between 1984 and 1989.

BENIGN TUMORS OF SURFACE EPITHELIUM

Squamous Cell Papilloma

Definition. Squamous cell papillomas are benign sessile and pedunculated tumors of the conjunctiva in which acanthotic squamous epithelium covers fibrovascular fronds.

Clinical Features. Conjunctival papillomas tend to be pedunculated in children and sessile in adults. Most are asymptomatic without associated conjunctivitis. Although pedunculated papillomas are located most frequently inferiorly in the fornix and sessile papillomas on the bulbar conjunctiva, both types may develop anywhere in the conjunctiva. Sessile papillomas can spread onto the cornea where they may interfere with visual acuity. The papillomas may be multifocal or bilateral. They are usually grayish red, fleshy, soft, pedunculated or sessile elevations with an irregular surface that sometimes is cauliflower-like. The vessels within the fibrovascular fronds appear as regularly spaced red dots through the translucent epithelium.

The clinical behavior of conjunctival papillomas is similar to papovavirus-induced verrucae of the skin, and it is presumed that papovavirus is implicated in the pathogenesis of both lesions. Human papilloma virus has been demonstrated in conjunctival specimens using the immunoperoxidase technique for genus-specific antigens and using hybridization techniques for human papilloma virus DNA sequences (5–7).

Conjunctival papillomas may recur after excision and multiple recurrences are not uncommon.

Pathologic Findings. The lesions can be divided into pedunculated and sessile types. Pedunculated papillomas are composed of multiple branching fronds emanating from a narrow base. Each frond has a central vascularized core surrounded by connective tissue in which acute and chronic inflammatory cells are often found. Sessile papillomas arise from a broad base with regularly spaced fibrovascular fronds. In both types, the fronds are covered by acanthotic, nonkeratinizing, goblet cell–containing stratified squamous epithelium that is not atypical (fig. 3-2). Koilocytosis has been observed in 60 percent of conjunctival papillomas (6). Several precancerous and carcinomatous lesions may also have a papillary configuration. Squamous papillomas that display cytologic atypia are best classified as dysplasias or carcinomas in situ. Very rare papillomas of the conjunctiva have an inverted growth pattern (4). These lesions invaginate into the underlying stroma instead of growing in the exophytic manner characteristic of other papillomas. This type of papilloma is far more common in the nose, paranasal sinuses, and lacrimal sac than in the conjunctiva.

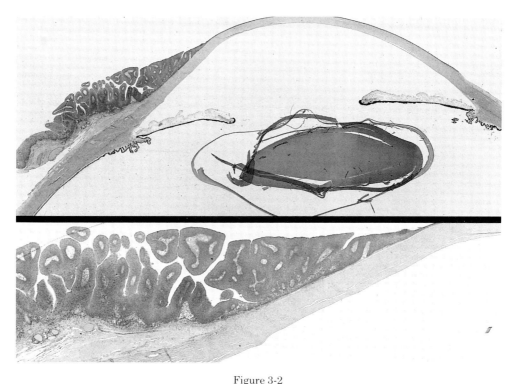

Figure 3-2
PAPILLOMA
Limbal tumor composed of fibrovascular fronds covered by squamous epithelium.

Keratotic Plaque

Leukoplakic lesions with little or no potential for carcinomatous change may develop in the bulbar or limbal conjunctiva. Histologically, these lesions lack the cytologic atypia of an actinic keratosis. The epithelial thickening is characterized mainly by acanthosis with hyperkeratosis. Keratotic plaques that develop in the interpalpebral area in patients with vitamin A–deficient xerosis are referred to as Bitot spots.

Pseudocarcinomatous Hyperplasia (Pseudoepitheliomatous Hyperplasia)

The conjunctival epithelium may become acanthotic, parakeratotic, or hyperkeratotic as a result of irritation initiated by preexisting stromal inflammation. The source of the inflammation may be infectious or irritation by lesions such as pinguecula and pterygia. The epithelial thickening and leukoplakia may clinically and histologically suggest a squamous cell carcinoma. Histologically, the acanthotic epithelium invading the stroma has a jagged border, with irregular masses of epithelial cells that often contain keratin cysts (figs. 3-3, 3-4). Pseudocarcinomatous hyperplasias that resemble keratoacanthomas of the skin may be observed in the conjunctiva (fig. 3-3). Mitotic figures may be numerous. A lack of nuclear atypia differentiates this tumor from squamous cell carcinoma. Invasion of inflammatory cells into the epithelium is characteristic of pseudocarcinomatous hyperplasia and is rare in squamous cell carcinoma.

Hereditary Benign Intraepithelial Dyskeratosis

Benign acanthosis of the conjunctiva and oral mucous membranes, with dyskeratosis of epithelial cells, occurs in Haliwa Indians. These individuals are descendants of white, American Indian, and black ancestors who lived in northeastern North Carolina. The disorder is inherited as an autosomal dominant trait with a high degree of penetrance. Affected individuals develop bilateral elevated plaques on the interpalpebral areas of the limbal conjunctiva, along with dilated vessels that cause the eyes to appear red. The epithelial

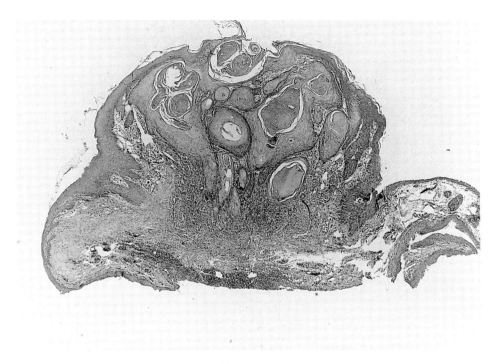

Figure 3-3
PSEUDOCARCINOMATOUS HYPERPLASIA
Excisional biopsy of a lesion that mimics a squamous cell carcinoma.

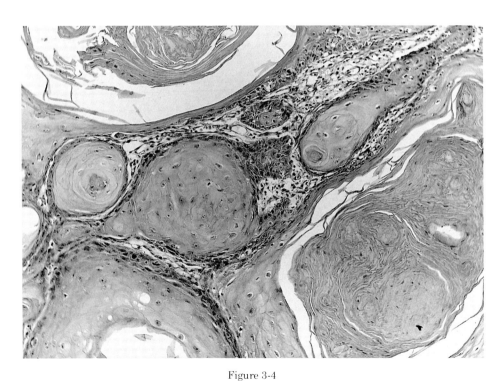

Figure 3-4
PSEUDOCARCINOMATOUS HYPERPLASIA
Higher magnification of the tumor in the previous figure shows the benign nature of the infiltrating squamous cells.

abnormality may extend around and onto the cornea. In mild cases the lesions are asymptomatic, but extensive lesions can involve most of the bulbar conjunctiva and cornea, resulting in corneal opacification and vascularization with marked loss of vision (8). Most patients complain of periodic photophobia and tearing, especially in the spring. Plaques also develop on the oral mucosa (9).

On histologic examination, the acanthotic conjunctival epithelium has prominent eosinophilic parakeratosis with individually keratinized cells in the germinal layers. The basal membrane is intact and nuclear atypia is absent. The stroma contains chronic inflammatory cells.

INTRAEPITHELIAL NEOPLASIA OF SURFACE EPITHELIUM AND RELATED LESIONS

Pinguecula, Pterygium, and Actinic Keratosis (Solar Keratosis)

Pingueculae and pterygia are not neoplasms but rather actinic degenerations of the stroma. Because they share a common etiology with, and represent precursor lesions of actinic keratosis, it is advantageous to discuss these actinically-related conditions as a group (10). Pingueculae are localized, yellow-gray, elevated masses close to the limbus on the nasal, temporal, or both sides of the cornea in the interpalpebral portion of the bulbar conjunctiva. Pingueculae located nasally are the most common. When the actinic degeneration extends from the limbus onto the cornea, the lesion is a pterygium.

Pingueculae and pterygia typically develop over a period of several years. Both are absent in infants and young children, and both occur more frequently and at younger ages in individuals living in areas with high levels of sunlight. They may become episodically inflamed, possibly as a result of irritation. Whereas pingueculae are innocuous, pterygia may interfere with visual acuity if they extend into the pupillary area of the cornea.

In both lesions, the superficial conjunctival stroma at the limbus undergoes degeneration with accumulation of amorphous, amphophilic staining, hyalinized, granular-appearing material interspersed with coiled or fragmented fibers resembling abnormal elastic tissue (elastotic degeneration). Ultrastructural studies

have shown that accumulated material consists of degenerated collagen, altered ground substance, osmiophilic granules, and large atypical elastic fibers (12). Often, the stromal fibroblasts are increased in number. In pterygia, there is an inflammatory pannus with destruction of the Bowman membrane. The degenerative elastotic material in the cornea often occurs as larger, spheroidal, basophilic hyalinized masses. The degenerative stromal material in the conjunctiva and cornea stains positively with Weigert and Verhoeff elastic tissue stains.

Actinic keratoses like pingueculae and pterygia are believed to be pathogenetically related to prolonged exposure of the conjunctiva to ultraviolet light (10). In geographic regions with high sunlight exposure and a rural population, actinic keratoses and the squamous cell carcinomas arising from them occur more frequently and in patients who are younger than in other parts of the world. Actinic keratoses usually develop slowly within the epithelium in the interpalpebral area overlying a preexisting pinguecula or pterygium. They are sharply circumscribed leukoplakic elevated plaques (fig. 3-5), which distinguishes them from dysplasias, which are flatter and less well-defined translucent lesions. Actinic keratoses do not differ in clinical appearance from other leukoplakic lesions that may be benign or malignant such as pseudocarcinomatous hyperplasia and squamous cell carcinoma.

Histologically, actinic keratoses are sharply demarcated plaques of acanthotic epithelium with parakeratosis and cytologic atypia overlying stroma that is damaged by elastotic degeneration (figs. 3-6–3-10). There is considerable variation in the degree of cytologic atypia, ranging in severity from mild acanthosis and parakeratosis (features that merge with those seen in benign keratotic plaques) to marked pleomorphism and dyskeratosis with abnormal mitoses (features that are characteristic of carcinoma); most pathologists grade the severity of the atypia in their diagnosis of actinic keratosis.

Dysplasia

In the conjunctiva, we recommend the use of "dysplasia" as a diagnostic term and not as a synonym for atypia. Dysplasias usually develop on the bulbar conjunctiva but differ from actinic keratoses in that they often occur outside the

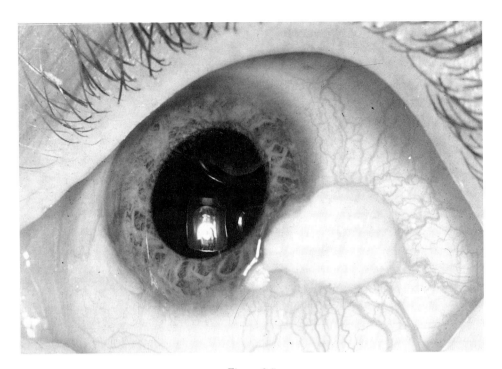

Figure 3-5
ACTINIC KERATOSIS
Elevated leukoplakic limbal tumor in the interpalpebral area.

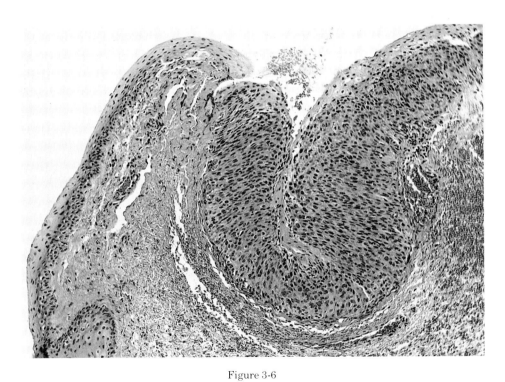

Figure 3-6
ACTINIC KERATOSIS
Sharply demarcated intraepithelial lesion with acanthosis, moderate atypia, parakeratosis, and subepithelial actinic elastosis.

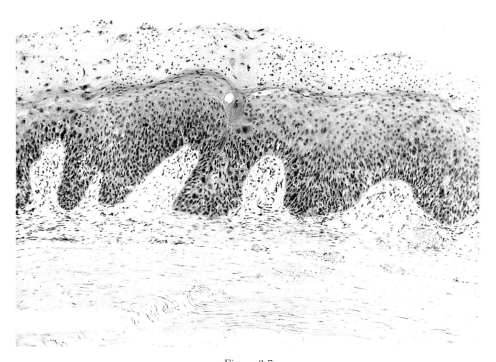

Figure 3-7
ACTINIC KERATOSIS
Intraepithelial lesion with severe atypia and parakeratosis involving the cornea.

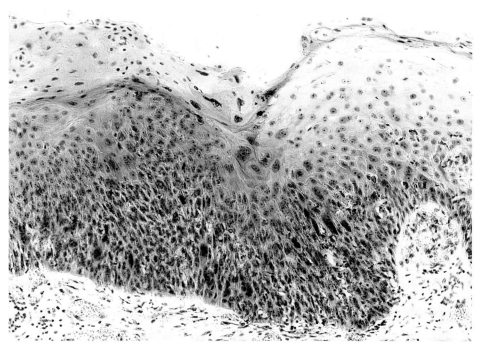

Figure 3-8
ACTINIC KERATOSIS
Higher magnification of the previous lesion.

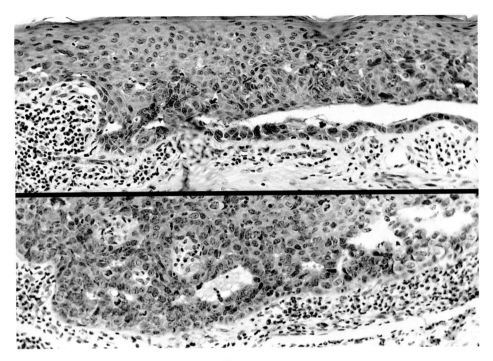

Figure 3-9
ACTINIC KERATOSIS
The lesion is acantholytic and there is a subepithelial lymphocytic infiltrate.

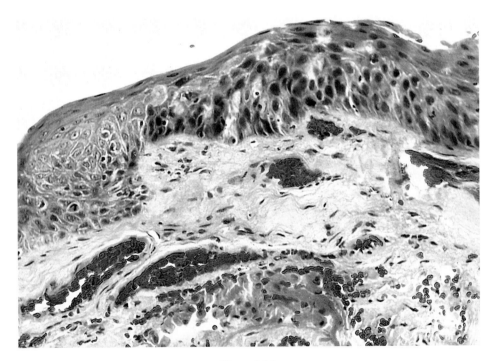

Figure 3-10
ACTINIC KERATOSIS
Atrophic lesion with atypia.

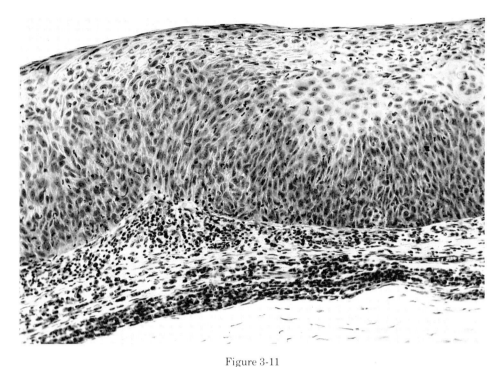

Figure 3-11
DYSPLASIA
Acanthotic lesion with moderate atypia involving half the thickness of the epithelium.

interpalpebral area. They are typically ill-defined lesions with a gelatinous appearance that blends with the surrounding normal conjunctiva. These lesions are often unrelated to actinic damage and are probably akin to the dysplasias that occur in non–sun-exposed mucous membranes. Human papilloma viruses 16 and 18 have been implicated in the pathogenesis of some of these lesions (11,13). Because their borders are often indistinct, dysplasias are more likely to be incompletely excised and more likely to recur than actinic keratoses. The risk of developing an invasive carcinoma is low but probably higher than with actinic keratosis.

Dysplasias are acanthotic lesions with cytologic atypia but little or no parakeratosis or hyperkeratosis (fig. 3-11). There is a gradual transition from normal conjunctiva to increasing acanthosis and atypia as one progresses towards the center of the lesion. Dysplasias are graded as mild, moderate, or severe depending on the degree of cellular atypia and disorganization of epithelial cell maturation. These changes are less severe than those of carcinoma in situ, in which the cellular atypia may be greater and the

cytologic abnormality always involves the full thickness of the epithelium.

Carcinoma in Situ

Carcinoma in situ represents the most malignant end of the spectrum of conjunctival dysplasias. We do not recommend using this term for actinic keratosis with severe atypia. Carcinoma in situ is placed in the malignant category in the WHO classification, but we consider it, like dysplasia, to be a precancerous lesion. We recommend classifying both dysplasias and carcinomas in situ as intraepithelial neoplasias. Like the dysplasias, carcinoma in situ usually remains confined to the epithelium and only infrequently becomes invasive. These lesions may undergo spontaneous regression (14). Therefore, the natural behavior of most of these lesions does not follow the course of a true invasive and metastasizing malignancy.

Carcinoma in situ may occur anywhere in the conjunctiva or cornea, but most often starts at the limbus. Most lesions have an opalescent papillary, rather than leukoplakic, clinical appearance. This reflects the lack of keratinization observed microscopically.

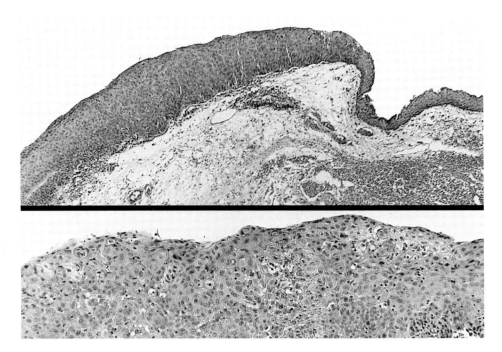

Figure 3-12
CARCINOMA IN SITU
Marked atypia involves the full thickness of the epithelium.

Carcinoma in situ is characterized histologically by acanthosis with total loss of normal cellular maturation and cytologic atypia affecting the full thickness of the epithelium. The neoplastic cells are often large and elongated, with their long axis oriented perpendicular to the basal lamina. Parakeratosis is minimal. Mitotic activity occurs in all layers (figs. 3-12–3-17).

MALIGNANT TUMORS OF SURFACE EPITHELIUM

Squamous Cell Carcinoma

Most squamous cell carcinomas arise from actinic keratoses in the interpalpebral area of the limbal conjunctiva and grow slowly in an exophytic, sometimes papillary fashion. These cancers are usually well differentiated and have a leukoplakic appearance. They vary in vascularity and amount of associated inflammation. Neglected lesions enlarge to fill the palpebral fissure, protrude between the lids, and extend posteriorly through the orbital septum to invade the orbit (16). In this country, squamous cell carcinoma of the conjunctiva is typically found in elderly people, but in parts of Africa, Asia, and Latin America these lesions arise with some frequency in young adults (19).

Squamous cell carcinomas that arise from dysplasias are likely to be poorly differentiated lesions. They lack keratinized cells and have a gelatinous, semitranslucent clinical appearance. Instead of creating an exophytic mass, these tumors are endophytic, invading into the cornea and sclera. Neglected tumors invade into the eye and posteriorly into the orbit. Human papilloma viruses have been implicated in the pathogenesis of some of these lesions (17).

In the United States, most squamous cell carcinomas of the conjunctiva tend to be only superficially invasive and to have a relatively benign clinical course (fig. 3-18). Intraocular invasion is uncommon. In a review of 27 cases, Iliff, Marback, and Green (16) found 3 patients with deep corneal invasion and 2 with intraocular extension (figs. 3-19, 3-20). Four patients had orbital invasion (fig. 3-20), and 2 had spread to regional lymph nodes (fig. 3-21). One patient died from metastatic tumor. The rarity of death

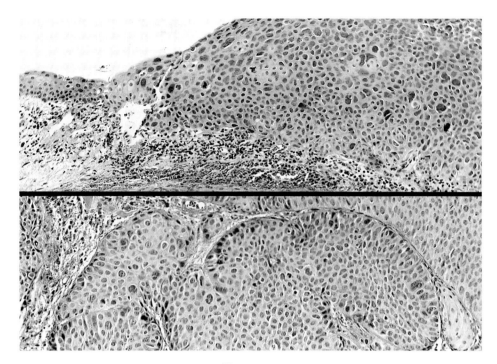

Figure 3-13
CARCINOMA IN SITU
Severe atypia with marked nuclear pleomorphism.

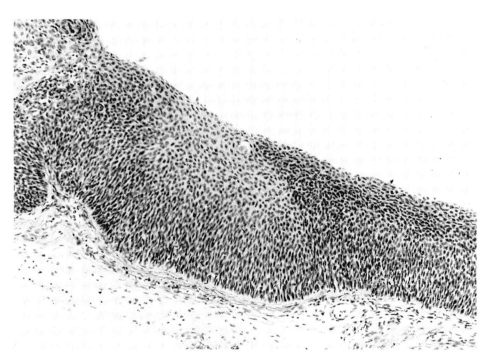

Figure 3-14
CARCINOMA IN SITU
Acanthotic lesion with loss of polarity and a high nuclear-cytoplasmic ratio.

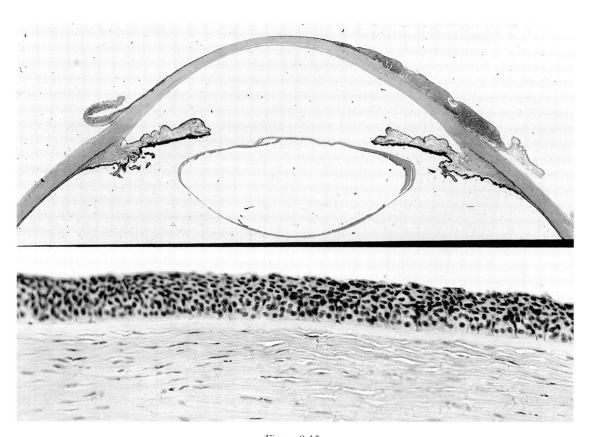

Figure 3-15
CARCINOMA IN SITU
Limbal lesion with extension onto the cornea.

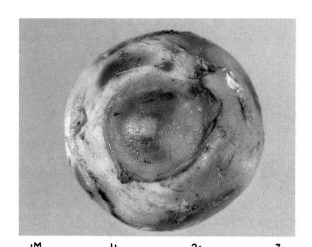

Figure 3-16
CARCINOMA IN SITU
Circumlimbal lesion with involvement outside the interpalpebral area.

caused by metastases was also noted by Zimmerman (20). ln his series of 87 cases of conjunctival squamous cell carcinoma, only 1 patient died from metastases (20). In cases received at the AFIP, advanced carcinomas requiring orbital exenteration because of deep invasion (fig. 3-22) are far more common in underdeveloped countries than in the United States.

Histologically, most conjunctival squamous cell carcinomas are well differentiated, with exophytic growth of atypical epithelial cells (fig. 3-18). In more advanced tumors, the substantia propria is usually inflamed and contains invading masses of atypical epithelial cells (fig. 3-22). There is great variation in the size, configuration, and degree of differentiation of the invading cells: hyperplastic and hyperchromatic cells, individually keratinized cells, concentric collections of keratinized cells (horn pearls), loss of cellular cohesiveness, and atypical mitotic figures may be seen.

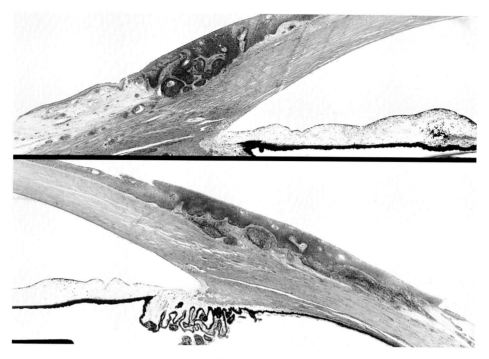

Figure 3-17
CARCINOMA IN SITU
Irregular acanthosis simulating invasion.

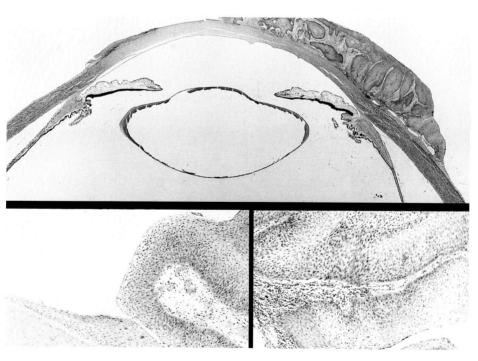

Figure 3-18
SQUAMOUS CELL CARCINOMA
Early invasive neoplasm with corneal involvement.

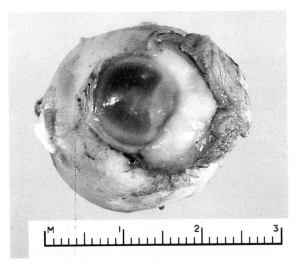

Figure 3-19
SQUAMOUS CELL CARCINOMA
Large limbal tumor has invaded into the anterior chamber.

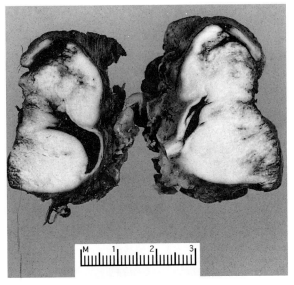

Figure 3-20
SQUAMOUS CELL CARCINOMA
Tumor has destroyed the eye and invaded the orbit.

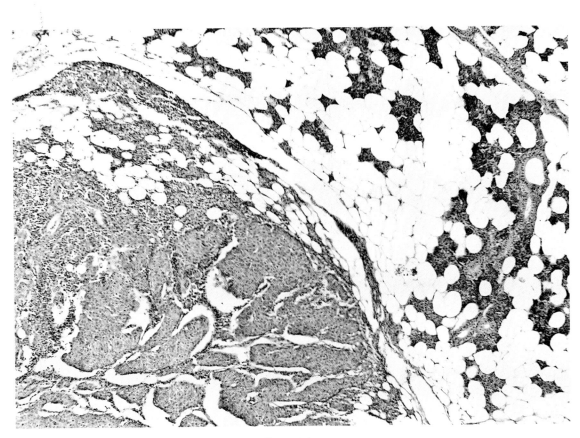

Figure 3-21
SQUAMOUS CELL CARCINOMA
Metastasis to preauricular node and parotid gland.

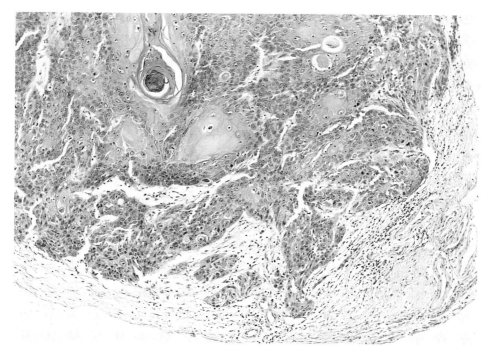

Figure 3-22
SQUAMOUS CELL CARCINOMA
Well-differentiated neoplasm with deep invasion.

Spindle cell variants of squamous cell carcinoma are occasionally encountered in the conjunctiva (15,18). Most spindle cell carcinomas of the skin have been attributed to prolonged actinic exposure, which is probably the most common cause of spindle cell carcinomas of the conjunctiva as well. These conjunctival tumors may behave in an aggressive fashion.

In routine histologic sections of spindle cell carcinoma of the conjunctiva, pleomorphic and hyperchromatic spindle-shaped cells may be difficult to distinguish from fibroblasts (figs. 3-23–3-25). Although they are typically superficial in location, their continuity with the overlying surface epithelium may not be evident. Such lesions have been mistaken for a fibrous histiocytoma or fibrosarcoma (pseudosarcoma). Occasionally, a transition from squamous to spindle cells is observed. Electron microscopic studies, which show the spindle cells to have frequent desmosomes and associated cytoplasmic tonofibril-like material, demonstrate the epithelial origin of this tumor. Immunohistochemical identification of

cytokeratin in the spindle cells is often easier than electron microscopy to confirm the epithelial nature of this tumor.

Mucoepidermoid Carcinoma

Malignant epithelial neoplasms composed of varying proportions of mucus-secreting cells, squamous cells, and intermediate cells (basal cells) are known as mucoepidermoid carcinomas. These tumors vary from conventional-appearing squamous cell carcinomas in which special stains (mucicarmine and Alcian blue) reveal scattered cells with intracytoplasmic mucin vacuoles to tumors that resemble adenocarcinoma (figs. 3-26–3-29).

Conjunctival mucoepidermoid carcinomas are uncommon and usually arise in elderly individuals, usually after the sixth decade of life (22,23), although one case was reported in a 36-year-old patient (21). They are more aggressive in their local behavior than conventional squamous cell carcinomas and tend to invade the

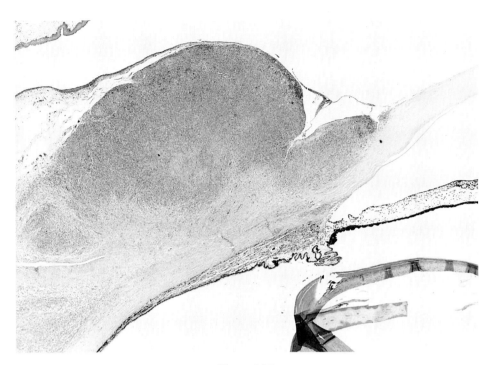

Figure 3-23
SQUAMOUS CELL CARCINOMA, SPINDLE CELL VARIANT
Large subepithelial tumor with deep scleral and corneal invasion.

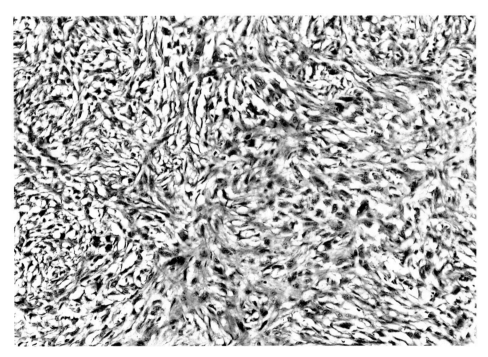

Figure 3-24
SQUAMOUS CELL CARCINOMA, SPINDLE CELL VARIANT
Higher magnification of neoplasm in the previous figure with a sarcomatous pattern.

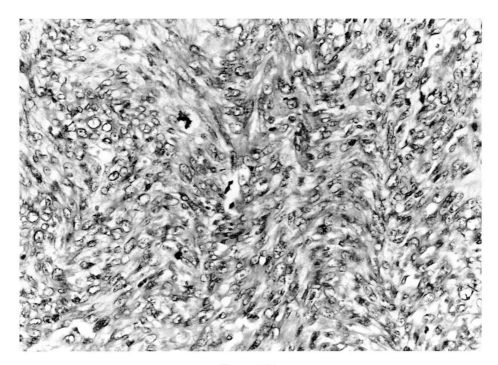

Figure 3-25
SQUAMOUS CELL CARCINOMA, SPINDLE CELL VARIANT
Another area of the neoplasm illustrated in figure 3-24 with a sarcomatous pattern.

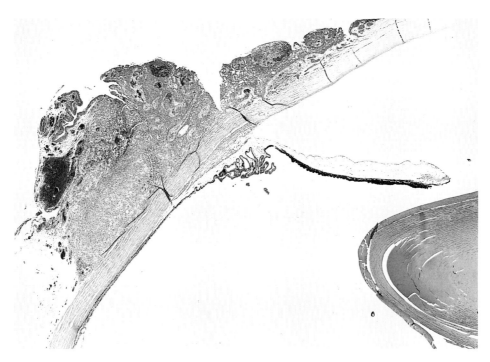

Figure 3-26
MUCOEPIDERMOID CARCINOMA
Limbal neoplasm with deep corneal invasion.

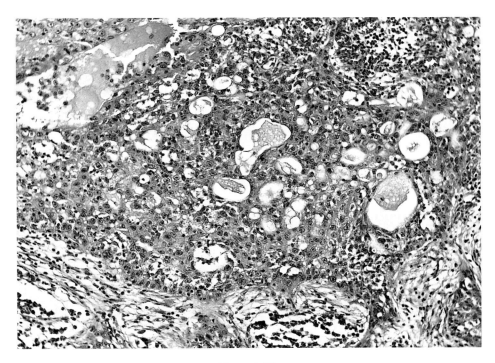

Figure 3-27
MUCOEPIDERMOID CARCINOMA

Higher power magnification of tumor in figure 3-26 showing neoplastic squamous cells with intracellular and extracellular vacuoles.

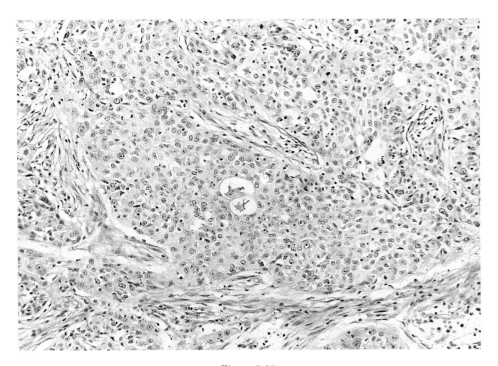

Figure 3-28
MUCOEPIDERMOID CARCINOMA

Islands of neoplastic squamous cells with scattered vacuoles. (Figures 3-28 and 3-29 are from the same lesion.)

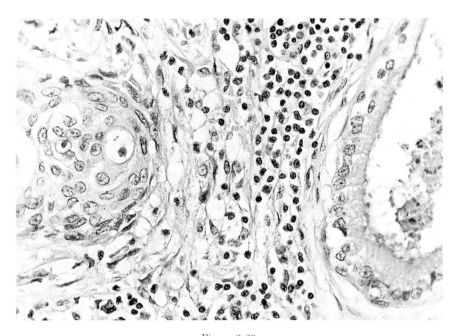

Figure 3-29
MUCOEPIDERMOID CARCINOMA
Infiltrating neoplasm with adjacent areas of squamous and glandular differentiation.

eye and orbit if incompletely excised. Most mucoepidermoid carcinomas arise in the limbal conjunctiva (fig. 3-26). Only one of the five cases studied by Rao and Font (22) originated outside the bulbar conjunctiva. This tumor arose in the lower conjunctival cul de sac and invaded the orbit. Mucin production may occur in only a small part of the tumor (23), and in some cases is not seen in the original lesion but in a recurrent lesion. In a few tumors, only the portion that invaded the eye exhibited mucin production, suggesting that the intraocular environment may induce this form of differentiation (23).

ADNEXAL TUMORS

Most tumors that arise in the adnexal structures of the eyelids, eyebrows, and orbit may also originate in the caruncle (e.g., pleomorphic adenoma, oncocytoma, sweat gland carcinoma, sebaceous gland carcinoma). This is not surprising, since the caruncle contains accessory lacrimal glands, sweat glands, sebaceous glands, and hair follicles. The most common malignant tumor of the caruncle is sebaceous gland carcinoma, which is discussed in the chapter, Tumors of the Eyelid.

Oncocytoma (Oncocytic Adenoma, Oxyphilic Adenoma)

The most common adnexal tumor of the caruncle is the oncocytoma (24). This tumor also develops in the lacrimal gland and lacrimal sac, as well as in other glandular and mucosal structures of the body. Conjunctival oncocytomas are usually asymptomatic, slowly enlarging swellings of the caruncle in older individuals. Biggs and Font (24) noted a predilection in women. Oncocytomas exhibit a variable histologic pattern in which the cells can be arranged either in sheets, cords, or nests and can also form ductal and cystic glandular structures (figs. 3-30–3-33). Occasional examples of oncocytic adenocarcinoma of the lacrimal sac and lacrimal gland have been observed.

The usual oncocytoma is composed of large cells with cytoplasm stuffed with eosinophilic granular material that electron microscopy reveals to be mitochondria. Oncocytic transformation is nonspecific and occurs in many glandular and mucosal structures throughout the body (25). It may represent an aging change since oncocytomas usually are found in individuals over 50. Caruncular lesions have been considered to originate from accessory lacrimal glands.

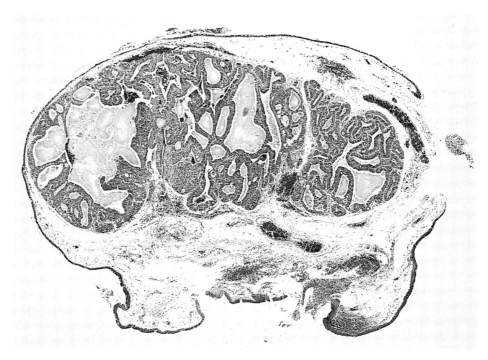

Figure 3-30
ONCOCYTOMA
Well-circumscribed, subepithelial, multiloculated cystadenomatous lesion.

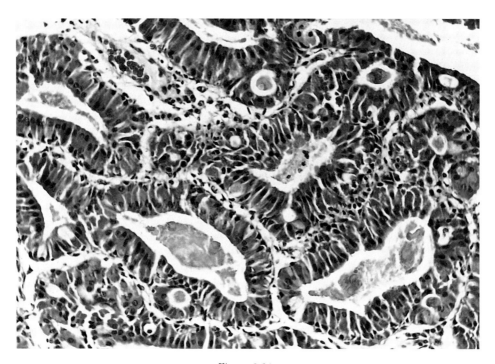

Figure 3-31
ONCOCYTOMA
Higher magnification of tumor in the previous figure showing tall columnar acidophilic cells lining glandular spaces.

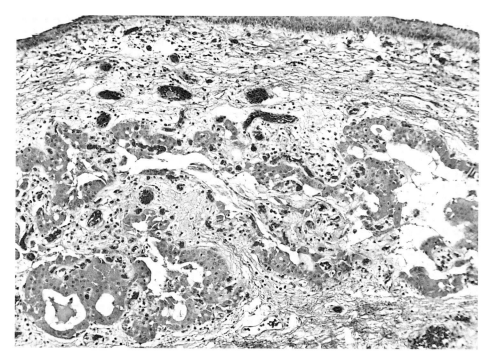

Figure 3-32
ONCOCYTOMA
Subepithelial glandular tumor.

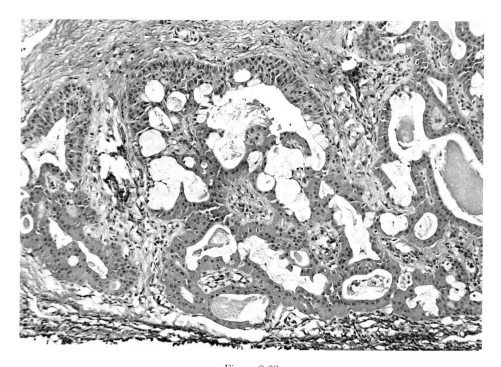

Figure 3-33
ONCOCYTOMA
Higher magnification of tumor in the previous figure showing glandular spaces lined by oncocytes and goblet cells.

TUMORS OF THE
MELANOCYTIC SYSTEM

The conjunctiva may be involved in a variety of melanocytic abnormalities. We use the term melanocytic to designate cells capable of producing melanin. These cells sometimes appear nonpigmented clinically or histologically because their melanosomes are either too few, too small, or too minimally melanized to be detected. Melanocytic cells may retain the melanin they produce (continent melanocytes) or they may discharge it into the cytoplasm of adjacent epithelial cells or subepithelial connective tissues (incontinent melanocytes). Free melanin granules may be phagocytosed by macrophages (melanophages). Blacks and other heavily pigmented individuals exhibit a striking tendency to develop significant degrees of melanotic pigmentation of lesions that are basically not melanocytic. A conjunctival papilloma, actinic keratosis, or carcinoma in a black patient may be deeply pigmented (secondary acquired melanosis).

Nevi

The melanocytic nevi of the conjunctiva are classified like those of the skin, with only minor modifications in terminology: intraepithelial (junctional), subepithelial (equivalent of dermal nevus), compound (intraepithelial plus subepithelial), spindle/epithelioid cell (juvenile melanoma or Spitz nevus), blue, and cellular blue.

Most conjunctival nevi are compound or subepithelial, and only in the young are pure intraepithelial nevi (junctional nevi) likely to be observed. Spindle/epithelioid cell, blue, and cellular blue nevi are rare on the conjunctiva. In patients with nevus of Ota, the discrete bluish episcleral spots may be considered special examples of blue nevi. A combination of an intraepithelial, subepithelial, or compound nevus with a blue or cellular blue nevus is a "combined nevus."

A problem in differentiating between a junctional nevus and acquired melanosis arises when only a small biopsy specimen is available for examination, and the clinical data are meager or not provided (26). A small biopsy specimen revealing nevoid melanocytes confined to nests along the basal layer of the conjunctival epithelium and no similar cells in the underlying substantia propria is more consistent with a junctional nevus. If, in addition, the specimen reveals individual enlarged melanocytes among the basal cells or scattered about the more superficial layers of the epithelium (pagetoid invasion), the possibility of primary acquired melanosis is more likely. A good summary of the clinical data is helpful. If the patient is a child or young adult who had the lesion since childhood, and if the lesion is localized, then a junctional nevus is almost certainly the correct diagnosis. On the other hand, if the patient is older and the lesion appeared and progressed insidiously to involve a large, diffuse, ill-defined area of which the biopsy specimen represents only a sample, then primary acquired melanosis is more likely.

Subepithelial and compound nevi of the conjunctiva are very similar in their clinical and histologic characteristics. If adequately sampled, most subepithelial nevi have a small junctional component. This component may be observed only within the subsurface inclusions of conjunctival epithelium found within the nevus. Inclusion of epithelium in the form of solid islands or cysts, is a frequently observed feature of compound and subepithelial nevi of the conjunctiva (figs. 3-34–3-37). It is not certain what these epithelial inclusions represent, but they may result from an anomalous development of the conjunctival epithelium that may be analogous to the hairy nevus of the skin. There may be great cytologic pleomorphism in conjunctival nevi (figs. 3-38, 3-39) and spindle- or epithelioid-shaped melanocytes characteristic of the Spitz nevi may be seen (27).

Subepithelial and compound nevi typically are tumors that elevate the conjunctival surface, whereas junctional nevi, like primary acquired melanosis, characteristically do not thicken the conjunctiva (26). The tumefaction is attributable to the space-occupying characteristics of the nevoid cells and the solid and cystic epithelial inclusions. A series of changes frequently occur in conjunctival nevi around the age of puberty. First, there is an increase in the size of the nevoid nests and epithelial inclusions. As the nevus becomes more prominent, it causes irritation with secondary inflammation. The inflammation sometimes causes increased pigmentation and the inflammatory cell infiltrate further increases the size and vascularity of the nevus. All these alterations provoke concern that a malignant melanoma

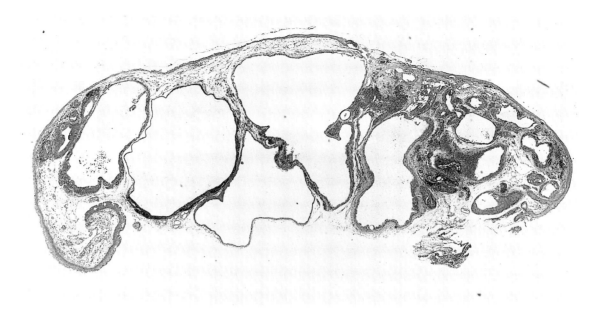

Figure 3-34
CYSTIC COMPOUND NEVUS
Melanocytic lesion with multiple large cysts.

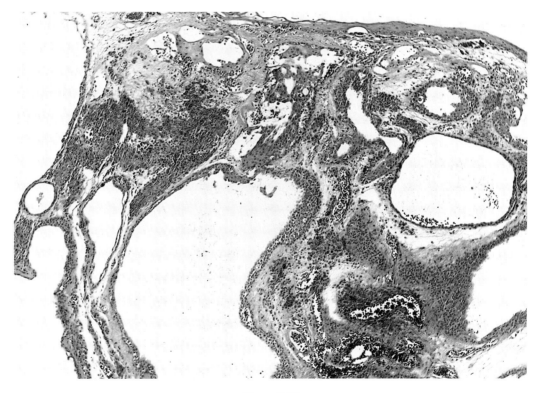

Figure 3-35
CYSTIC COMPOUND NEVUS
Higher magnification of nevus in the previous figure shows collections of nevoid cells in the junctional area around the cystic spaces.

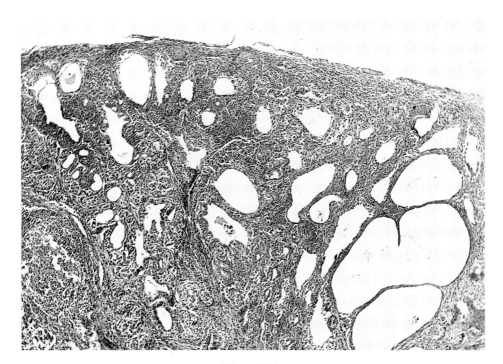

Figure 3-36
CYSTIC COMPOUND NEVUS
Sheets of melanocytes with variable-sized cysts.

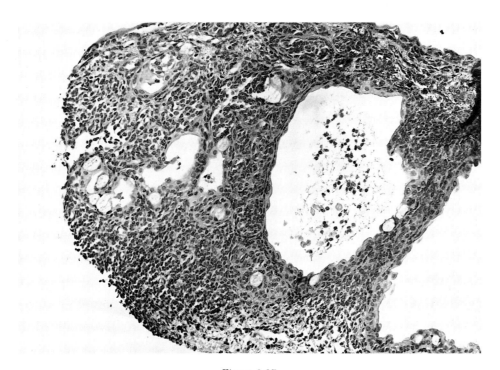

Figure 3-37
CYSTIC COMPOUND NEVUS
Diffuse proliferation of melanocytes, with cysts lined by conjunctival epithelium with goblet cells.

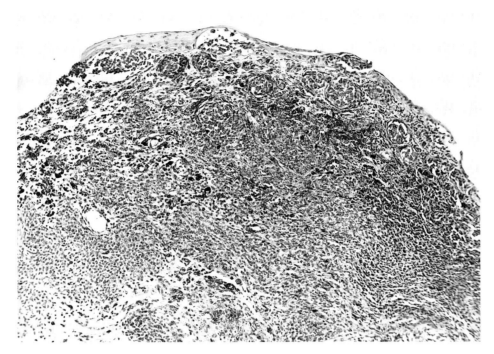

Figure 3-38
ATYPICAL COMPOUND NEVUS
Atypical melanocytes in the junctional area mature with smaller and less hyperchromatic nuclei as they extend deeper into the substantia propria.

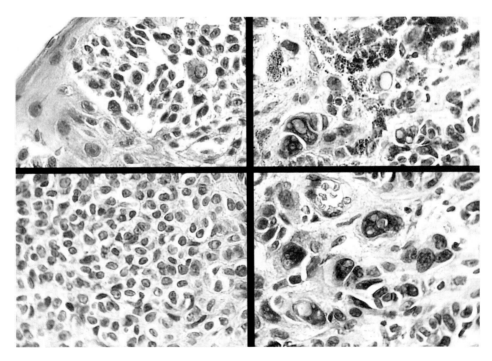

Figure 3-39
COMPOUND NEVUS
Variability in cytology within the benign lesion.

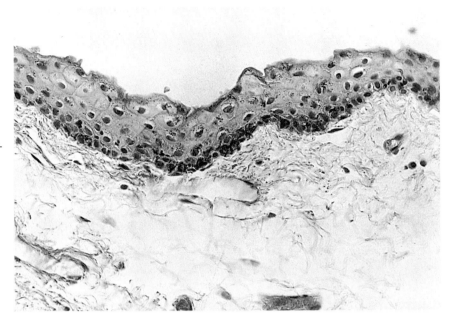

Figure 3-40
EPHELIS
Increased melanocytic activity in the basal cell layer.

arose from the nevus, resulting in a large number of benign conjunctival nevi being excised around the age of puberty.

Pigmentation is variable in conjunctival nevi. Some nevi are totally amelanotic and when small, the epithelial inclusions may predominate. As they enlarge or become inflamed, they may be confused with epithelial lesions. Occasionally, as a nonpigmented nevus becomes inflamed, it may become so vascular that it is mistaken for an angiomatous tumor. Because of these problems, it is likely that the pathologist will receive biopsies of unsuspected conjunctival nevi and must pick out small nests of nevoid cells against a background of inflammatory cells, inclusions of proliferated epithelial cells, and engorged blood vessels in order to make the correct diagnosis (26).

Melanosis

Melanosis refers to excessive melanotic pigmentation. Classification is based on three main considerations: whether the abnormality is congenital or acquired, whether the melanosis is epithelial or subepithelial, and whether the melanosis is primary or secondary. All of the congenital melanoses are primary and they are divided into epithelial and subepithelial types. All of the acquired melanoses are epithelial and they are divided into primary and secondary types. Thus

a good history and a careful clinical biomicroscopic examination are essential for accurate classification.

Epithelial Congenital Melanosis. An *ephelis* (freckle) is a discrete stationary lesion characterized by the presence of melanin mainly in the basal layers of the conjunctival epithelium. Typically, it is present since birth or early childhood. The melanocytes in an ephelis are not atypical and this lesion is not a precursor of malignant melanoma (fig. 3-40).

Subepithelial Congenital Melanosis. Technically this is not a lesion of the conjunctiva, since the abnormal melanocytes are situated in the sclera and episclera deep to the substantia propria of the conjunctiva. But because it is observed through the conjunctiva, it is in the differential diagnosis of pigmented conjunctival tumors and discussed here.

Subepithelial congenital melanosis has two main forms based on clinical findings. When only the ocular tissues are affected, the condition is termed *ocular melanocytosis* or *melanosis oculi*. This is characterized by a congenital increase in the number, size, and pigmentation of melanocytes of the uvea associated with an increased number of pigmented melanocytes in the sclera and episclera. It is almost invariably a unilateral abnormality. Heterochromia iridis with episcleral pigmentation in the more heavily pigmented

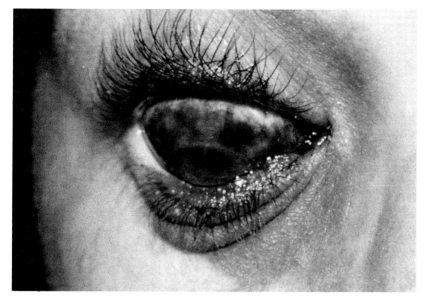

Figure 3-41
NEVUS OF OTA
Congenital subepithelial melanosis involving skin, eyelid, and sclera.

eye is a visible clinical sign of melanosis oculi. In some patients, increased pigmentation of the iris, choroid, and sclera is confined to a sector of the eye, with other areas of the eye uninvolved.

In the other main form of subepithelial congenital melanosis, called *oculodermal melanocytosis* or *nevus of Ota* (fig. 3-41), the ocular manifestations are accompanied by ipsilateral melanosis of the deep dermal tissues of the lids, periocular facial skin, or both. Rarely, bilaterality may be observed but in such cases there is usually asymmetry in the severity of involvement. Oculodermal melanocytosis is more common in Asians and blacks, while the pure ocular form is more common in whites. Both conditions may be associated with melanosis of the orbital tissues or melanosis of the meninges of the optic nerve or brain.

Subepithelial congenital melanosis does predispose to the development of malignant melanoma. Owing to the rarity of malignant melanoma in nonwhite individuals, there have been only a few reports of malignant change in the nevus of Ota (29). Any of the affected tissues in these forms of congenital melanosis may spawn a malignant melanoma, but most melanomas arise in the uveal tract. The second most frequent site is the orbit.

In both forms of congenital subepithelial melanosis, the affected tissues are a characteristic slate blue–gray, in contrast with the yellow-brown to brown-black of intraepithelial forms of melanosis. Histologically, individual and small clusters of melanocytes are interspersed with the connective tissue of the sclera, episclera, and dermis of the eyelid.

Secondary Melanosis. Bilateral acquired melanoses are almost always secondary. They are attributable to racial, metabolic, or toxic factors and do not predispose to the development of malignant melanoma. By far the most frequent of these is the acquired melanosis of the limbal and perilimbal conjunctival epithelium of blacks, which in heavily pigmented individuals is generally considered a normal aspect of aging (fig. 3-42). Unilateral acquired melanosis of the conjunctival epithelium may develop as a reaction secondary to some other primary lesion or may arise without apparent cause.

Unilateral secondary acquired melanosis, like bilateral melanosis, is observed most frequently in nonwhite patients. It is associated with any subepithelial or epithelial mass. Subepithelial lesions that elevate the conjunctival surface and irritate the overlying epithelium, such as a cyst, foreign body, or mound of scar tissue, may induce melanosis in the epithelium. In melanosis, melanocytes that lie dormant within the normal epithelium are stimulated to proliferate, migrate, and produce melanin. Secondary melanosis assumes its greatest clinical significance when primary epithelial tumors of black patients are affected; papillomas, actinic keratoses,

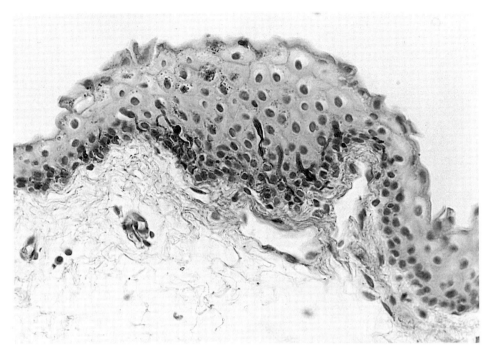

Figure 3-42
RACIAL MELANOSIS
Dendritic melanocytes are present.

squamous cell carcinomas, and mucoepidermoid carcinomas of the conjunctiva in blacks have been mistaken for malignant melanomas (28).

Primary Acquired Melanosis (Atypical Melanocytic Hyperplasia, Malignant Melanoma in Situ, Benign Acquired Melanosis, Precancerous Melanosis). Primary acquired melanosis is a unilateral neoplastic melanocytic proliferation within the conjunctival epithelium, observed most often in white patients. In clinicopathologic studies of skin (32), similar lesions have been subdivided into several entities carrying different prognostic and therapeutic implications: *Hutchinson freckle* or *lentigo maligna, superficial spreading melanoma in situ, acrolentiginous melanosis,* and *dendritic-lentiginous melanosis*. Of these, lentigo maligna most frequently involves the skin of the face, including the skin of the eyelid. In such cases there may be associated conjunctival involvement. Apart from this condition, it is seldom possible to subdivide acquired melanosis into the distinct clinicopathologic categories used in dermal pathology (34,35). Ackerman (30) has taken the opposite approach and advocated that both cutaneous and conjunctival acquired melanoses should be diagnosed as melanoma in situ. We do not advocate this approach because historically, primary acquired melanosis of the conjunctiva has been overtreated; follow-up data indicate that only one third of biopsied conjunctival primary acquired melanoses progress to melanoma and that the probability of progression is related to the degree of atypia of the melanocytes (33).

Clinical Features. Primary acquired melanosis typically begins insidiously in middle age or later as a subtle, yellow-brown stippling within the epithelium (fig. 3-43). Although bulbar conjunctival involvement is most common, any part of the conjunctiva, including the non-exposed fornical, palpebral, and canthal regions, may be affected. When the palpebral conjunctiva at the lid margin or canthal regions is affected, the melanosis often extends onto the adjacent epidermis. The lesion is usually flat, which distinguishes it from nevi and melanomas, which are elevated (fig. 3-44). When elevated lesions develop in primary acquired melanosis, they are

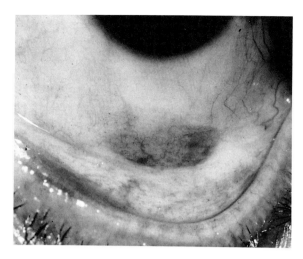

Figure 3-43
PRIMARY ACQUIRED MELANOSIS
Flat, diffuse pigmentation of the fornix and palpebral conjunctiva. (Figures 3-43 and 3-44 are from the same patient.)

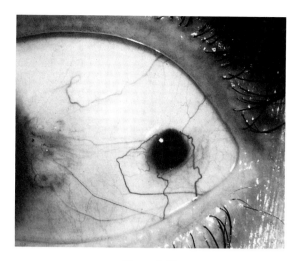

Figure 3-44
MALIGNANT MELANOMA
Nodular, elevated, heavily pigmented lesion adjacent to an area of primary acquired melanosis.

usually a sign of malignancy; in rare cases, discrete nodular masses composed entirely of inflammatory cells may simulate a malignant melanoma (36).

The evolution of primary acquired melanosis is unpredictable. It often progresses slowly, but may wax and wane. Spontaneous disappearance of pigmentation may be observed in one area, while a simultaneous increase of pigmentation may develop in another. Clinical evaluation by simple inspection and slitlamp examination may not reveal the full extent of the melanosis. By use of ultraviolet light (Wood lamp), areas of subclinical melanosis may be identified, extending far beyond the edges of the obvious lesion. The rate of progression is extremely variable but typically is measured in years. In a series of 41 cases of biopsied primary acquired melanosis, 13 (32 percent) progressed to malignant melanoma, but none of the other patients developed a malignant melanoma in a 10-year follow-up (35).

Pathologic Findings. The histologic features of primary acquired melanosis are extremely variable, not only in different cases but in different areas within a lesion. The melanocytes vary in size, shape, and atypia. There may be small polyhedral cells with no atypia, spindle-shaped cells with moderate atypia, or large highly atypical epithelioid cells (figs. 3-45–3-49).

The pattern of involvement also varies. Individual melanocytes may line up along the basal lamina of the epithelium (figs. 3-45, 3-46), form nests of melanocytes extending into the epithelium (fig. 3-47), invade the epithelium in a pagetoid fashion (fig. 3-48), or completely replace the epithelium with atypical melanocytes mimicking an in situ carcinoma (fig. 3-49). In a study from the AFIP (35), two histologic features were found to be very useful in predicting which lesions would most likely spawn a malignant melanoma. When melanocytes invaded the epithelium in a pagetoid fashion or replaced the epithelium (figs. 3-48, 3-49), the risk of melanoma was 90 percent; when they were confined to the basal layer of the epithelium (figs. 3-45, 3-46), the risk of that lesion developing into a melanoma was 20 percent. Seventy-five percent of tumors that contained epithelioid cells progressed to melanoma (fig. 3-48). Lesions in which no or only minimal atypia could be detected (figs. 3-45, 3-46) did not progress to melanoma.

Because histologic examination provides significant prognostic information, biopsy of conjunctival lesions with primary acquired melanosis is often essential for clinical management. The conjunctival epithelium, when involved by primary acquired melanosis, is friable and conjunctival biopsies must be handled carefully.

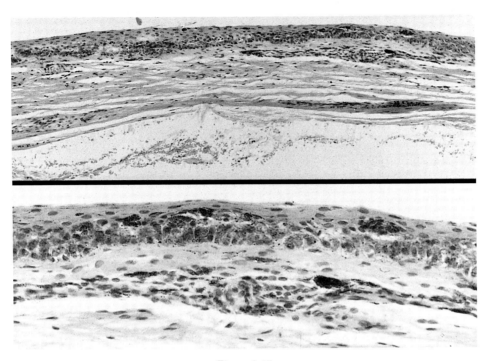

Figure 3-45
PRIMARY ACQUIRED MELANOSIS, WITHOUT ATYPIA
The melanocytic hyperplasia is confined to the basilar layer.

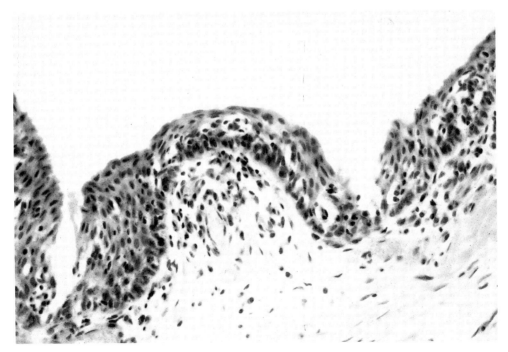

Figure 3-46
PRIMARY ACQUIRED MELANOSIS, WITH MINIMAL ATYPIA
Mildly atypical melanocytes are present in the basilar layer.

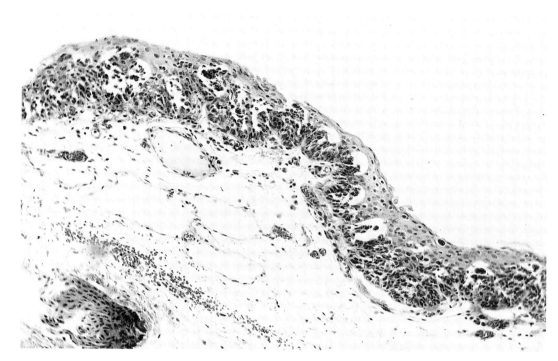

Figure 3-47
PRIMARY ACQUIRED MELANOSIS, WITH MODERATE ATYPIA
Nests of atypical melanocytes extend throughout the thickness of the epithelium.

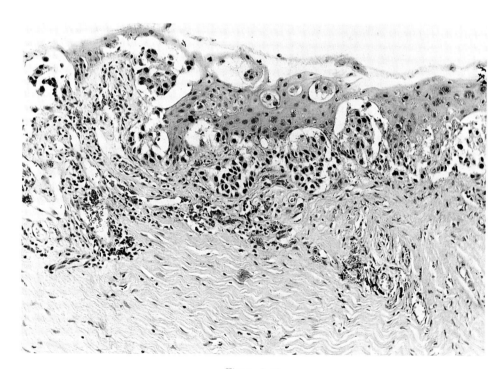

Figure 3-48
PRIMARY ACQUIRED MELANOSIS, WITH SEVERE ATYPIA
Nests and individual epithelioid melanocytes extend throughout the thickness of the epithelium in a pagetoid fashion.

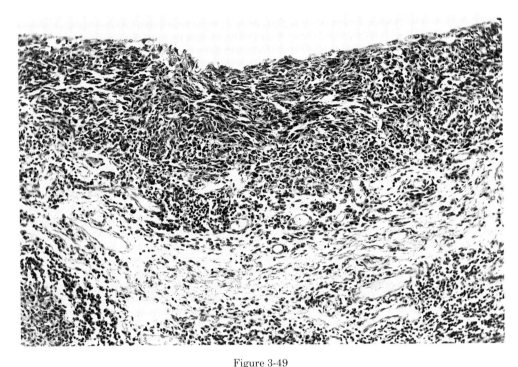

Figure 3-49
PRIMARY ACQUIRED MELANOSIS, WITH SEVERE ATYPIA AND EARLY INVASIVE MELANOMA
Spindle-shaped malignant melanocytes completely replace the conjunctival epithelium, with minimal invasion of the inflamed substantia propria.

All lesions, especially those with the histologic features indicative of high risk, should be considered for resection, if feasible. Brownstein and co-workers (31) found that subtotal excision combined with cryotherapy provided effective therapy for extensive lesions that could not be completely resected.

Histologic studies of acquired melanosis of the conjunctiva have shown an associated nevus in at least 20 percent of the cases (35). In some cases, the nevus was recognized clinically long before the onset of acquired melanosis, but often the nevus escaped attention and was discovered only as an "incidental finding" during microscopic examination of the resected lesion. Because of the frequency with which nevi are present within areas of acquired melanosis, with or without malignant melanoma, it appears that there is a causal relationship. It is possible that the presence of a nevus predisposes the conjunctiva to the development of both acquired melanosis and malignant melanoma. The presence of a nevus, however, does not significantly increase the chances of melanoma developing in acquired melanosis or affect the prognosis once a melanoma has developed.

MALIGNANT MELANOMA

Conceptually, the development of malignant melanomas of the conjunctiva includes three groups: melanomas derived from primary acquired melanosis (figs. 3-43, 3-44, 3-50, 3-51), those derived from preexisting nevi, and those that develop de novo from apparently normal conjunctiva (figs. 3-52–3-57)(48). This schema is an oversimplification because it does not consider melanomas that develop with a nevus associated with primary acquired melanosis. Additionally, there are some practical problems in the use of such a pathogenetic classification. To properly classify a melanoma, a reliable clinical history of the evolution of the process, an equally good description of the results of clinical examination, and adequate tissue to study histologically are needed. If a wide rim of surrounding conjunctiva is not excised with the melanoma, primary acquired melanosis surrounding the

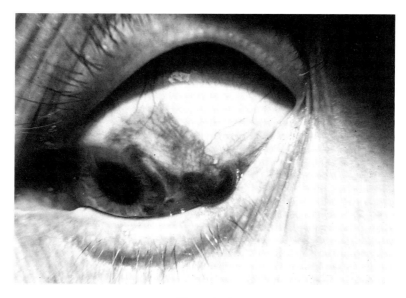

Figure 3-50
MALIGNANT MELANOMA ARISING IN PRIMARY ACQUIRED MELANOSIS
An elevated melanotic nodule arose in an area of flat melanosis.

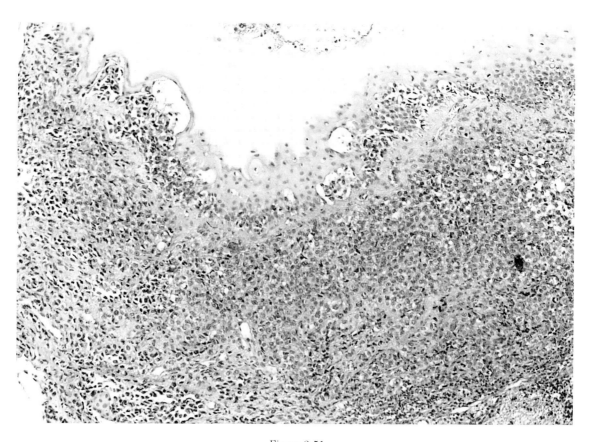

Figure 3-51
MALIGNANT MELANOMA ARISING IN PRIMARY ACQUIRED MELANOSIS
Anaplastic melanocytes are present within nests in the epithelium and infiltrate the substantia propria.

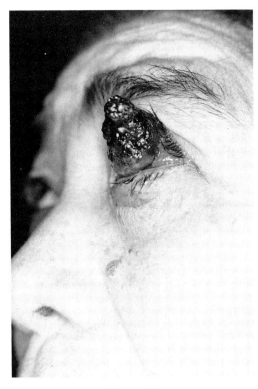

Figure 3-52
MALIGNANT MELANOMA
Large neglected melanoma protrudes between eyelids.
(Figures 3-52–3-54 are from the same patient.)

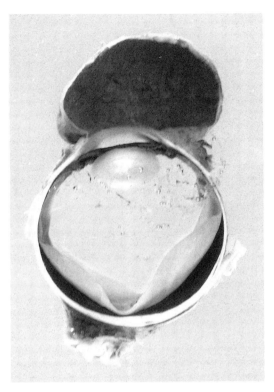

Figure 3-53
MALIGNANT MELANOMA
Large heavily pigmented nodule covers the cornea .

melanoma may escape recognition histologically (fig. 3-51), and the malignant melanoma may be inappropriately considered a melanoma having arisen de novo. Large melanomas (figs. 3-52–3-56) may destroy the nevus or primary acquired melanosis from which they arose and be incorrectly classified as a de novo melanoma. Although the presence or absence of a nevus or primary acquired melanosis in a conjunctival melanoma does not appear to be a significant factor affecting survival, we believe that the pathologist should be concerned with detecting primary acquired melanosis because its presence doubles the risk of melanoma recurrence following excision (39).

Clinical Features. Most conjunctival malignant melanomas occur in adults and two thirds of these arise in acquired melanosis. For these reasons, any change in a pigmented lesion of the conjunctiva, particularly growth with increasing elevation, should be suspected of being a malignant melanoma and treated accordingly (41).

Pathologic Findings. The definition of a malignant melanoma requires that atypical melanocytes invade from the epithelium into the substantia propria of the conjunctiva. Because atypical melanocytes come in a wide spectrum of cytologic types, they may be difficult to recognize. Most easily recognized are the large bizarre epithelioid cells (figs. 3-54, 3-56). Smaller polyhedral melanoma cells (fig. 3-51) can be difficult to distinguish from benign nevus cells. When they are observed, the presence of mitotic activity, lack of maturation, and infiltrative growth at the deep margin are helpful in differential diagnosis. Spindle-shaped melanoma cells (fig. 3-49) are often amelanotic and they may induce a desmoplastic stroma. They tend to be more locally invasive than other melanomas, involving nerves and extending posteriorly into the orbit. Such orbit tumors can be difficult to differentiate from malignant schwannomas.

At times, because of the complete absence of pigmentation, the melanocytic nature of a lesion may be totally unsuspected by the clinician and

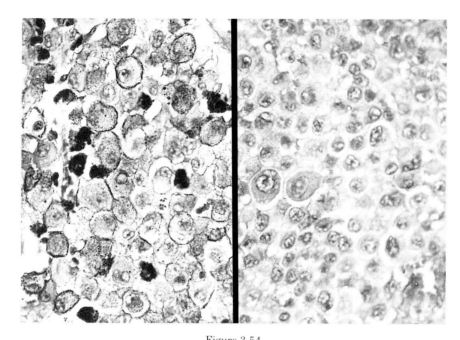

Figure 3-54
MALIGNANT MELANOMA
Large heavily pigmented epithelioid cells with prominent nucleoli lack cohesion. (Bleached preparation on right.)

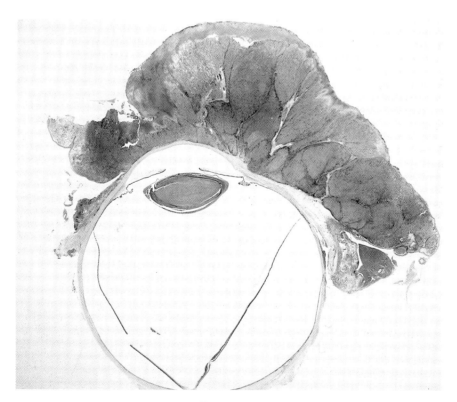

Figure 3-55
MALIGNANT MELANOMA
Large exophytic tumor covers the conjunctiva and cornea.

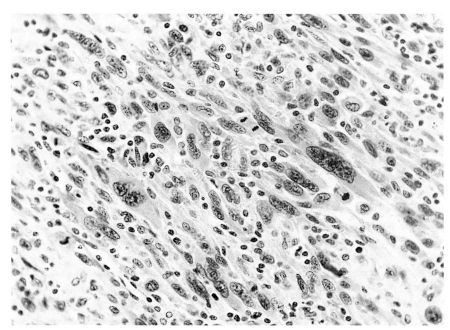

Figure 3-56
MALIGNANT MELANOMA
Higher power magnification of tumor in figure 3-55 showing highly pleomorphic cytologic features.

very difficult to establish beyond reasonable doubt by light microscopy of routinely stained sections. In such cases certain silver stains (Fontana and Warthin-Starry methods) may be very helpful in making fine melanin granules visible by light microscopy. Positive immunoperoxidase staining for HMB-45 and S-100 and negative staining for cytokeratin provide a reliable method for distinguishing melanocytes from epithelial cells (42).

Prognosis. The thickness of the melanoma of the conjunctiva, as in the skin, is the most important prognostic feature (figs. 3-49, 3-53, 3-55, 3-57). Because the conjunctival epithelium is thinner than the epidermis and has a simpler architecture, the Breslow method (37) must be modified slightly for conjunctival tumors: the full thickness from the surface of the epithelium to the tumor's deepest level of invasion is measured histologically, using a calibrated micrometer grid. Silvers and co-workers (46) found that a thickness of about 1.8 mm separated most lethal from nonlethal conjunctival melanomas. Recent studies have confirmed that there is a relationship between increasing tumor thickness and fatal outcome (39,40,47), but Folberg et al. (39) found that even with flat melanomas measuring less than 0.8 mm in thickness, one cannot entirely exclude the possibility of a lethal outcome. Craw-

ford (38) also described a flat malignant melanoma that metastasized and killed the patient. One explanation for a lethal course from a minimally invasive conjunctival melanoma is that the conjunctival lymphatic channels are situated very close to the epithelium (fig. 3-58).

Folberg and co-workers (39) found that histologic examination of melanomas that develop in primary acquired melanosis provided prognostic information in addition to the thickness of the tumor. Melanomas that were more likely to metastasize did one or more of the following: involved the nonbulbar conjunctiva, invaded the sclera or orbit, infiltrated the epithelium with a pagetoid or in situ–like pattern, or recurred. A better prognosis was associated with melanomas that were confined to the bulbar conjunctiva (fig. 3-50) or with an inflammatory infiltrate (fig. 3-49) around the invasive tumor. A favorable prognosis was noted with limbal lesions (40) and a poor prognosis with extension of primary acquired melanosis with melanoma to involve the skin margin of the eyelid (44). Increased mitotic activity is also an adverse risk factor (45).

It is clear from their behavior that conjunctival melanomas have more in common with cutaneous than with uveal melanomas. In sharp contrast with uveal melanomas, which almost never metastasize to the regional lymph nodes,

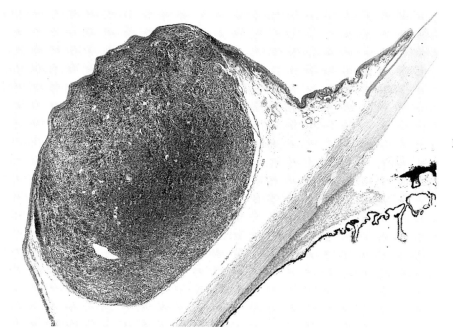

Figure 3-57
MALIGNANT MELANOMA
Nodular tumor at limbus.

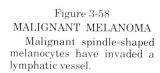

Figure 3-58
MALIGNANT MELANOMA
Malignant spindle-shaped melanocytes have invaded a lymphatic vessel.

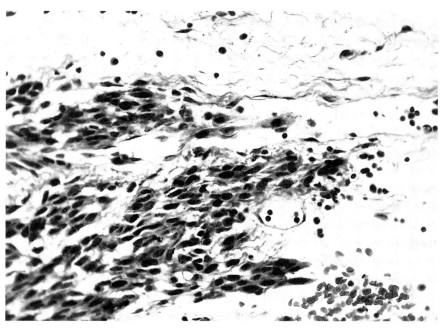

conjunctival melanomas share with cutaneous melanomas the ability to invade lymphatics (fig. 3-58) and spread initially to the regional lymph nodes (fig. 3-59). The preauricular and intraparotid nodes are more often affected than the submandibular and cervical lymph nodes. Lymphatic spread to regional nodes indicates a poor prognosis, but it does not always herald widespread dissemination or a lethal outcome. We have seen several cases of malignant melanoma metastatic to preauricular lymph nodes, not followed by further spread or death after simple excision, even though no radical surgery or supplemental therapy was employed.

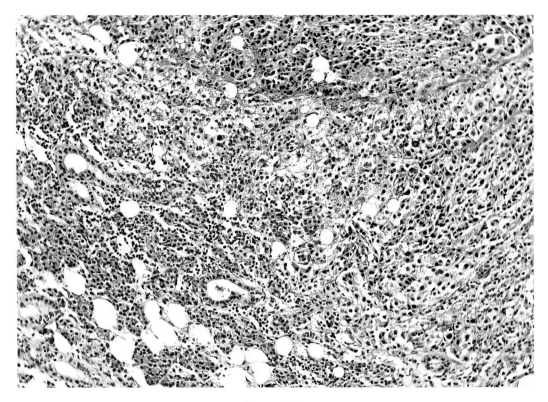

Figure 3-59
MALIGNANT MELANOMA
Malignant epithelioid melanocytes have metastasized to a parotid lymph node.

Robertson and co-workers (43) reported an unusual mode of spread of primary acquired melanosis with melanoma to the nasal cavity and paranasal sinuses. We have observed primary acquired melanosis of the conjunctiva that invaded the epithelium of the lacrimal drainage system in a pagetoid fashion; this was probably the route of metastasis in the cases of Robertson et al. When examining exenteration specimens for primary acquired melanosis with melanoma, we recommend that the pathologist sample the lacrimal drainage system.

SOFT TISSUE, LYMPHOID, HEMATOPOIETIC, AND HISTIOCYTIC TUMORS

Although conjunctival involvement of most of these tumors is adequately discussed in the chapter, Tumors of the Orbit, Kaposi sarcoma more frequently involves the conjunctiva than the orbit or eyelid.

Kaposi Sarcoma

Until recently, Kaposi sarcoma of the conjunctiva was considered to be a rare disease, primarily occurring in older individuals with similar lesions of the skin of the legs (53). This tumor has now been observed frequently in the conjunctiva of young individuals with AIDS (49,52). The relationship between Kaposi sarcoma and immunodeficiency is now well documented, but the pathogenic mechanism is still poorly understood. The conjunctival lesions usually involve the palpebral or fornical conjunctiva. In immunodeficient individuals, the sarcoma usually develops after a prolonged period of multiple opportunistic infections; however, on occasion, the conjunctival lesion may be one of the earliest clinical manifestations of AIDS.

Dugel et al. (49) examined 18 conjunctival Kaposi sarcoma lesions related to AIDS. These lesions were classified into three types. Type I and type II tumors were patchy and flat (less than

3 mm in height) and of less than 4 months' duration. Type III tumors were nodular (fig. 3-60) and elevated (greater than 3 mm in height), and longer than 4 months' duration. Histologically, type I consisted of thin, dilated vascular channels lined by flat endothelial cells with lumina containing erythrocytes. Type II featured plump, fusiform, endothelial cells, often with hyperchromatic nuclei, foci of immature spindle cells, and occasional slit vessels. Type III was characterized by large aggregates of densely packed spindle cells with hyperchromatic nuclei, occasional mitotic figures, and abundant slit spaces often containing erythrocytes (figs. 3-61, 3-62). A characteristic finding in Kaposi sarcoma is the presence of multiple, small, PAS-positive intracellular hyaline globules (figs. 3-63, 3-64) that are believed to be degenerated erythrocytes (50,51). Immunohistochemistry has confirmed that the spindle-shaped cells are of endothelial origin (51). Type I lesions are impossible to distinguish from granulation tissue without clinical correlative data.

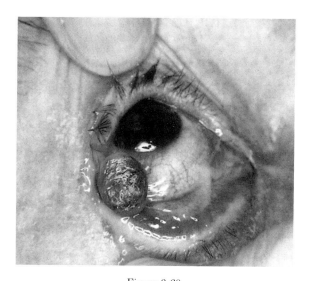

Figure 3-60
KAPOSI SARCOMA
Elevated nodule arising from the fornix. (Figures 3-60–3-62 are from the same lesion.)

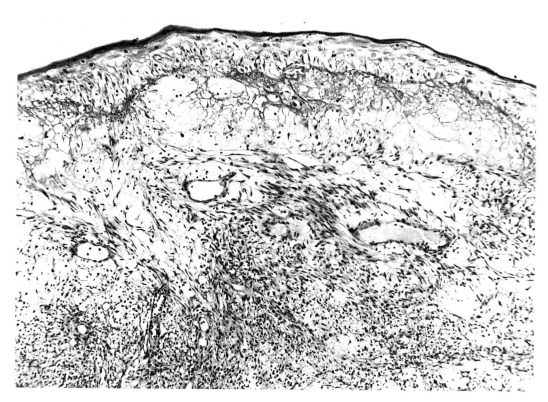

Figure 3-61
KAPOSI SARCOMA
Subepithelial proliferation of spindle-shaped cells and vessels.

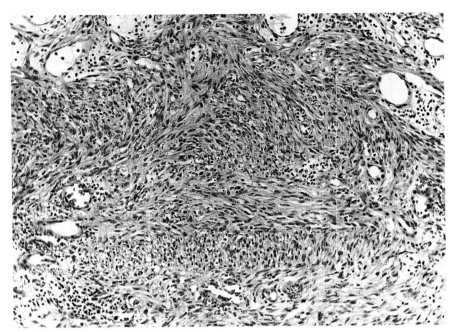

Figure 3-62
KAPOSI SARCOMA
Biphasic subepithelial neoplasm composed of solid and edematous areas.

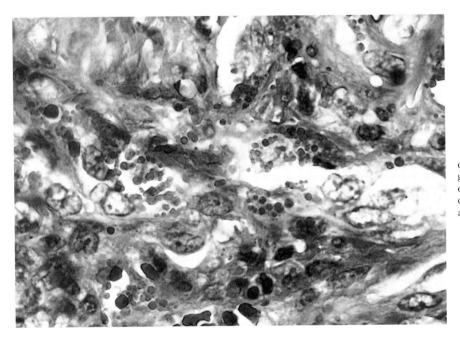

Figure 3-63
KAPOSI SARCOMA
Swollen endothelial cells contain numerous hyaline globules that represent degenerated fragments of erythrocytes. (Figures 3-63 and 3-64 are from the same patient.)

CHORISTOMAS

Epibulbar dermoid tumors arising within the limbal and canthal portions of the conjunctiva are classified as choristomas because they contain displaced epithelial, mesenchymal, and dermal elements normally not found in these areas. The lesions are present at birth and have little or no growth potential. Three types are generally recognized: the solid limbal dermoid, the more diffuse dermolipoma, and the complex choristoma that varies in its content and configuration. All types can occur either as isolated ocular lesions or in association with anomalies affecting other tissues (Goldenhar syndrome, mandibulofacial dysostosis, neurocutaneous syndrome) (54).

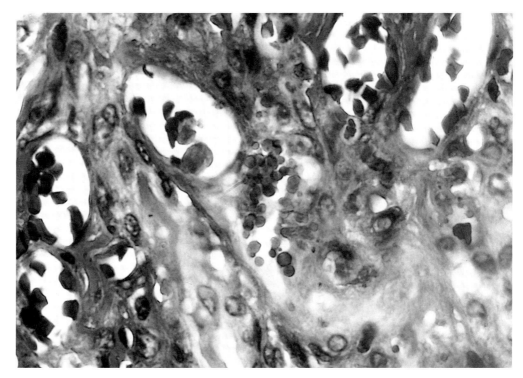

Figure 3-64
KAPOSI SARCOMA
Enlarged endothelial cell contains a cluster of hyaline globules that represent degenerated fragments of erythrocytes.

Limbal Dermoid

Dermoids occurring at the limbus are usually well circumscribed, firm, and solitary. They vary in size, configuration, and color from small (2 to 3 mm), slightly elevated, whitish nodules to large (12 to 15 mm), round, tan tumors that protrude through the palpebral aperture and interfere with lid closure. Occasionally, more than one is found. Most are located inferiorly and temporally. The occasional coexistence of lid colobomas suggests that the pathogenesis of limbal dermoids may be related in part to aberrant development of the lids, with displacement of lid elements to the limbus. Rarely, inferotemporal limbal dermoids occur as part of a complex choristomatous malformation associated with aberrant fetal fissure closure (55).

Histologically, limbal dermoids are covered by stratified squamous epithelium, which often has a granular layer and produces keratin. The stroma is composed of dense collagenous tissue interspersed with pilosebaceous units and sweat glands (figs. 3-65, 3-66). Occasionally, when other choristomatous elements, like lobules of lacrimal gland (fig. 3-67) and cartilage (fig. 3-68), are present the lesions are classified as complex choristomas (55). When adipose tissue is present they are classified as dermolipomas.

Dermolipoma

Most dermolipomas are yellowish tan, soft, fusiform tumors, usually localized to the temporal aspect of the conjunctiva near the lateral canthus. They may be lobulated and often extend superiorly and posteriorly between the lateral and superior rectus muscle, where they lie close to the lacrimal gland; they also may extend posteriorly into the orbit or anteriorly toward the cornea.

Histologically, the epithelium is of the stratified squamous type and may be partially keratinized. The stroma contains bundles of dense collagen similar to that seen in limbal dermoids; pilosebaceous structures are usually absent. When these lesions contain cartilage or lacrimal gland acini (figs. 3-67, 3-68), they are classified as complex choristomas.

91

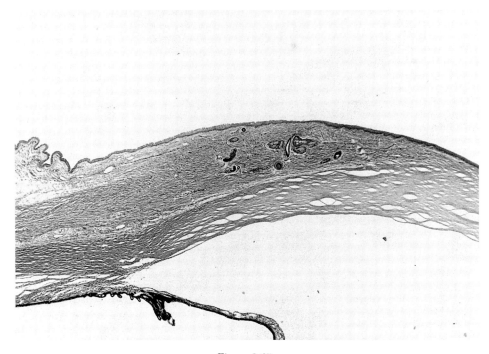

Figure 3-65
LIMBAL DERMOID
Subepithelial fibrous tissue resembling reticular dermis with skin appendages.

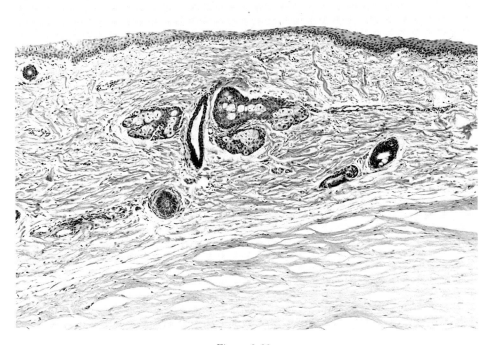

Figure 3-66
LIMBAL DERMOID
Higher power magnification showing pilosebaceous units.

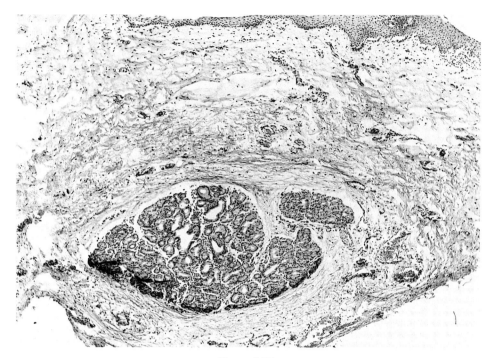

Figure 3-67
COMPLEX CHORISTOMA
Island of lacrimal gland tissue within a limbal dermoid.

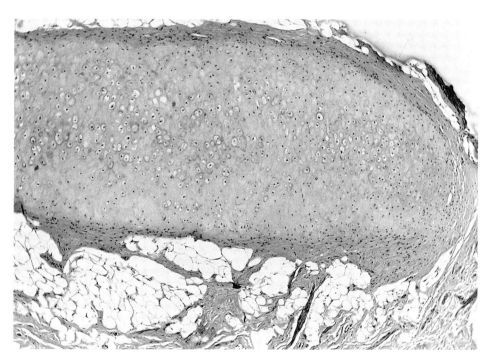

Figure 3-68
COMPLEX CHORISTOMA
Island of cartilage within a limbal dermoid.

REFERENCES

General References

Jakobiec FA, Iwamoto T. The ocular adnexa: lids, conjunctiva and orbit. In: Fine BS, Yanoff M, eds. Ocular histology: a text and atlas. 2nd ed. Hagerstown, Md.: Harper & Row, 1979:289–342.

Spencer WH, Zimmerman LE. Conjunctiva. In: Spencer WH, ed. Ophthalmic pathology. An atlas and textbook. 3rd Ed. Philadelphia: WB Saunders, 1985:109–177.

Classification and Frequency

1. Burnier MN Jr, Belfort R Jr, Rigueiro MP, et al. Malignant tumors of the conjunctiva. Arch I P B 1988;30:203–8.
2. _____, Belfort R Jr, Rigueiro MP, et al. Benign tumors of the conjunctiva. Arch I P B 1988;30:190–3.
3. Garner A. The pathology of tumours at the limbus. Eye 1989;3(Pt 2):210–7.

Squamous Cell Papilloma

4. Jakobiec FA, Harrison W, Aronian D. Inverted mucoepidermoid papillomas of the epibulbar conjunctiva. Ophthalmology 1987;94:283–7.
5. Mäntyjärvi M, Syrjänen S, Kaipiainen S, Mäntyjärvi R, Kahlos T, Syrjänen K. Detection of human papillomavirus type 11 DNA in a conjunctival squamous cell papilloma by in situ hybridization with biotinylated probes. Acta Ophthalmol (Copenh) 1989;67:425–9.
6. McDonnell JM, McDonnell PJ, Mounts P, Wu TC, Green WR. Demonstration of papillomavirus capsid antigen in human conjunctival neoplasia. Arch Ophthalmol 1986;104:1801–5.
7. Naghashfar Z, McDonnell PJ, McDonnell JM, Green WR, Shah KV. Genital tract papillomavirus type 6 in recurrent conjunctival papilloma. Arch Ophthalmol 1986;104:1814–5.

Hereditary Benign Intraepithelial Dyskeratosis

8. von Sallman L, Paton D. Hereditary benign intraepithelial dyskeratosis. I. Ocular manifestations. Arch Ophthalmol 1960;63:421–9.
9. Witkop CJ, Shankle DH, Graham JB, et al. Hereditary benign intraepithelial dyskeratosis. II. Oral manifestations and hereditary transmission. Arch Pathol 1960;70:696–711.

Intraepithelial Neoplasia

10. Clear AS, Chirambo MC, Hutt MS. Solar keratosis, pterygium, and squamous cell carcinoma of the conjunctiva in Malawi. Br J Ophthalmol 1979;63:102–9.
11. Lauer SA, Malter JS, Meier JR. Human papillomavirus type 18 in conjunctival intraepithelial neoplasia. Am J Ophthalmol 1990;110:23–7.
12. Ledoux-Corbusier M, Danis P. Pinguecula and actinic elastosis. An ultrastructural study. J Cutan Pathol 1979;6:404–13.
13. McDonnell JM, McDonnell PJ, Sun YY. Human papillomavirus DNA in tissues and ocular surface swabs of patients with conjunctival epithelial neoplasia. Invest Ophthalmol Vis Sci 1992;33:184–9.
14. Morsman CD. Spontaneous regression of a conjunctival intraepithelial neoplastic tumor. Arch Ophthalmol 1989;107:1490–1.

Squamous Cell Carcinoma

15. Huntington AC, Langloss JM, Hidayat AA. Spindle cell carcinoma of the conjunctiva. An immunohistochemical and ultrastructural study of six cases. Ophthalmology 1990;97:711–7.
16. Iliff WJ, Marback R, Green WR. Invasive squamous cell carcinoma of the conjunctiva. Arch Ophthalmol 1975;93:119–22.
17. McDonnell JM, McDonnell PJ, Stout WC, Martin WJ. Human papillomavirus DNA in a recurrent squamous carcinoma of the eyelid. Arch Ophthalmol 1989;107:1631–4.
18. Ni C, Liu SL, Zhong CS. Spindle cell carcinoma of cornea and conjunctiva with pseudosarcomatous metaplasia. Light microscopic, electron microscopic and immunohistochemical findings in 2 patients. Chin Med J (Engl) 1989;102:387–91.
19. Templeton AC. Tumors of the eye and adnexa in Africans of Uganda. Cancer 1967;20:1689–98.
20. Zimmerman LE. Squamous cell carcinoma and related lesions of the bulbar conjunctiva. In: Boniuk M, ed. Ocular and adnexal tumors: new and controversial aspects. St. Louis: CV Mosby, 1964:49–74.

Mucoepidermoid Carcinoma

21. Margo CE, Weitzenkorn DE. Mucoepidermoid carcinoma of the conjunctiva: report of a case in a 36-year-old with paranasal sinus invasion. Ophthalmic Surg 1986;17:151–4.
22. Rao NA, Font RL. Mucoepidermoid carcinoma of the conjunctiva: a clinicopathologic study of five cases. Cancer 1976;38:1699–709.
23. Searl SS, Krigstein HJ, Albert DM, Grove AS Jr. Invasive squamous cell carcinoma with intraocular mucoepidermoid features. Conjunctival carcinoma with intraocular invasion and diphasic morphology. Arch Ophthalmol 1982;100:109–11.

Oncocytoma

24. Biggs SL, Font RL. Oncocytic lesions of the caruncle and other ocular adnexa. Arch Ophthalmol 1977;95:474–8.
25. Hamperl H. Benign and malignant oncocytoma. Cancer 1962;15:1019–27.

Nevi

26. Folberg R, Jakobiec FA, Bernardino VB, Iwamoto T. Benign conjunctival melanocytic lesions. Clinicopathologic features. Ophthalmology 1989;96:436–61.
27. Kantelip B, Boccard R, Nores JM, Bacin F. A case of conjunctival Spitz nevus: review of literature and comparison with cutaneous locations. Ann Ophthalmol 1989;21:176–9.

Congenital and Secondary Melanosis

28. Jauregui HO, Klintworth GK. Pigmented squamous cell carcinomas of the cornea and conjunctiva. Cancer 1976;38:778–88.

29. Nik NA, Glew WB, Zimmerman LE. Malignant melanoma of the choroid in the nevus of Ota in a black patient. Arch Ophthalmol 1982;100:1641–3.

Primary Acquired Melanosis

30. Ackerman AB, Sood R, Koenig M. Primary acquired melanosis of the conjunctiva is melanoma in situ. Mod Pathol 1991;4:253–63.
31. Brownstein S, Jakobiec FA, Wilkinson RD, Lombardo J, Jackson WB. Cryotherapy for precancerous melanosis (atypical melanocytic hyperplasia) of the conjunctiva. Arch Ophthalmol 1981;99:1224–31.
32. Clark WH Jr. A classification of malignant melanomas in man correlated with histogenesis and biologic behavior. In: Montagner W, Hu F, eds. Advances in biology of the skin. The pigmentary system, Vol. 8. London: Pergamon Press, 1967:621–1967.
33. Folberg R, Jakobiec FA, McLean IW, Zimmerman LE. Is primary acquired melanosis of the conjunctiva equivalent to melanoma in situ? Mod Pathol 1992;5:2–8.
34. _____, McLean IW. Primary acquired melanosis and melanoma of the conjunctiva: terminology, classification, and biologic behavior. Hum Pathol 1986; 17:652–4.
35. _____, McLean IW, Zimmerman LE. Primary acquired melanosis of the conjunctiva. Hum Pathol 1985;16:129–35.
36. Jakobiec FA, Folberg R, Iwamoto T. Clinicopathologic characteristics of premalignant and malignant melanocytic lesions of the conjunctiva. Ophthalmology 1989;96:147–66.

Malignant Melanoma

37. Breslow A. Tumor thickness, level of invasion and node dissection in stage I cutaneous melanoma. Ann Surg 1975;182:572–5.
38. Crawford JB. Conjunctival melanomas: prognostic factors a review and an analysis of a series. Trans Am Ophthalmol Soc 1980;78:467–502.
39. Folberg R, McLean IW, Zimmerman LE. Malignant melanoma of the conjunctiva. Hum Pathol 1985; 16:136–43.
40. Fuchs U, Kivelä T, Liesto K, Tarkkanen A. Prognosis of conjunctival melanomas in relation to histopathological features. Br J Cancer 1989;59:261–7.
41. Jakobiec FA, Folberg R, Iwamoto T. Clinicopathologic characteristics of premalignant and malignant melanocytic lesions of the conjunctiva. Ophthalmology 1989;96:147–66.
42. McDonnell JM, Sun YY, Wagner D. HMB-45 immunohistochemical staining of conjunctival melanocytic lesions. Ophthalmology 1991;98:453–8.

43. Robertson DM, Hungerford JL, McCartney A. Malignant melanomas of the conjunctiva, nasal cavity, and paranasal sinuses. Am J Ophthalmol 1989;108:440–2.
44. _____, Hungerford JL, McCartney A. Pigmentation of the eyelid margin accompanying conjunctival melanoma. Am J Ophthalmol 1989;108:435–9.
45. Seregard S, Kock E. Conjunctival malignant melanoma in Sweden 1969-91. Acta Ophthalmol (Copenh) 1992;70:289–96.
46. Silvers D, Jakobiec FA, Freeman T, et al. Melanoma of the conjunctiva: a clinicopathologic study. In: Jakobiec FA, ed. Ocular and adnexal tumors. Birmingham: Aesculapius Publishing Company, 1978:583–599.
47. Uffer S. Melanomes malins de la conjonctive: etude histopathologique. Klin Monatsbl Augenheilkd 1990; 196:290–4.
48. Zimmerman LE. The histogenesis of conjunctival melanomas: the first Algernon B. Reese Lecture. In: Jakobiec FA, ed. Ocular and adnexal tumors. Birmingham: Aesculapius Publishing Company, 1978:600–30.

Kaposi Sarcoma

49. Dugel PU, Gill PS, Frangieh GT, Rao NA. Ocular adnexal Kaposi's sarcoma in acquired immunodeficiency syndrome. Am J Ophthalmol 1990;110:500–3.
50. Fukunaga M, Silverberg SG. Hyaline globules in Kaposi's sarcoma: a light microscopic and immunohistochemical study. Mod Pathol 1991;4:187–90.
51. Kao GF, Johnson FB, Sulica VI. The nature of hyaline (eosinophilic) globules and vascular slits of Kaposi's sarcoma. Am J Dermatopathol 1990;12:256–67.
52. Palestine AG, Rodrigues MM, Macher AM, et al. Ophthalmic involvement in acquired immunodeficiency syndrome. Ophthalmology 1984;91:1092–9.
53. Weiter JJ, Jakobiec FA, Iwamoto T. The clinical and morphologic characteristics of Kaposi's sarcomas of the conjunctiva. Am J Ophthalmol 1980;89:546–52.

Choristoma (Dermoid)

54. Goldenhar M. Associations malformatives de l'oeil et de l'orielle, en particulier le syndrome epibulbaire-appendices auriculaires-fistula auris congenita et ses relations avec la dysostose mandibulofaciale. J Genet Hum 1952;1:243–82.
55. Pokorny KS, Hyman BM, Jakobiec FA, Perry HD, Caputo AR, Iwamoto T. Epibulbar choristomas containing lacrimal tissue. Clinical distinction from dermoids and histologic evidence of an origin from the palpebral lobe. Ophthalmology 1987;94:1249–57.

❖ ❖ ❖

4
TUMORS OF THE RETINA

ANATOMY AND HISTOLOGY

The retina is formed from the neuroectodermal (medulloepithelial) cells lining the floor of the primitive forebrain. These cells proliferate outward as a diverticulum. The proliferation continues until the diverticulum forms the single-layered optic vesicle that is connected to the forebrain by the optic stalk. Invagination of the optic vesicle produces a two-layered structure, the optic cup. The cells of these two primitive neuroectodermal layers come to lie in apposition, apex-to-apex, forming a pigmented outer layer and a nonpigmented inner layer. Thus, the retinal pigment epithelium is derived from the outer wall of the optic cup and the multilayered neurosensory retina is derived from the inner wall.

Retinal Pigment Epithelium

The retinal pigment epithelium (RPE) is a single layer of polygonal cells of uniform size (16 μm in diameter) and regular arrangement. In the foveal region, the RPE cells are taller, narrower, and darker. This epithelium extends from the edge of the optic disc to the ora serrata. From that point forward in the eye, the RPE is continuous with the pigmented epithelium of the ciliary body. Internally, microvilli at the apex of the RPE cells interdigitate with the photoreceptors; externally, the base of the RPE cells is attached to the Bruch membrane. The epithelial cells have a round nucleus that is situated near the base, and melanin granules that are concentrated in the apical portion of the cell.

Being derived from the outer layer of the optic vesicle, the RPE cells are melanin producing and not of neural crest origin. Thus, in the eye there are two embryologic classes of melanocytes: those derived from the neural crest and those derived from the neuroepithelium of the optic cup. There are also morphologic differences between these two classes of melanocytes. Melanocytes in the uvea derived from the neural crest are dendritic or spindle shaped in contrast to the pigmented epithelia of the retina, ciliary body,

and iris. Furthermore, melanosomes in the pigmented epithelial cells are larger and more oval than uveal melanocytes.

The lateral surfaces of adjacent RPE cells are joined to each other by junctional complexes near the apical surface. These junctions prevent diffusion of substances between the choroid and subretinal space and form part of the blood-retinal barrier. The basal surface of each cell has a convoluted cell membrane with several infoldings. The basal plasma membrane is separated from the basal lamina by a narrow space; the basal lamina forms the inner most layer of the Bruch membrane. The apical surface of each cell has long villi that interdigitate with the rod and cone outer segments of the photoreceptors. The cytoplasm of the RPE cells contains abundant smooth endoplasmic reticulum, and there is an active lysosomal system which digests phagocytized rod outer segments. With increasing age, lipofuscin accumulates in the cytoplasm.

Sensory (Neural) Retina

The sensory retina is a delicate, transparent layer not firmly attached to the underlying RPE. Separation of these two layers (retinal detachment) can occur in vivo or as an artifact in the pathology laboratory. The retina is maintained in position by several factors: intraocular pressure, interdigitation between the photoreceptor outer segments and the RPE villi, gylcosaminoglycans surrounding the photoreceptors, and an active transport system that removes fluid from the subretinal space. At the internal surface of the retina, the basal lamina of the retinal Müller cells forms the internal limiting membrane. In young persons, the internal limiting membrane is firmly bound to the vitreous by collagenous filaments. With increasing age, the connections between the two become tenuous.

The retina is composed of layers of neurons that are connected to each other by synapses between axons and dendrites. The neurons are supported by astrocytes. Müller cells are specialized astrocytes that span the full thickness of the retina. The sensory retina is made up of nine

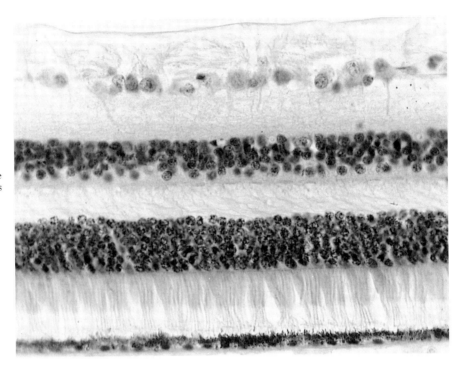

Figure 4-1
NORMAL RETINA
Nonmacular area of the retina composed of nine layers and the RPE.

layers (fig. 4-1). From outside inward, these layers are rods and cones, external limiting membrane, outer nuclear layer, outer plexiform layer, inner nuclear layer, inner plexiform layer, ganglion cell layer, nerve fiber layer, and internal limiting membrane.

Layer of Rods and Cones. These have a palisaded arrangement. The rods are slender and cylindrical and their length corresponds to the thickness of the entire layer. The cones are flask-shaped and shorter than the rods. Each rod and cone is composed of an outer and inner segment. The outer segment contains the discs and the inner segment contains numerous mitochondria; the cones contain more mitochondria than the rods. Different areas of the retina contain different proportions of rods and cones. At the fovea (the center of the macula) only cones are found, and these are long and slender, resembling rods. Glycosaminoglycans produced by the RPE, the photoreceptor cells, and possibly the Müller cells surround the rod and cone outer and inner segments and also the villi of the RPE.

External Limiting Membrane. This is not a true membrane but a continuous layer of junctional complexes (zonula occludens) uniting the Müller cells to the photoreceptor cell inner segments. The Müller cells extend fine cytoplasmic

processes externally between the inner segments of the rod and cone photoreceptors for a short distance.

Outer Nuclear Layer. This is composed of eight or nine layers of densely staining nuclei of the photoreceptor cells. Rods and cones can be identified on the basis of nuclear morphology. The smaller, more densely staining nuclei belong to the rods; the larger nuclei, that tend to lie just within the external limiting membrane, belong to the cones. Occasionally, cone nuclei are displaced into the rod and cone layer as a normal variation.

Outer Plexiform Layer. The synapses between the cells of the outer and inner nuclear layers are here. There is a loose network of axons from photoreceptor cells of the outer nuclear layer and dendrites of bipolar and horizontal cells of the inner layer. The Müller cells fill all the space between the processes. In the macular region, where the axons and dendrites of the outer plexiform layer are elongated and radiate outward from the foveal region, the outer plexiform layer is thickened, forming the fiber layer of Henle.

Inner Nuclear Layer. This is thinner than the outer nuclear layer and consists of the nuclei of Müller cells and three types of neurons. The bipolar cells have dendrites that are in contact with the axons of the photoreceptor cells in the outer plexiform layer. Their axons extend into the inner plexiform layer, forming synapses with the dendrites of the ganglion cells and with the amacrine cells. The horizontal cells have long and arborizing processes in the outer plexiform layer that synapse with the rod and cone axons, and adjacent bipolar cells. The amacrine cells are pear shaped and lie at the inner aspect of the inner nuclear layer. They synapse widely with the dendrites of the ganglion cells and with the bipolar axons in the internal plexiform layer. The Müller cells send cellular processes internally to produce the basement membrane material of the internal limiting membrane and externally to form the zonula occludens of the external limiting membrane.

Inner Plexiform Layer. A fine reticulum of axons and dendrites, this layer is composed of the synapses of the bipolar cells, the amacrine cells, and the ganglion cells.

Ganglion Cell Layer. This is composed of a row of ganglion cells separated from each other by the cytoplasmic extensions of the Müller cells, astrocytes, and blood vessels. The nuclei of astrocytes are found in the ganglion cell layer. The ganglion cells are multipolar, with large nuclei and prominent Nissl granules. Their long axons extend along the nerve fiber layer of the retina and form the optic nerve. The ganglion cell layer is a single nuclear layer, except in the macular region, where the ganglion cells are more numerous and form a layer two to eight nuclei thick.

Nerve Fiber Layer. This consists of the axons of the ganglion cells. These axons extend to the brain via the optic nerve. This layer is thickest near the optic disc because of the accumulation of the fibers in this area as the axons converge on the optic disc.

Internal Limiting Membrane. This is a very delicate basement membrane structure applied to flat, footplate-like extensions of the Müller cells. In fact, the internal limiting membrane represents the basal lamina of the Müller cells. It is absent or greatly attenuated at the optic nerve head, in the foveola, and over major retinal vessels. The fine collagenous fibers from the cortical vitreous are attached to and blend with this basal lamina. Rare macrophages or fibroblastic cells of the cortical vitreous may also be present along the inner surface of the internal limiting membrane. These cells with reniform nuclei have been called hyalocytes.

Table 4-1

EQUIVALENT ANATOMIC, HISTOLOGIC, AND CLINICAL TERMS

Anatomic	Histologic	Clinical
Area centralis	Macula	Posterior pole
Fovea centralis	Fovea centralis	Macula
Foveola	Foveola	Fovea

In order to provide maximal visual acuity, several modifications in the retinal architecture have taken place at the macular region. See Table 4-1 for the equivalent clinical, anatomic, and microscopic terms.

Anatomically, the area centralis is a region measuring 5.85 mm in diameter that corresponds to the clinical posterior pole and to the histologic macula. The histologic macula is defined as the area of the retina where more than one layer of ganglion cells can be found. In the center of the histologic macula is a pit or depression, slightly oval in shape, measuring about 1.5 mm in its horizontal diameter, which corresponds to the fovea centralis (fig. 4-2). There are no retinal vessels in the fovea centralis to hinder vision and although there are no rods, the cones are modified so that they resemble rods. The external segments of the cones are long and approach the apical side of the RPE cells. The abundance of these specialized cones in this region forms a forward, bow-shaped configuration called the umbo. Both the ganglion cell and inner nuclear layers disappear within the fovea centralis. In the center of the fovea centralis, comprising the foveal floor, is a deeper, red, disc-shaped area, the foveola. Histologically, only photoreceptor cells are present here. Maximal resolution is obtained in the foveola because each cone is united with a single bipolar cell and a single ganglion cell.

The retina terminates at the ora serrata. From this point forward, the neurosensory retina is continuous with the nonpigmented epithelium of the ciliary body. At the periphery of the retina, the external segments of the rods and cones disappear and the inner segments become deformed bulbous structures. There is a relative increase in the number of rods, astrocytes, and Müller cells in the far periphery, as compared with the equatorial region.

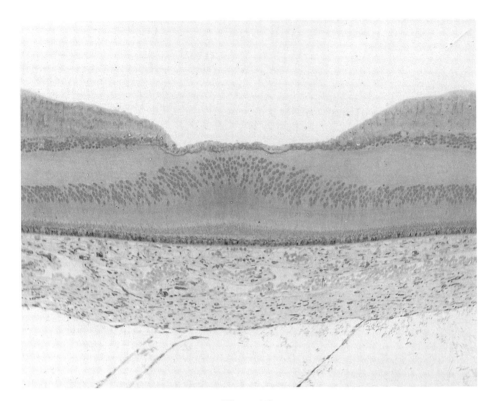

Figure 4-2
NORMAL ANATOMIC FOVEA
The ganglion cell and nerve fiber layers are absent.

The blood supply to the retina is via the central retinal vessels that enter and leave the eye through the optic nerve head. Four main branches of the central retinal artery and vein supply and drain blood. These small retinal arteries do not have an internal elastic lamina. Arterioles branch quickly to form a capillary net that is spread densely throughout the retina, except in the fovea and around the arteries, where capillary free zones are present. The retinal capillaries have a 1 to 1 ratio of pericytes and endothelial cells. The endothelial cells of the retinal vessels have tight junctions (zonula occludens) between them, which prevents diffusion between the vascular lumen and the extracellular space of the retina. These tight junctions, along with the junctions between RPE cells, form the blood-retinal barrier. Blood vessels are present only in the inner half of the retina. The layers of the retina external to the inner nuclear layer derive nutrition and oxygen from the choriocapillaris layer of the choroid.

CLASSIFICATION AND FREQUENCY

Retinoblastoma is the most common intraocular tumor of childhood and the most common tumor of the retina (Table 4-2). The prevalence of tumors and pseudotumors of the retina reported in the Armed Forces Institute of Pathology (AFIP) Registry of Ophthalmic Pathology (ROP) is similar to that reported from Brazil (1), but in Brazil the ratio of retinoblastomas to melanomas is much greater. In African countries with predominately black populations, retinoblastoma is far more common than any other intraocular tumor (2). *Pseudoretinoblastomas* are lesions that clinically mimic retinoblastoma. They may be called *pseudogliomas* by ophthalmologists, which is a holdover from the time retinoblastoma was considered a glioma of the retina. Coats disease, which probably represents a vascular malformation, is the most common pseudoretinoblastoma (Table 4-2). *Malignant lymphoma* of the central nervous system is the second most prevalent neoplasm affecting the retina.

Table 4-2

TUMORS AND PSEUDOTUMORS OF THE NEUROSENSORY RETINA*

Type of Tumor	Number of Cases
Retinoblastoma	188
Pseudoretinoblastoma	
Coats disease	17
Toxocara endophthalmitis	5
Persistent hyperplastic primary vitreous	6
Capillary hemangioma of von Hippel	4
Cavernous hemangioma	1
Astrocytoma	1
Astrocytic hamartoma (tuberous sclerosis)	1
Malignant lymphoma	14
Leukemia	3

* Frequency distribution of 235 tumors in the AFIP Registry of Ophthalmic Pathology collected between 1984 and 1989.

Statistics concerning tumors of the retina are complicated by several factors. In series based on clinical experience, the frequency of pseudotumors is higher because these are usually managed without the need for a pathologic specimen (3). Also, retinoblastomas that are detected early and treated by radiation, photocoagulation, or cryotherapy often are not confirmed histopathologically (4).

RETINOBLASTOMA, RETINOCYTOMA, AND PSEUDORETINOBLASTOMA

Retinoblastoma is a rare malignant tumor with a prevalence of about 1/23,000 live births in England (60), 1/16,000 in Holland (61), and 1/20,000 in Japan (21). The conquest of retinoblastoma in the developed countries of the world provides a model for what can be achieved through research and education (84). In 100 years, retinoblastoma has changed from an almost uniformly fatal disease to one in which 95 percent of patients are cured. Recently, the genetic cause of retinoblastoma was found to be the loss of both alleles of a normal tumor suppressor gene (the RB gene) on the long arm of chromosome 13 (see fig. 4-4). This gene, classified as a recessive oncogene or antioncogene (13), has

been cloned (27,41). Researchers have discovered that mutations of the RB gene play a role in the development of a wide variety of cancers in addition to retinoblastoma (14,57).

James Wardrop (9) is credited with establishing retinoblastoma as an entity in 1809. He advocated enucleation as treatment but he never achieved a cure. Wardrop steadfastly maintained that his failures were attributable to the advanced stage of the disease at the time of enucleation and to the fact that the optic nerve was always involved.

Rudolph Virchow (9) considered the tumor a glioma of the retina, and because of his influence, this remained its most widely used name for many years. Flexner in 1881 and Wintersteiner in 1897 described and illustrated the characteristic rosettes, which have been given their names. Influenced by these rosettes, Flexner suggested that the tumor be called neuroepithelioma of the retina, which was also the term used by Wintersteiner in the title of his monograph. Over the years, many names have been proposed but in 1926 the American Ophthalmological Society adopted the term retinoblastoma, which had been suggested by Verhoeff in 1922 (9). More recently, this name was advocated by the World Health Organization.

Retinoblastomas vary greatly in differentiation and this is in part responsible for the many different names proposed for them. Flexner-Wintersteiner rosettes were considered the highest degree of differentiation prior to 1969, when Tso et al. (75) described cytologically benign cells in retinoblastomas. They observed foci of benign-appearing cells that individually or in small bouquet-like clusters (fleurettes) exhibited photoreceptor differentiation (74,76). In most instances, such areas of benign-appearing tumor cells represented only a small component within an otherwise typical retinoblastoma, but rare tumors were composed entirely of cells with benign cytologic features (76). In 1983 Margo et al. (47) introduced the term retinocytoma for these tumors. This classification was patterned after neural tumors of the pineal gland: *pineoblastoma* for the malignant group and *pineocytoma* for the more highly differentiated, comparatively benign group (59).

Based on long-term clinical observations, Gallie et al. (28) introduced a new name, *retinoma*, for small, often partially calcified retinal tumors exhibiting no growth. Although they studied 36 eyes with such lesions clinically, none was examined histologically. It seems clear, however, that the tumors they studied are identical to the retinocytomas of Margo.

Epidemiology and Genetics. Retinoblastoma is worldwide in distribution, affecting all racial groups without sex predilection. Analysis of data from the Netherlands (61), Japan (21), and the United States (71) has shown that the incidence of retinoblastoma has not changed in the past 10 to 20 years. Schipper (61) showed that from 1920 through 1969 there was no change in the proportion of bilateral cases in the Netherlands, which remained at about 33 percent. In Japan, 34 percent of the cases were bilateral (21). In cases from the ROP obtained between 1922 and 1959, the prevalence of bilateral retinoblastoma was 21 percent (38).

The incidence of retinoblastoma decreases with age, with the majority of cases being diagnosed before 3 years. Retinoblastoma has been observed in both premature babies and in infants born at term. In a series of 760 cases on file in the ROP, only 5 patients were over 10 years of age (84); the tumor rarely occurs in adults.

Retinoblastoma can arise either as a germinal (heritable) mutation or a somatic (nonheritable) mutation. Multiple primary retinoblastomas, whether in one or both eyes, always result from a germinal mutation. Median age at diagnosis of bilateral retinoblastoma is significantly lower than for unilateral retinoblastoma (38). For a population of patients with retinoblastoma, Knudson (37) plotted the proportion of patients that were still unaffected versus patient age. He found a simple exponential relationship for bilateral cases, implying that a single event in addition to the germline mutation is required to produce the tumors. The relationship of age and disease for patients with unilateral retinoblastoma was more complex, suggesting that tumorigenesis involves more than one event. From such data, Knudson formulated his "two hit hypothesis." He postulated that the development of any retinoblastoma requires two complementary tumor-inducing events to convert a normal retinal cell into a neoplastic cell. In cases of heritable retinoblastoma, the first mutation is in the germ cell and therefore every cell in the patient has the first hit. The second hit occurs in the somatic cell

that will give rise to the retinoblastoma. In nonheritable retinoblastoma both hits must occur in the same somatic cell, which explains why patients with nonheritable retinoblastoma are older than those with the heritable type.

With a germinal mutation, every cell of the body has one mutant allele of the retinoblastoma (RB) protein gene or one hit in Knudson's theory. Because there are at least 200 million cells in the developing retina, the chance of at least one cell developing the second hit is high even though the probability of the second mutation occurring in any given cell is very low. Only 5 to 10 percent of patients who are carriers of a mutation of the RB gene do not develop a retinoblastoma, 25 to 35 percent have unilateral retinoblastoma, and 60 to 75 percent have bilateral tumors. Knudson (37) estimated that the mean number of tumors in patients carrying the retinoblastoma mutation is between three and four. In Japan, the average number of tumors in cases of bilateral retinoblastoma is 3.7 (21), which is consistent with Knudson's estimate.

Another major difference between patients with heritable and nonheritable retinoblastomas is that survivors of the heritable type are highly susceptible to the development of other nonocular cancers (6,22,24,42,57). Based on data from the AFIP ROP on patients with bilateral retinoblastoma, Roarty et al. (57) estimated that the 30-year cumulative incidence rate for nonocular tumors was 26 percent, which is in general agreement with data from large tumor registries from around the world (22,24,42). For patients who received radiation, the 30-year incidence rate was 35 percent and 6 percent for those who did not receive radiation therapy. The most common tumors developing both within and outside the field of radiation were sarcomas (Table 4-3), with osteogenic sarcomas most prevalent. Osteosarcoma of the lower extremities occurs 500-fold more frequently in survivors of bilateral retinoblastoma than in children who are not carriers of the mutant retinoblastoma gene. Intracranial tumors, which closely resemble retinoblastoma, occur far more frequently in the pineal or parasellar locations in patients with heritable retinoblastoma than in other patients (11,43,85). The association of these intracranial tumors with bilateral retinoblastoma is called *trilateral retinoblastoma*.

Table 4-3

**SECOND TUMORS DEVELOPING
IN AND OUT OF THE FIELD*
OF IRRADIATION IN
RETINOBLASTOMA SURVIVORS****

Type of Tumor	Number of Patients Developing Tumors		
	In Field	Out of Field	Total
Osteogenic sarcoma	4	1	5
Chondrosarcoma	1	0	1
Sarcoma, spindle cell type	2	0	2
Melanoma	1	3	4
Sebaceous carcinoma	2	0	2
Transitional cell carcinoma	1	0	1
Squamous cell carcinoma	1	1	2
Carcinoma, undifferentiated	1	0	1
Undifferentiated malignancy	0	1	1
Myxoma	1	0	1
Leukemia	0	1	1
Pineoblastoma	0	2	2
Neuroblastoma	0	1	1
Astrocytoma	0	1	1
Brain tumor, unknown type	0	1	1
TOTAL	14	12	26

*"Out of the field" includes tumors in nonirradiated patients.
**From reference 57.

The genetic classification of retinoblastoma has changed with a better understanding of the genetic defects responsible for tumorigenesis. Retinoblastoma is inherited as an autosomal dominant disease but is recessive at the cellular level: the mutation responsible for the development of retinoblastoma is recessive, occurring in a gene located at the q14 locus of chromosome 13 (13). This gene normally produces a phosphoprotein (RB protein) that regulates cell division by binding to DNA (40). Several cell lines of retinoblastoma, osteosarcoma, synovial sarcoma, and breast carcinoma have failed to produce RB protein (40,78) and replacement of the mutant RB gene in cultured human cancer cells has resulted in suppression of the neoplastic phenotype (40,44). It is interesting that the mechanism by which adenovirus and SV40 virus produce transformation in tissue cultured cells is by binding to and inactivating normal RB protein (40).

Familial cases represent heritable retinoblastoma in which there is another affected family member. Less than 10 percent of the cases of retinoblastoma in the ROP are familial, and in some underdeveloped countries where there are virtually no survivors, there are no familial cases. The rest of the cases are sporadic, but this is a heterogeneous group: about one fourth are heritable tumors in patients with new germinal mutations; the remainder are nonheritable tumors derived from somatic mutations in retinal cells. Analysis of DNA polymorphism within the retinoblastoma gene is now being used to predict the risk of heritable retinoblastoma (82).

Chromosomal deletion retinoblastoma represents a subclass of patients with heritable retinoblastoma in which the germinal mutation affects more than the retinoblastoma gene. These patients have a measurable defect in one of the long arms of chromosome 13 involving the q14 band. In addition to retinoblastoma, these children typically have various somatic and mental developmental abnormalities (80,83). When the q14 band is not included in the deleted segment, there is no retinoblastoma. This observation directed attention to the 13q14 band as the locus for the RB gene (fig. 4-3). This is the least common form of retinoblastoma. Deletions within the retinoblastoma gene are more frequent. Analysis of DNA in one series of 49 retinoblastomas revealed deletions within the RB gene in 12 tumors (18).

Clinical Features. The clinical manifestations of retinoblastoma vary with the stage of the disease. In the past in the United States and Europe (fig. 4-4), and currently in underdeveloped regions (fig. 4-5), far advanced retinoblastoma with extraocular extension was the rule and treatment was largely palliative. Common presenting features included a fungating mass prolapsed through a corneal perforation, proptosis caused by massive posterior orbital invasion, buphthalmos from advanced secondary glaucoma, neurological manifestations related to brain or leptomeningeal involvement, and enlarged preauricular or submandibular lymph nodes from metastasis. Before the turn of the century advanced retinoblastoma was common in Europe and North America. With improvement in the general medical education of the public, greater physician awareness of the early signs of retinoblastoma, and increased availability of eye

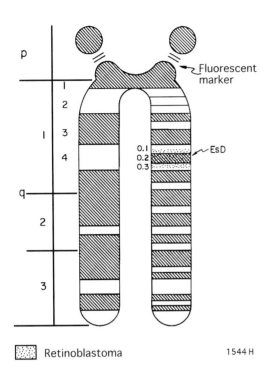

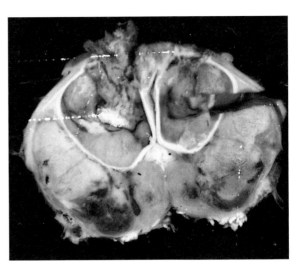

Figure 4-4
RETINOBLASTOMA

Far advanced tumor with massive extraocular extension
that was typical of cases seen in the United States and
Europe at the beginning of this century. This was the first
surgical specimen submitted to the Army Medical Museum
(1917, AFIP accession number 6) and it was originally misdiagnosed as melanosarcoma in a 6-year-old black child.

Figure 4-3
RETINOBLASTOMA

Diagram of chromosome 13 illustrating site of retinoblastoma gene near site of esterase D gene at the q14 band.

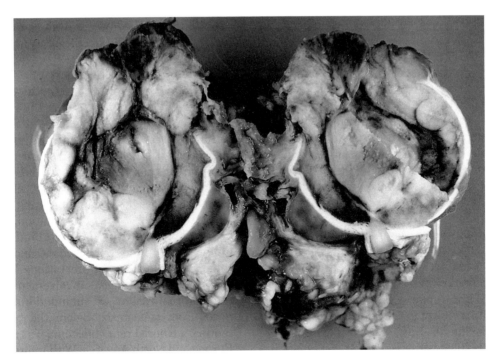

Figure 4-5
RETINOBLASTOMA

Far advanced tumor from an African patient that has destroyed the anterior segment of the eye with extraocular extension.

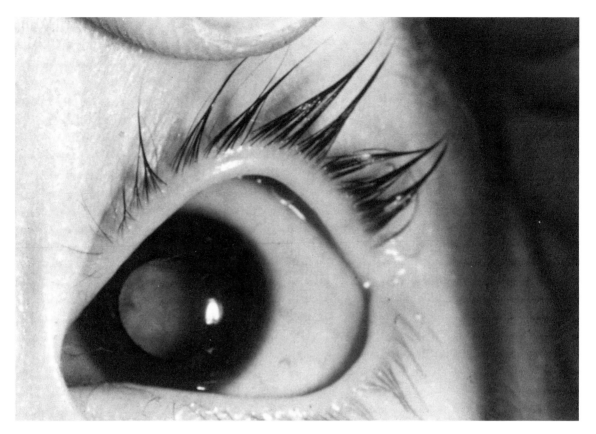

Figure 4-6
RETINOBLASTOMA
Leukocoria caused by retinal tumor.

care, advanced cases are now seldom seen in these areas. In Shields' review of 60 consecutive new cases seen between 1974 and 1978 (62), none of the retinoblastomas had extraocular extension, buphthalmos, or manifestations of metastatic disease. In four cases, the tumor was asymptomatic, having been discovered on a routine examination.

Today, most retinoblastomas are discovered when someone, usually a parent, notices the abnormal appearance of one or both pupils (fig. 4-6). In Shields' review, 90 percent of patients had leukocoria. The pupil usually appeared white, pink, or grayish yellow. Strabismus was present in 35 percent of the cases (fig. 4-7). Other presenting signs observed in a very few cases included a dilated fixed pupil, hyphema, and heterochromia iridis. In a series from Japan (21), leukocoria was the initial manifestation in 60 percent of the patients and strabismus in 13 percent.

Leukocoria is usually the consequence of a retrolental mass, but a discrete intraretinal tumor situated at the posterior pole may also reflect light back, producing a white pupil. Obviously, all leukocorias are not indicative of a retinoblastoma since this symptom is present in a broad spectrum of developmental, inflammatory, degenerative, and other pathologic conditions. Computed tomography (CT) aids in determining the size and location of the retinoblastoma (figs. 4-8, 4-9) and can be used to detect macroscopic extraocular extension; microscopic spread within the optic nerve beyond the lamina cribrosa is not detectable with CT (33).

Recently, small, often calcified tumors (pl. IIIA) typically found in eyes retaining useful vision have been identified as retinocytomas (12, 28,47). These tumors, although smaller, have an ophthalmoscopic appearance similar to retinoblastomas that were treated by radiation and had

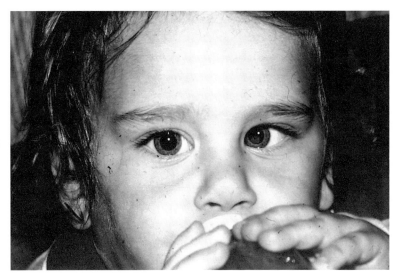

Figure 4-7
RETINOBLASTOMA
Strabismus without leukocoria is an early clinical symptom.

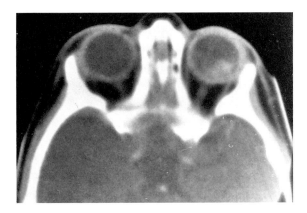

Figure 4-8
RETINOBLASTOMA
Computed tomograph of ovoid retinal tumor.

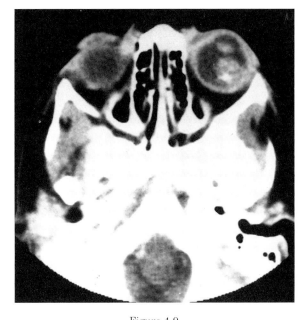

Figure 4-9
RETINOBLASTOMA
Computed tomograph of round retinal tumor with foci of calcification.

regressed. Some authors consider retinocytomas to be spontaneously regressed retinoblastomas (5,8). We do not favor this interpretation because spontaneous regression usually occurs in a larger tumor and results in phthisis bulbi (15). Gallie and co-workers (28) described the clinical appearance of retinocytoma as a comparatively small, homogeneous, translucent, gray, slightly elevated plaquoid mass, with functional retinal blood vessels looping into the mass in 90 percent of cases. Within the mass are opaque, white calcified flecks (pl. IIIA) having the appearance of cottage cheese (78 percent of cases) and in areas underlying or adjacent to the tumor there is proliferation and migration of retinal pigment epithelium (56 percent of cases).

Retinocytomas usually occur in a functional eye with clear media and no retinal detachment. They may be observed unilaterally in nongenetic cases or bilaterally in genetically determined cases of retinoblastoma (28). Eagle et al. (25) described a retinocytoma that remained stationary for 3 years and then grew rapidly. Histologic examination revealed a typical retinocytoma except in the area where the growth occurred. In

PLATE III

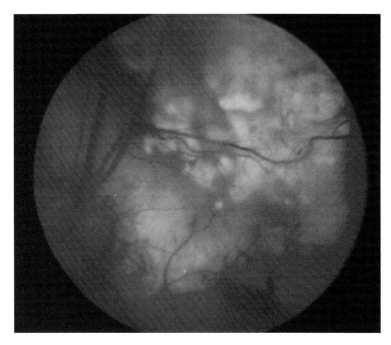

A. RETINOCYTOMA

Fundus photograph of translucent intraretinal tumor with focal opacified areas representing calcification.

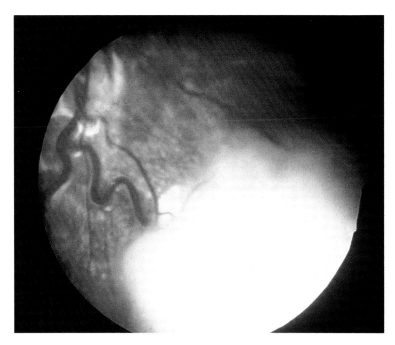

B. ENDOPHYTIC RETINOBLASTOMA

Fundus photograph of fluffy white retinal tumor that has grown into the vitreous. Retinal vessels are obscured by the tumor.

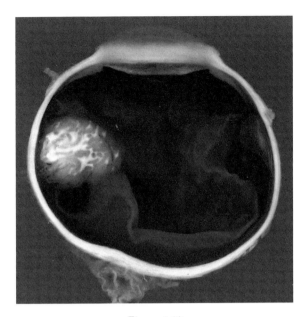

Figure 4-10
RETINOBLASTOMA
Small retinal tumor with large whitish areas of necrosis.

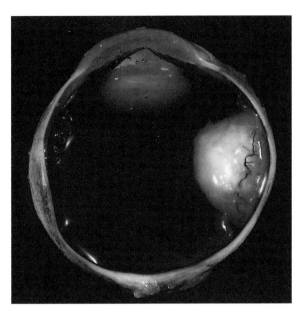

Figure 4-11
RETINOBLASTOMA
Small retinal tumor with foci of calcification.

this location the cytology was that of a poorly differentiated retinoblastoma, suggesting malignant transformation of the benign retinocytoma. This scenario may explain the rare retinoblastomas that occur in adults.

Pathologic Findings. The gross features of intraocular retinoblastoma are dependent on the growth pattern of the tumor. Five growth patterns are recognized: endophytic, exophytic, mixed endophytic-exophytic, diffuse infiltrating, and complete spontaneous regression. These explain certain clinical variations as well as differences in intraocular and extraocular spread.

Endophytic retinoblastomas (pl. IIIB, figs. 4-10, 4-11) grow mainly from the inner surface of the retina into the vitreous. Thus, on ophthalmoscopic examination, the tumor is viewed directly. Retinal vessels are typically lost from view as they enter the tumor. As endophytic tumors grow large and become friable, tumor cells are shed into the vitreous where they grow into separate tiny spheroidal masses that appear as fluff balls or cotton balls. The spheroidal masses of tumor can mimic inflammatory conditions such as mycotic or nematodal endophthalmitis. Tumor cells in the vitreous may seed onto the inner surface of the retina (fig. 4-12) and invade into the retina.

It is important to distinguish multicentric retinoblastoma (fig. 4-13) from retinal seeding (fig. 4-12) because the presence of multiple tumors indicates a germinal mutation. While this distinction is frequently difficult or impossible to make, there are some clues that are helpful. If the tumor lies mainly on the inner surface of the retina rather than within it, or if the tumor cell clusters are seen within the vitreous, retinal seeding is suggested.

Tumor cells in the vitreous may also spread into the posterior chamber and then into the anterior chamber by aqueous flow (figs. 4-14, 4-15). Secondary deposits on the lens, zonular fibers, ciliary epithelium, iris, corneal endothelium, and trabecular meshwork may be observed and tumor cells may follow the aqueous outflow pathways out of the eye. In such cases, anterior segment changes may be misinterpreted clinically as granulomatous iridocyclitis.

Exophytic retinoblastomas (pls. IVA–C) grow primarily from the outer retinal surface towards the choroid, producing first an elevation and then a detachment of the retina. On ophthalmoscopic examination, the tumor is viewed through the retina and the retinal vessels course over it. As the tumor grows larger, it may give rise to total

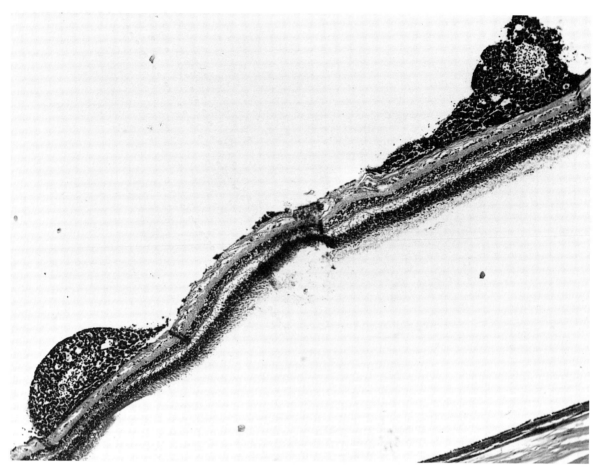

Figure 4-12
RETINOBLASTOMA
Nodules of neoplastic cells seeding onto the inner surface of the retina.

retinal detachment and tumor cells may escape into the subretinal exudate. Secondary implants then develop on the outer retinal surface where they can invade into the retina or the inner surface of the RPE. The implants then replace the RPE and eventually infiltrate through the Bruch membrane into the choroid (fig. 4-16). From the choroid, tumor cells escape along ciliary vessels and nerves into the orbit and conjunctiva. From there they gain access to blood vessels and lymphatics and metastasize.

Mixed endophytic-exophytic tumors are probably more common than either type alone, especially among larger tumors. The combined features of both endophytic and exophytic growth characterize these tumors.

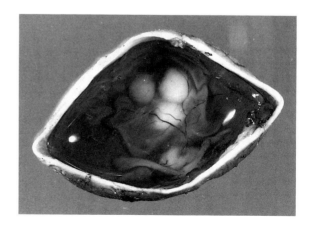

Figure 4-13
MULTICENTRIC RETINOBLASTOMA
Three small tumors have arisen in the retina.

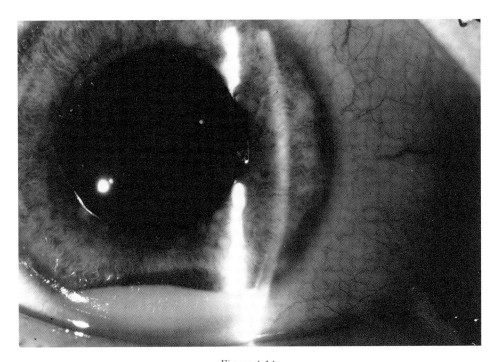

Figure 4-14
RETINOBLASTOMA
Slitlamp photograph of neoplastic cells infiltrating the anterior chamber and mimicking inflammation (pseudohypopyon).

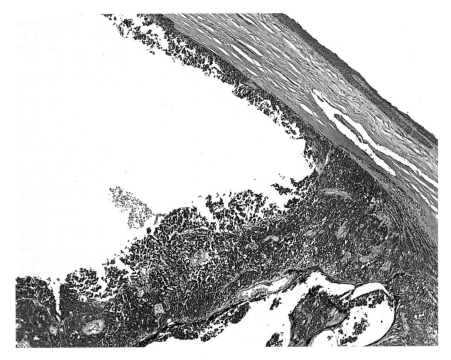

Figure 4-15
RETINOBLASTOMA
Neoplastic cells involving anterior chamber, iris, and angle structures (pseudohypopyon).

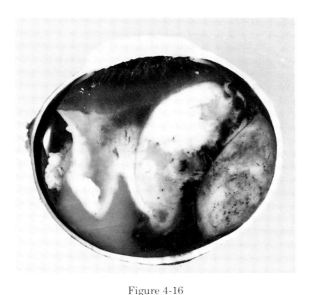

Figure 4-16
RETINOBLASTOMA
Large area of choroidal invasion adjacent to partially necrotic retinal tumor.

Diffuse infiltrating retinoblastomas are the least common and often present the greatest difficulty in clinical diagnosis (46,55,64). These tumors grow diffusely within the retina without greatly thickening it. Tumor cells are discharged into the vitreous, often seeding the anterior chamber and producing a pseudohypopyon. Because of the absence of a mass this type of retinoblastoma masquerades as a retinitis, vitritis, or *Toxocara* endophthalmitis. With anterior chamber involvement, hyperacute iritis with hypopyon, juvenile xanthogranuloma, or tuberculosis may be suspected (64).

Complete spontaneous regression (figs. 4-17–4-20) is believed to occur more frequently in retinoblastoma than in any other malignant neoplasm (28). Typically, there is a severe inflammatory reaction followed by phthisis bulbi (15). The mechanism or mechanisms by which regression occurs are unknown. In several cases of bilateral retinoblastoma from the AFIP ROP there was total necrosis and phthisis bulbi on one side, and a viable tumor massively filling the eye and invading the orbit on the other side (15). Such cases would seem to exclude the possibility of a systemic mechanism for tumor necrosis: production of antibodies against the tumor, a circulating toxin, or hypercalcemia. Occlusion of the central retinal artery has been observed in eyes with necrotic retinoblastoma, but whether this occurs before or after the tumor becomes necrotic cannot be established.

Histologically, retinoblastomas are essentially malignant neuroblastic tumors that may arise in any of the nucleated retinal layers. The predominant cell has a large basophilic nucleus of variable size and shape and scanty cytoplasm (fig. 4-21). Mitotic figures are typically numerous. The tumor cells have a striking tendency to outgrow their blood supply. Characteristically, especially in large tumors, sleeves of viable cells are present along dilated blood vessels (pl. IVC, figs. 4-22–4-26). If the tumor cells are displaced more than 90 to 110 μm from the vessel, they undergo ischemic coagulative necrosis (17,61). Although this is a relatively constant finding, Burnier et al. (17) demonstrated an inverse relationship between the thickness of the cuff and the mitotic activity within the cuff. A cuff thickness of 100 μm represents the approximate distance that oxygen can diffuse before it is completely consumed in rapidly growing neoplasms.

When viable tumor cells are shed into the vitreous or subretinal fluid, they may grow into spheroidal aggregates with diameters that rarely exceed 1 mm (61). The more peripherally situated cells derive their nutrition from the vitreous or subretinal fluid and the more central cells undergo necrosis. This represents the opposite situation from the cuffs of viable tumor cells that surround the vessels in retinoblastomas. If viable cells in the vitreous or subretinal space become attached to the retina, they gain oxygen from the retinal vasculature and stimulate the proliferation of capillaries from the retina into the tumor. Similarly, tumor cells in the subretinal exudate may seed onto the inner surface of the RPE, remaining viable by deriving nutrition from the choriocapillaris.

Almost without exception, the tumor's intrinsic blood vessels cannot keep pace with the proliferation of neoplastic cells. At this stage, the growth rate of the tumor is limited by the ability of the tumor to induce new vessel formation. This results in extensive areas of coagulative necrosis. Foci of calcification occur frequently within these areas (fig. 4-26). In most instances, the necrotic portions of retinoblastomas do not provoke much of an inflammatory response. With marked necrosis, the DNA liberated from the tumor's nuclei may

PLATE IV

A. EXOPHYTIC RETINOBLASTOMA
Fundus photograph of retinal tumor that has grown into the subretinal space. Retinal blood vessels pass over the tumor.

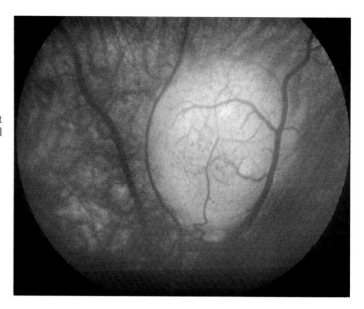

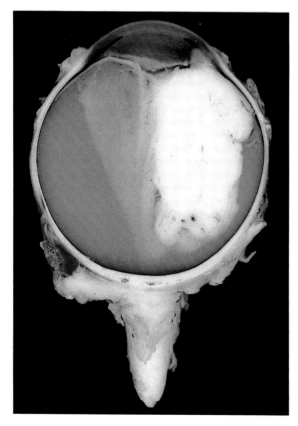

B. RETINOBLASTOMA
Large exophytic white tumor with foci of calcification producing total exudative retinal detachment. (Plates B and C are from the same patient.)

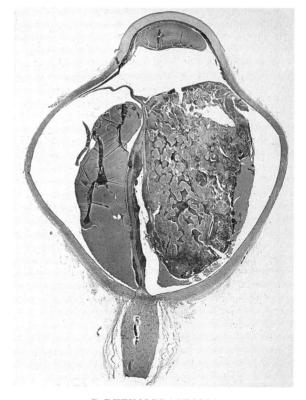

C. RETINOBLASTOMA
Total retinal detachment and collapse of the anterior chamber caused by a partially necrotic tumor with viable cells surrounding blood vessels in a sleeve pattern. There is no invasion of choroid, sclera, or optic nerve.

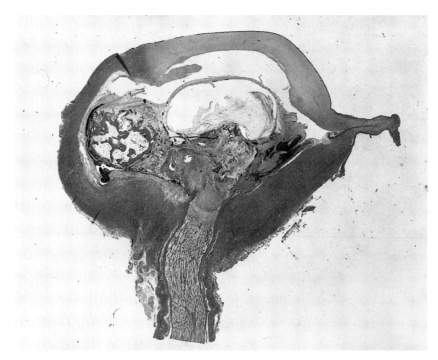

Figure 4-17
SPONTANEOUS REGRESSION OF RETINOBLASTOMA
Within this phthisical eye, the intraocular contents are disorganized with areas of calcification and ossification. (Figures 4-17–4-19 are from the same patient.)

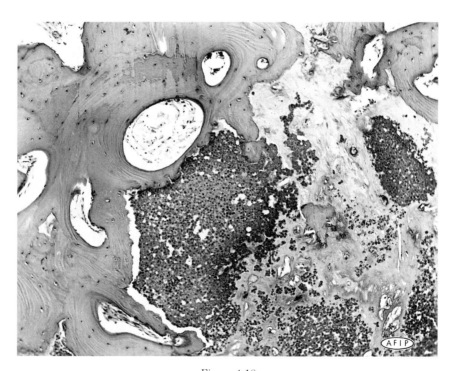

Figure 4-18
SPONTANEOUS REGRESSION OF RETINOBLASTOMA
Higher power magnification of eye seen in previous figure showing osseous metaplasia and calcified tumor cells.

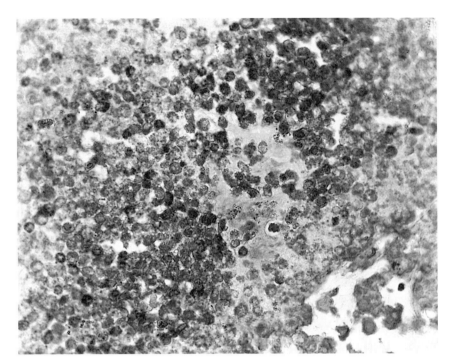

Figure 4-19
SPONTANEOUS REGRESSION OF RETINOBLASTOMA
Higher power magnification of fossilized neoplastic cells.

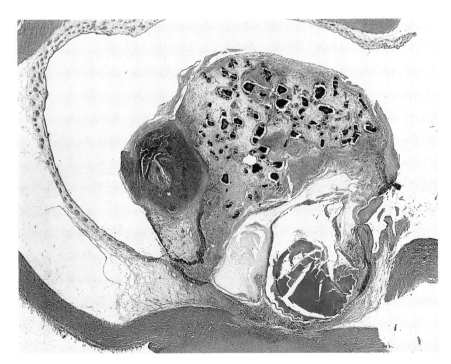

Figure 4-20
SPONTANEOUS REGRESSION OF RETINOBLASTOMA
Massive gliosis of retina, with large dilated blood vessels adjacent to foci of calcified neoplastic cells.

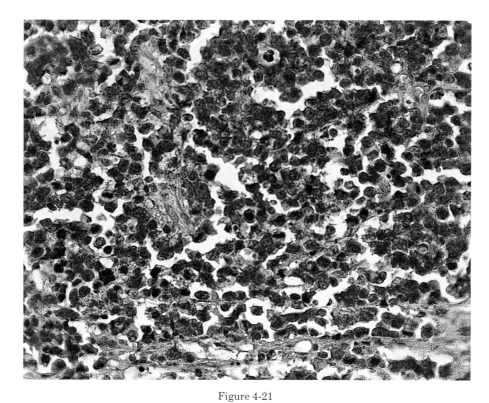

Figure 4-21
RETINOBLASTOMA
Poorly differentiated area of uniform cells with large hyperchromatic nuclei and numerous mitotic figures.

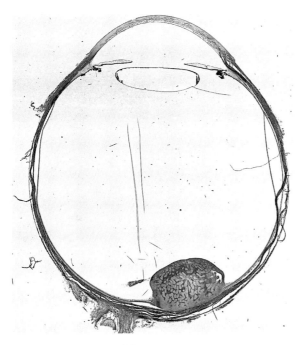

Figure 4-22
RETINOBLASTOMA
Small endophytic tumor.

become absorbed preferentially in the walls of blood vessels (fig. 4-27) and by the internal limiting membrane of the retina, giving a deep blue (hematoxylinophilic) or Feulgen-positive stain to these tissues (16). Similar basophilic staining is seen in the lens capsule, vessels in the iris, or the tissues adjacent to the Schlemm canal, indicating that some of the disintegrated DNA escapes into the aqueous.

The formation of Flexner-Wintersteiner rosettes (fig. 4-28) is highly characteristic of retinoblastomas. Pineoblastoma and medulloepithelioma are the only other neoplasms in which we have observed these rosettes. The Flexner-Wintersteiner rosette represents differentiation by the tumor, but the cells of the rosettes are not benign. Characteristically, Flexner-Wintersteiner rosettes are found within areas of undifferentiated malignant cells exhibiting mitotic activity, and the cells that form the rosettes may also contain mitotic figures. Some rosettes are incompletely formed and the cells blend with the surrounding undifferentiated cells.

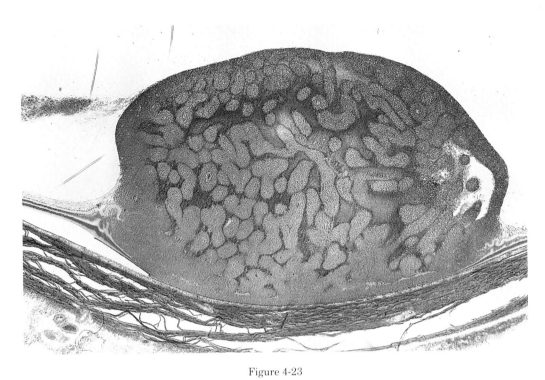

Figure 4-23
RETINOBLASTOMA
Higher magnification of neoplasm seen in figure 4-22 showing viable cells surrounding blood vessels and forming sleeves.

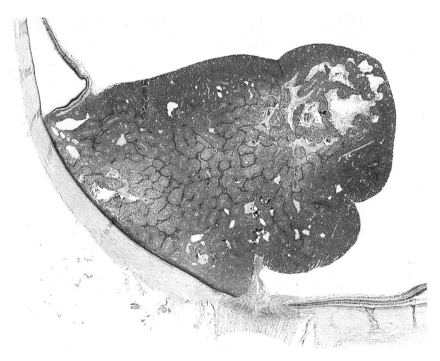

Figure 4-24
RETINOBLASTOMA
Endophytic tumor adjacent to optic nerve head with sleeve pattern.

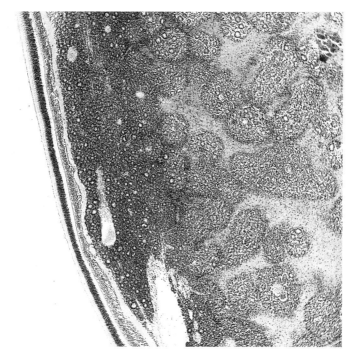

Figure 4-25
RETINOBLASTOMA
Area of tumor with sleeve pattern and Flexner-Wintersteiner rosettes.

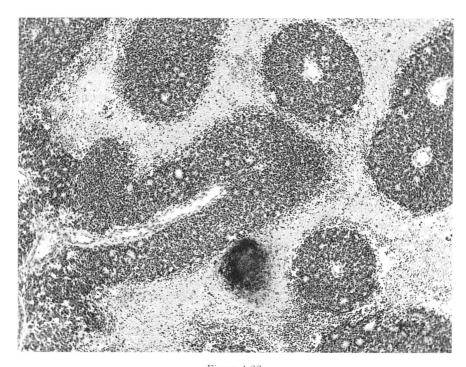

Figure 4-26
RETINOBLASTOMA
Area of tumor with Flexner-Wintersteiner rosettes within sleeves of viable cells and calcification within the necrotic area.

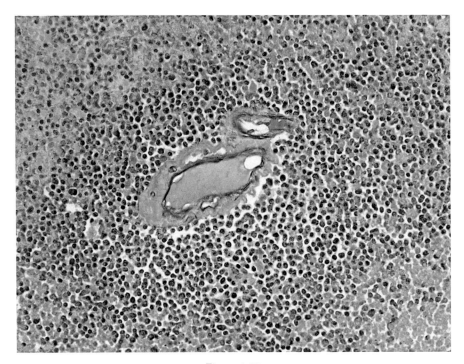

Figure 4-27
RETINOBLASTOMA
Basophilic staining representing DNA deposition in the walls of blood vessels. The tumor cells have undergone necrosis with many pyknotic or coagulated nuclei.

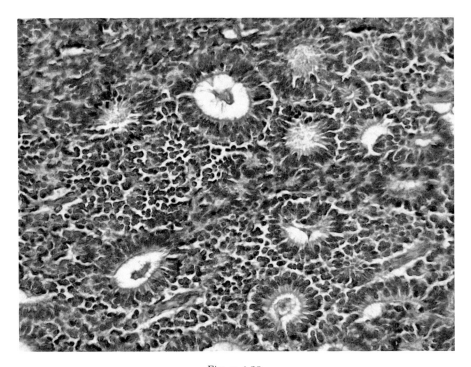

Figure 4-28
RETINOBLASTOMA
Well-differentiated area containing Flexner-Wintersteiner rosettes.

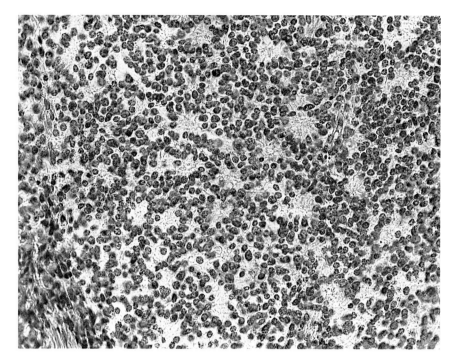

Figure 4-29
RETINOBLASTOMA
Area containing Homer Wright rosettes.

The typical Flexner-Wintersteiner rosette (fig. 4-28) is lined by tall cuboidal cells that circumscribe an apical lumen. The basal ends of the cells that form the rosettes contain the nuclei. The apical ends of the cuboidal cells are held together by terminal bars and the cells may have apical cytoplasmic projections into the lumen of the rosette. Electron microscopy has demonstrated that these projections represent primitive inner and outer segments and, therefore, these cells represent an attempt by the tumor to form photoreceptor cells (73). Alcian blue and colloidal iron stains reveal a coating of hyaluronidase-resistant acid mucopolysaccharide in the lumina of the rosettes that has similar staining characteristics to the glycosaminogycan matrix that surrounds the rods and cones of the retina (84). Tso and co-workers (73) described several additional ultrastructural features that the cells forming Flexner-Wintersteiner rosettes share with retinal photoreceptors: zonula occludens that form a luminal limiting membrane analogous to the cellular junctions that form the outer limiting membrane of the retina, cytoplasmic microtubules, cilia with the 9+0 pattern, and

lamellated membranous structures resembling the discs of rod outer segments. Immunohistochemical and lectin histochemical studies have also supported the concept that retinoblastomas arise from undifferentiated retinal cells that may differentiate into photoreceptor-like cells (23,36,79).

Homer Wright rosettes (fig. 4-29) are less common in retinoblastomas than Flexner-Wintersteiner rosettes. Because they are found in a variety of neuroblastic tumors, they are less specific for retinoblastoma. The Homer Wright rosette was first described in sympathicoblastomas. They are also highly characteristic of cerebellar medulloblastomas (59). In these rosettes, the cells are not arranged about a lumen but instead send out cytoplasmic processes that form a tangle within the center of the rosette.

Glial differentiation (fig. 4-30) has been described in retinoblastomas (39,51,72), but in our experience it is difficult to differentiate from reactive gliosis. More convincing support for the concept that retinoblastoma cells can differentiate towards both neurons and glia is provided by studies of undifferentiated retinoblastoma cells

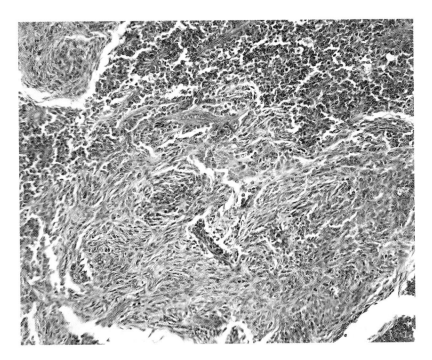

Figure 4-30
RETINOBLASTOMA
Area containing spindle-shaped glia.

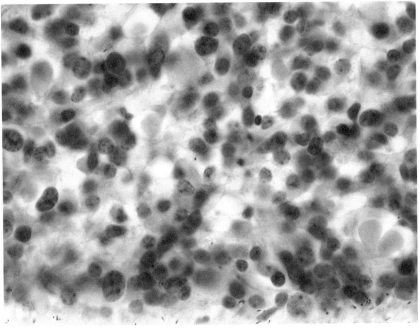

Figure 4-31
RETINOBLASTOMA
Benign cytology in area of photoreceptor differentiation with fleurettes consisting of small clusters of eosinophilic bulbous processes that extend into a lumen.

in tissue culture. Variations in the composition of culture media induced the undifferentiated cells to undergo neuronal differentiation with the formation of neuritic-type processes and rosettes, and other alterations in the culture media produced glial differentiation (19).

In 1970, Tso et al. (76) reported that 18 of 300 retinoblastomas (6 percent) treated by enucle-

ation had foci of cytologically benign cells with features of photoreceptors (figs. 4-31–4-33). In most of these 18 tumors, the areas exhibiting photoreceptor differentiation could easily be spotted at low magnification as discrete, comparatively eosinophilic islands standing out in contrast to the much more intensely basophilic portions of the tumor. The tumor cells that exhibited

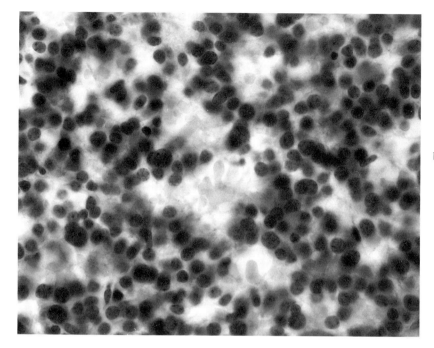

Figure 4-32
RETINOBLASTOMA
Multiple fleurettes within an area of
benign-appearing differentiated cells.

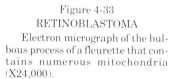

Figure 4-33
RETINOBLASTOMA
Electron micrograph of the bul-
bous process of a fleurette that con-
tains numerous mitochondria
(X24,000).

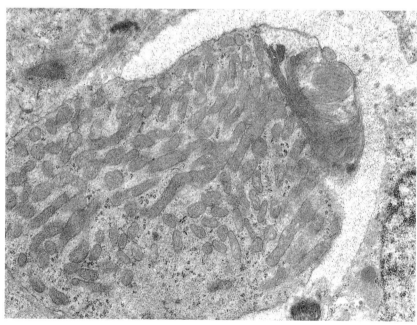

photoreceptor differentiation had more abundant cytoplasm and smaller, less basophilic nuclei that were much less densely packed. In these
areas, mitotic figures were uncommon, necrosis
was absent, and scattered deposits of calcium
were occasionally present. Individual cells and
clusters of cells with long cytoplasmic processes
stained brightly with eosin. The cytoplasmic processes projected through a fenestrated membrane and often fanned out like a bouquet of
flowers (hence the name "fleurette") (figs. 4-31,
4-32). Electron microscopy revealed that the
cells of the fleurettes contain structures that
resemble retinal cones (74). The bulbous eosinophilic processes contain numerous mitochondria
(fig. 4-33), which resemble cone inner segments.

121

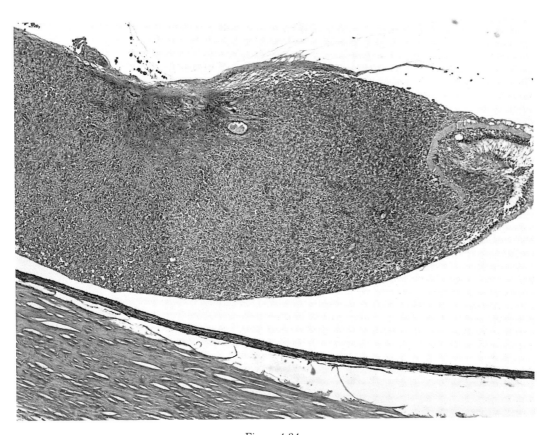

Figure 4-34
RETINOCYTOMA
Tumor confined to the retina is composed of uniform cells without necrosis.

In a subsequent study, Tso et al. (77) examined retinoblastomas in 54 eyes enucleated after having been irradiated. Only 42 eyes contained viable tumor cells and 17 of these tumors (40 percent) exhibited photoreceptor differentiation. In 7 cases, the residual tumor was composed entirely of cells showing photoreceptor differentiation. Consequently, these investigators suggested that tumors containing such benign components might be incompletely radioresponsive because, as a general rule, benign and highly differentiated tumors are more radioresistant. Follow-up information was obtained in 13 of the 17 cases; there was only one tumor death. Despite uncontrolled tumor growth, the parents of this child refused to permit enucleation. The patient died of intracranial extension of the retinoblastoma. Histologic study of this tumor revealed areas of undifferentiated retinoblastoma and areas of benign-appearing cells that exhibited photoreceptor differentiation.

Histologically, totally benign-appearing tumors (figs. 4-34, 4-35) have been described in eyes not irradiated prior to enucleation; they have been designated as retinocytomas (47). Glial differentiation has been described in these benign variants of retinoblastoma (47,68), but it is difficult to be certain whether this represents reactive gliosis from the adjacent retina or glial differentiation of tumor cells.

In phthisical eyes with totally necrotic "regressed" retinoblastomas, it may be difficult to diagnose the retinoblastoma. Histologic examination reveals dense calcification in a tumor that exhibits complete coagulative necrosis (see figs. 4-17–4-20). Under high magnification, the ghostly outlines of fossilized tumor cells can usually be seen. Further confusion is created by exuberant reactive proliferation of RPE cells, ciliary epithelial cells, and glial cells, and by ossification.

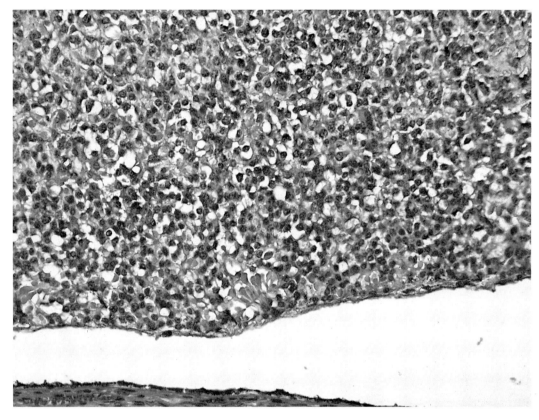

Figure 4-35
RETINOCYTOMA
Higher magnification of tumor in figure 4-34 showing cells with small round nonhyperchromatic nuclei, no mitotic activity, and scattered fleurettes.

Extraocular Extension and Metastasis. Most retinoblastomas exhibit the relentlessly progressive, rapidly invasive growth that is characteristic of blastic tumors of childhood. If left untreated, they usually fill the eye and completely destroy the internal architecture of the globe (fig. 4-36). The most common method of spread is by invasion through the optic disc into the optic nerve (figs. 4-37–4-40). Once in the nerve, the tumor spreads directly along the nerve fiber bundles back towards the optic chiasm or infiltrates through the pia into the subarachnoid space. From the subarachnoid space tumor cells are carried via the circulating cerebrospinal fluid to the brain and spinal cord. Once the tumor has invaded the choroid (figs . 4-16, 4-41), it may then spread into the orbit via the scleral canals or by massively replacing the sclera (figs. 4-4, 4-5, 4-36). Approximately 6 months are required from the time the retino-

blastoma produces its first symptoms to the time it invades outside the eye (26). Extraocular invasion dramatically increases the chances of hematogenous dissemination and permits access to conjunctival lymphatics and metastasis to regional lymph nodes.

Retinoblastomas metastasize in four ways: direct infiltration, dispersion, hematogenous dissemination, and lymphatic spread.

Direct infiltrative spread occurs along the optic nerve from the eye to the brain. Once the orbital soft tissues are invaded, the tumor spreads directly into the orbital bones, through the sinuses into the nasopharynx, or via the various foramina into the cranium. Dispersion of tumor cells occurs after cells in the optic nerve have invaded the leptomeninges and gained access to the circulating subarachnoid fluid. This occurs without involvement of the cut end of the optic nerve. Flow of cerebrospinal fluid carries

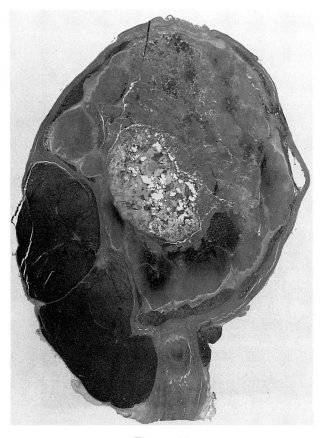

Figure 4-36
RETINOBLASTOMA
Large tumor fills the globe with massive choroidal and extraocular invasion.

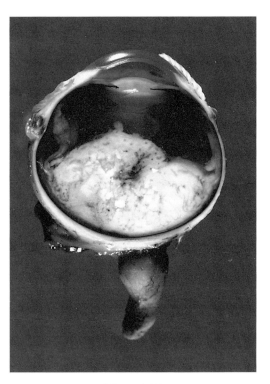

Figure 4-37
RETINOBLASTOMA
Large exophytic tumor with enlargement of optic nerve due to invasion.

Figure 4-38
RETINOBLASTOMA
Tumor invading just the optic nerve head.

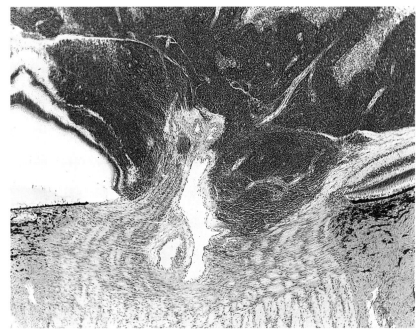

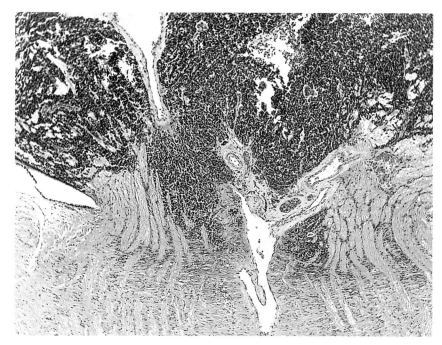

Figure 4-39
RETINOBLASTOMA
Tumor invading the optic nerve
to the level of the lamina cribrosa.

Figure 4-40
RETINOBLASTOMA
Tumor invading the optic nerve
parenchyma posterior to the lamina
cribrosa but not reaching the level of
surgical transection.

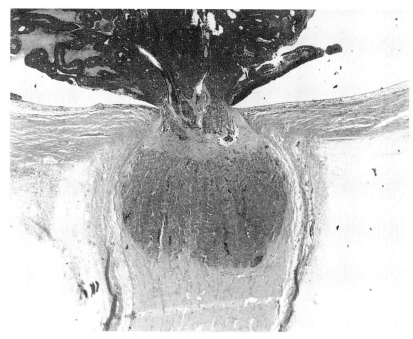

tumor cells from the eye to the brain and spinal cord, and we have even observed spread to the optic nerve on the opposite side. Hematogenous dissemination leads to widespread metastasis to the lungs, bones, brain, and other viscera. Extraocular invasion and, to a lesser degree, choroidal invasion increase the risk for hematogenous spread. Lymphatic spread occurs in those cases with anteriorly

located or massive extraocular extension. There are no intraocular or orbital lymphatic channels, but the bulbar conjunctiva and eyelids are richly supplied with lymphatic vessels.

When metastasis occurs, it is generally within the first year or two following treatment. Kopelman et al. (38) found that the median time to death in patients with fatal retinoblastoma was

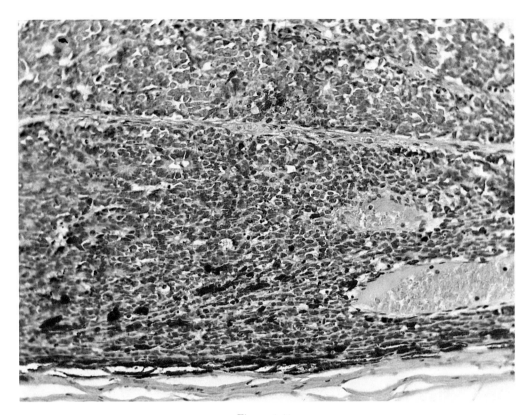

Figure 4-41
RETINOBLASTOMA
Tumor has invaded the full thickness of the choroid.

6.4 months in unilateral cases and 14.2 months in bilateral cases. In contrast, Gamel et al. (29) estimated the median time to death for patients with metastatic uveal melanoma to be 7.2 years. Late death from metastasis, which occurs so frequently following enucleation for uveal melanoma, is so rare after treatment for retinoblastoma that when metastasis is suspected, the question of an independent new primary tumor must be considered. Hematogenous metastasis from retinoblastoma is characteristically widespread, but unlike uveal melanoma, is frequently preceded by spread to regional lymph nodes. The brain may be selectively affected when spread occurs via the optic nerve. Invasion of leptomeninges of the optic nerve typically gives rise to a thick accumulation of tumor cells in the meninges along the basilar surface of the brain and in the ventricles, which can be detected by CT (50).

As is typical of metastatic lesions, metastatic retinoblastoma appears much less differentiated than the intraocular primary tumor. Rosettes,

which are often numerous and highly organized in the primary tumor, are difficult to find and poorly formed in metastatic lesions. Fleurettes are never observed.

The primary retinoblastomas observed in the pineal and parasellar sites of patients with trilateral retinoblastoma (11,38) have been confused with metastatic retinoblastoma, but in contrast with the latter, these tumors are solitary and not accompanied by other tumors as would be expected with metastatic disease. They often appear several years after the successful treatment of the intraocular tumor and may be far more differentiated with numerous rosettes, fleurettes, and individual cells exhibiting the photoreceptor differentiation than would be expected in a metastatic tumor. In addition to intracranial primary retinoblastomas, similar retinoblastoma-like tumors have been observed in many locations in patients with heritable retinoblastoma including the orbit, nasopharynx, trunk, and extremities.

Recurrence of retinoblastoma in the orbit following enucleation is almost always the result of tumor cells that were left untreated in the orbit. This may be the result of subclinical orbital involvement that escaped histopathologic recognition, but more frequently it is a consequence of incomplete removal of the orbital component or invasion of the optic nerve beyond the plane of surgical transection. Rarely, orbital recurrence is the result of lymphatic or hematogenous spread to the bony walls or soft tissues of the orbit to the lids.

Unsuspected Retinoblastoma. Stafford and co-workers (69), in their analysis of 618 histologically proven cases for which adequate clinical data were available, found that almost 15 percent had been misdiagnosed initially. In 6.6 percent of the cases, the incorrect initial diagnosis led to a delay in enucleation while treatment was given for panophthalmitis, endophthalmitis, tuberculosis, or other forms of uveitis. In another 8.3 percent, a variety of noninflammatory, nonneoplastic conditions had been diagnosed. Shields et al. (67) described 5 patients with retinoblastoma that presented with orbital cellulitis, without extraocular extension of the tumor. In all 5 cases, the retinoblastoma had undergone extensive necrosis. Delays in enucleation were associated with a much greater mortality than in the cases in which a correct initial diagnosis was followed promptly by enucleation. Kopelman et al. (38) found that death was 2.5 times more frequent in patients with clinically undiagnosed retinoblastoma.

Differential Diagnosis. Data from the ROP describing 56 eyes enucleated because of clinical suspicion of retinoblastoma between 1974 and 1980 (48) showed that 15 (27 percent) had nonneoplastic lesions such as Coats disease, other retinal detachments, glaucoma, etc. Because the AFIP receives the majority of its eye cases from nonteaching hospitals, this experience can be considered representative of the average state-of-the-art ophthalmologic diagnosis in the United States. As might be expected, in those institutions with specialists in ocular oncology, the frequency of simulating lesions in enucleated eyes is significantly less (58,62).

The entities most frequently misdiagnosed as retinoblastoma clinically are not easily confused with retinoblastoma on histopathologic examination. An exception is medulloepithelioma. *Toxocara* endophthalmitis, persistent hyperplastic primary vitreous, and Coats disease account for approximately 60 percent of pseudoretinoblastomas (62). These lesions have a number of histopathologic features in common, so that differentiating between the different pseudoretinoblastomas may be a problem for the pathologist. For example, all three may have a retinal detachment and both persistent hyperplastic primary vitreous and *Toxocara* endophthalmitis may have retrolenticular fibrosis.

Toxocara Canis Endophthalmitis. Endophthalmitis caused by larvae of the nematode *Toxocara canis* is almost always a disease of children but is never present at birth. Frequently, there is a history of the child eating dirt or playing with puppies. In humans, the ingested eggs hatch in the intestine. The larvae penetrate the intestinal mucosa, enter the circulatory system, and locate in any organ of the body (54). Characteristically, the ocular lesions are painless, often without external signs or symptoms of inflammation. The larvae usually do not invoke an inflammatory response until they die and then a characteristic eosinophilic abscess forms around the degenerating organism. The most frequent histologic finding is a low-grade sclerosing vitreitis that has caused a total retinal detachment (pls. VA, B) and less commonly, *Toxocara* larvae produce a more localized retinochoroidal lesion. Plasma cells are the most common inflammatory cell in the infiltrate. Because of the small size of the organism (20 by 400 µm), the *Toxocara* larvae and the characteristic eosinophilic abscesses are not always seen on routine sections of the globe. Eosinophils may be rare unless the section is close to a degenerating *Toxocara* larva. Antigen-antibody complexes may be deposited around the organism (the Splendore-Hoeppli phenomenon) (pl. VIA) (54).

Persistent Hyperplastic Primary Vitreous. This is a congenital anomaly of the primary vitreous (31). The vascular components of the primary vitreous consist of the hyaloid, its branches, and the posterior portion of the tunica vasculosa lentis. They begin forming in the third week of intrauterine life and normally regress during the third trimester. By birth all of the vessels in the vitreous normally disappear. In persistent hyperplastic primary vitreous (PHPV) these vessels persist after birth and are

PLATE V
TOXOCARA CANIS ENDOPHTHALMITIS

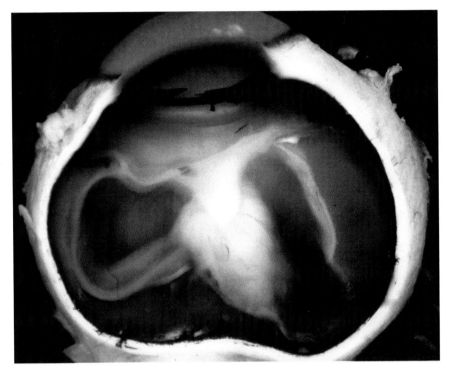

A. Whitish sclerotic vitreous mass causing traction total retinal detachment.

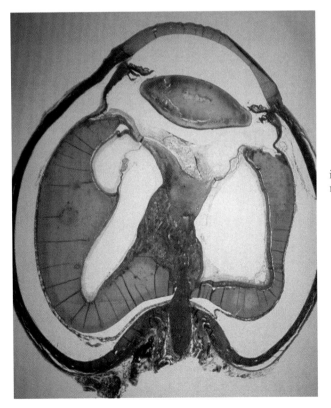

B. Trichrome stain of mass seen in A demonstrating collagen in the vitreous mass and exudative total retinal detachment.

PLATE VI

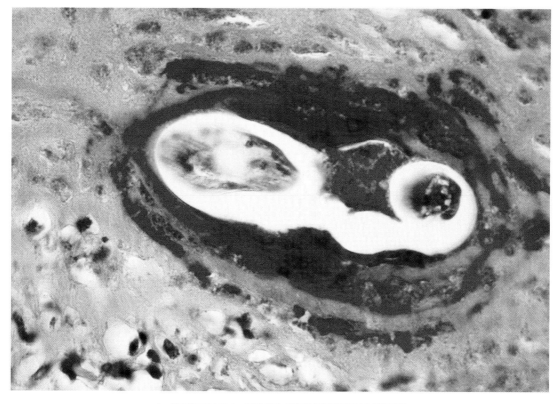

A. *TOXOCARA CANIS* ENDOPHTHALMITIS

Higher power magnification of vitreous mass in plate V showing a larva surrounded by acidophilic material (Splendore-Hoeppli phenomenon) and scattered eosinophils.

B. PERSISTENT HYPERPLASTIC
PRIMARY VITREOUS

Mild microphthalmos with persistent hyaloid artery extending from the optic nerve head to a white retrolental mass.

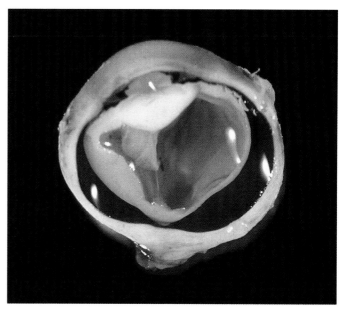

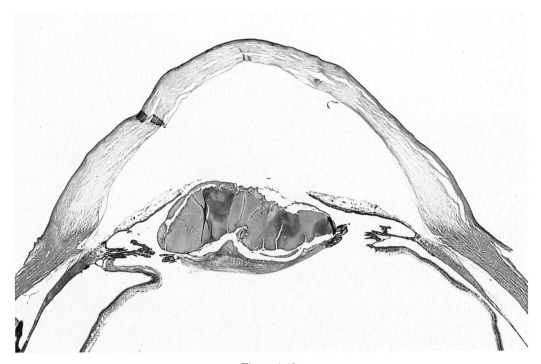

Figure 4-42
PERSISTENT HYPERPLASTIC PRIMARY VITREOUS
Retrolental mass with rupture of posterior lens capsule and anterior insertion of the retina. The epithelium in the pars plana of the ciliary body is absent.

associated with proliferation of mesenchymal tissue (31). The mesenchymal tissue has a loose embryonic appearance that is very different from the dense fibrous scar tissue of *Toxocara* endophthalmitis; inflammatory cells are usually absent. Most often, the mass of mesenchymal tissue (pls. VIB, VIIA, figs. 4-42, 4-43) is located directly behind the lens and is firmly adherent to the posterior lens capsule, which may rupture (pl. VIIB) with formation of a posterior subcapsular cataract. Less commonly, the mass of mesenchymal tissue is located at the optic nerve head. There is often an associated retinal detachment and retinal dysplasia (pl. VIIA) may also be present. The retinal detachment can be detected with ultrasound or CT (fig. 4-44). The normal position of the ora serrata of the retina is displaced anteriorly so that in some sectors the ciliary epithelium of the pars plana is absent (fig. 4-42). The ciliary processes are elongated and drawn into the retrolental mass. In rare cases, there may be adipose tissue in the retrolental mass of PHPV (31). Only in a few cases has PHPV been described in association with retinoblastoma (53).

Coats Disease. Coats disease differs from *Toxocara* endophthalmitis and PHPV in that there is almost never vitreous fibrosis or vascularization (20). Coats disease is characterized by a peripheral area of retinal vascular telangiectasis (pls. VIIIA–C). The telangiectatic vessels typically leak large amounts of exudate that accumulate in the outer retinal layers and subretinal space (pl. VIIIC) leading to a total retinal detachment (pl. VIIIB, fig. 4-45). The exudate is periodic acid–Schiff (PAS) positive and rich in lipid. Foamy macrophages and cholesterol clefts frequently accumulate in the subretinal exudate. Whereas *Toxocara* endophthalmitis and PHPV mimic endophytic retinoblastoma, Coats disease mimics exophytic retinoblastoma.

Treatment. The management of retinoblastoma is complex and the best treatment for each patient must be determined on an individual basis. The method of treatment should depend on the size and extent of the tumor, whether there is bilateral involvement, and the general health of the patient (62). The age of the patient is also an important consideration because younger

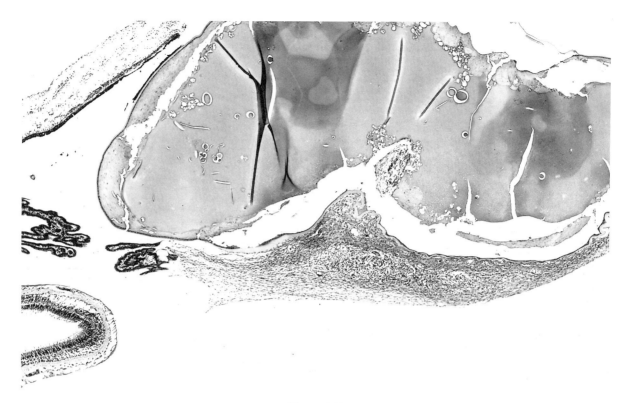

Figure 4-43
PERSISTENT HYPERPLASTIC PRIMARY VITREOUS
Higher magnification of the retrolental fibrovascular mass seen in previous figure showing cataractous changes and elongation of ciliary processes.

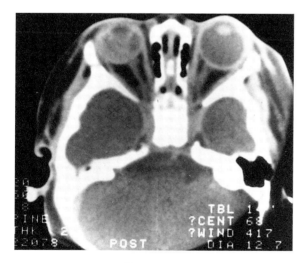

Figure 4-44
PERSISTENT HYPERPLASTIC PRIMARY VITREOUS
Computed tomograph showing microphthalmic eye with total retinal detachment.

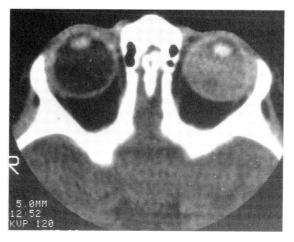

Figure 4-45
COATS DISEASE
Computed tomograph showing increased density within eye.

PLATE VII
PERSISTENT HYPERPLASTIC PRIMARY VITREOUS

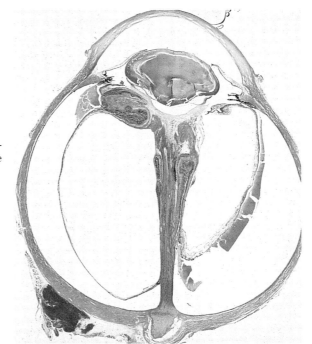

A. Falciform fold of detached dysplastic retina encircles the persistent hyaloid artery that extends from the optic nerve head to the retrolental mass.

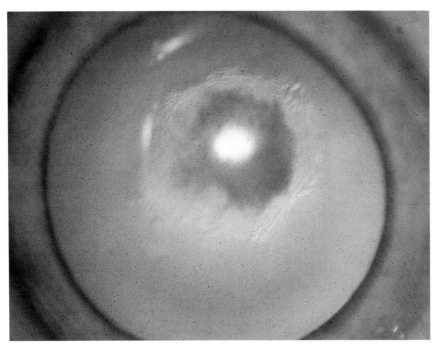

B. Wrinkling and rupture of the posterior lens capsule caused by a hemorrhagic retrolental mass.

PLATE VIII
COATS DISEASE

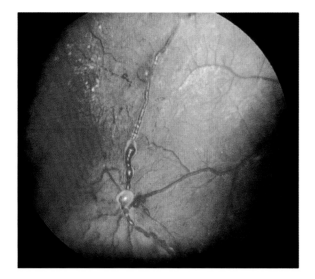

A. Fundus photograph of telangiectatic vessels on the surface of the detached retina.

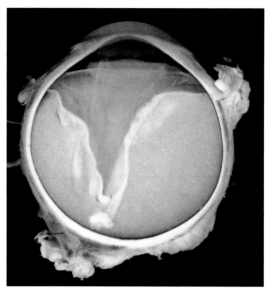

B. Total retinal detachment with subretinal exudate containing cholesterol crystals and a fibrous nodule in the posterior pole.

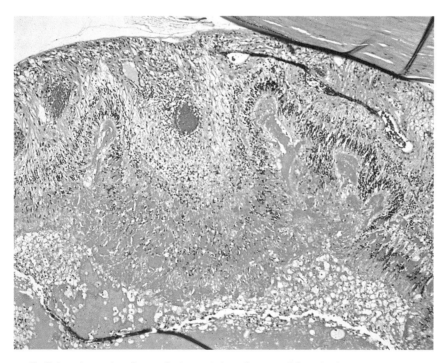

C. Telangiectasia of vessels in peripheral area of detached and gliotic retina with intraretinal and subretinal exudation.

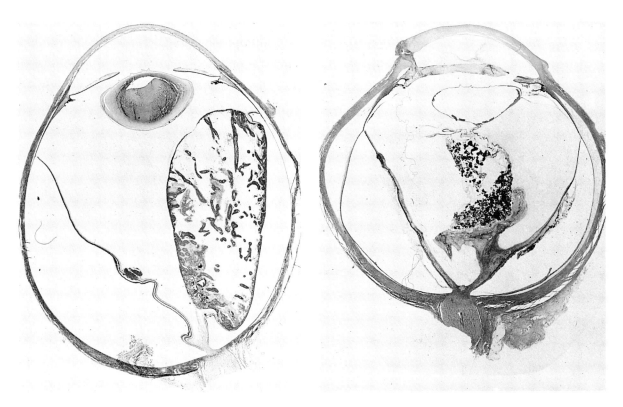

Figure 4-46
BILATERAL RETINOBLASTOMA

The patient died of an intracranial tumor.
Left: Left eye containing multicentric tumor without optic nerve invasion.
Right: Right eye containing regressed tumor after radiation therapy without optic nerve invasion.

patients are more likely to have a germinal mutation and are more likely to develop additional retinoblastomas (7). Enucleation is the most commonly employed treatment modality but in the United States (66) and Great Britain (60) the proportion of patients with retinoblastoma treated by enucleation is decreasing. For small tumors, photocoagulation and cryotherapy may be employed (63,65); for medium tumors there is plaque irradiation (10) or external beam irradiation (62); for large tumors, enucleation; for tumors with extraocular extension, enucleation combined with radiation and chemotherapy (34); for orbital recurrence, radiation and chemotherapy (32); and for metastatic retinoblastoma, chemotherapy (35). Only with modern chemotherapy have patients survived with extraorbital metastasis of retinoblastoma (30,81).

Prognosis. There are many risk factors affecting prognosis but the most important is the extent of invasion by the retinoblastoma. Kopel-

man et al. (38) in an analysis of cases from the ROP found that the extent of invasion into the optic nerve and through the ocular coats were the two most important predictors of patient outcome. The importance of extraocular invasion as the most important predictor of death is supported by a number of studies (21,32,45,52,70). When the data were evaluated by multivariate analysis, bilaterality was the only variable that proved to be more significantly associated with a fatal outcome than in univariate analysis, suggesting that bilaterality is related to death for reasons unrelated to the primary tumor. In some of these cases the cause of death was attributed to spread of retinoblastoma to the brain, yet there was no optic nerve invasion (fig. 4-46). We believe that new intracranial primary tumors (trilateral retinoblastomas) are responsible for the deaths in these cases.

A problem with this study is that it was based on cases of retinoblastoma that were treated prior

Table 4-4

PROGNOSTIC FACTORS DETERMINED BY LOGISTIC REGRESSION*

Variable	Odds Ratio	P
Invasion of ocular coats		
Into choroid	2.9	<0.0001
Into sclera	9.1	<0.0001
Into orbit	37.6	<0.0001
Invasion of optic nerve		
Resected	4.4	<0.0001
Unresected	13.3	<0.0001
Bilaterality	2.9	0.0001
Pre-1963 American cases	4.1	<0.0001

*514 American cases obtained prior to 1963 and 460 German cases obtained after 1962 (from reference 49).

to 1962 and the possibility exists that more modern treatment could affect the results. Because most of the more recent cases in the ROP are from less developed countries where it is impossible to obtain follow-up data, McLean et al. (49) compared 514 cases of retinoblastoma from the ROP obtained between 1917 and 1962 (mean, 1945) with 460 cases from Germany obtained between 1963 to 1986 (mean, 1976). The cause-specific survival rate, in which only deaths attributed to spread or metastasis of the retinoblastoma were considered, was lower in the older sample from the United States (66 percent at 5 years) than in the German sample (93 percent at 5 years). Invasion of the ocular coats and invasion into the optic nerve were the most significant prognostic factors in both samples. A multivariate logistic model using seven variables (post-1962 German versus pre-1963 ROP cases, unilateral versus bilateral, invasion of choroid, invasion of sclera, invasion of orbit, invasion of retrolaminar optic nerve, and invasion of the resected margin of the optic nerve) described well the observed mortality patterns (Table 4-4). In the absence of other risk factors, there were no deaths in the German series and eight deaths in the series from the ROP. Because metastasis of retinoblastoma is unlikely in the absence of extraocular invasion, many oncologists no longer recommend lumbar puncture and

bone marrow aspiration in patients with retinoblastoma confined within the eye (56).

We reviewed 12 cases of fatal unilateral retinoblastoma from the ROP in which the tumor was confined to the eye without invasion into the optic nerve or sclera. In half the cases there was choroidal invasion. In 8 cases, 4 with choroidal invasion and 4 without choroidal invasion, there was orbital recurrence which preceded the development of distant metastasis. These histories suggest that there was probably microscopic extraocular spread that was not detected by histologic examination. This emphasizes the importance of extraocular invasion as the pathway of metastasis of retinoblastoma and the great need for careful histologic examination aimed at the detection of this invasion.

GLIAL TUMORS AND TUMOR-LIKE CONDITIONS

Astrocytoma

As astrocytes are normally present in the retina, it is to be expected that an astrocytoma can develop from these cells. Such tumors do occur but they are rare (88). Ulbright et al. (90) reviewed 42 cases of histologically documented astrocytic tumors of the retina. Twenty-four patients (57 percent) had tuberous sclerosis, 6 patients (14 percent) had neurofibromatosis, and 12 patients (29 percent) were otherwise normal. Patients with tuberous sclerosis often had multiple tumors, peripheral tumors, or tumors that contained giant astrocytes. Approximately half of the patients with tuberous sclerosis have retinal glial hamartomas (89).

Clinically, the early lesions are rather flat and translucent. Older lesions tend to calcify, and may be confused with retinoblastoma.

Histologically, the astrocytomas of the retina are always benign neoplasms usually composed of elongated fibrous (pilocytic) astrocytes containing small oval nuclei. Their cytoplasmic processes interlace to form a fine meshwork. Usually, the tumor is confined to the retina. It does not destroy the internal limiting membrane of the retina or infiltrate other structures. Rare giant cell (gemistocytic) astrocytomas have been observed (86,87). These commonly involve the optic nerve head, occasionally becoming quite large and calcified, and may lead to loss of vision.

Massive Gliosis

Reactive gliosis in the central nervous system typically is not a space occupying lesion. Gliosis of the retina is a major exception to this rule (see fig. 4-20). Glial proliferation of the retina may occur as both a reparative or a degenerative pathologic process. Reactive fibroglia proliferate after microinfarctions, retinitis, longstanding retinal detachment, central retinal vein occlusion, and diabetic retinopathy. In most of these conditions, the glial proliferation is usually confined to the retinal layers. Massive gliosis occurs when reactive gliosis forms a tumor. This reactive process may fill the entire eye, simulating a neoplasm (91). Massive gliosis is more likely to occur if the underlying pathologic process occurs in childhood and there is a long time-interval between the pathologic insult and enucleation.

Histologically, these areas of gliosis are composed of interweaving bundles of spindle shaped astrocytes, with uniform nuclei and abundant, pale, eosinophilic cytoplasm. Numerous dilated, thick-walled blood vessels and abundant fibrillary material are observed throughout the lesion. Calcification and ossification may also occur in longstanding lesions.

VASCULAR TUMORS AND TUMOR-LIKE CONDITIONS

Angiomatosis Retinae (Hemangioblastoma, Capillary Hemangioma, von Hippel-Lindau Syndrome)

Angiomatosis retinae, although considered a hamartomatous lesion, usually is not discovered until early adult life. These benign angioblastic retinal tumors are similar to cerebellar hemangioblastomas. Horton and co-workers (95) studied 50 patients with von Hippel-Lindau syndrome and found retinal angiomatosis in 58 percent and cerebellar hemangioblastomas in 36 percent. Other frequently occurring manifestations included renal cell carcinoma in 28 percent and pheochromocytoma in 10 percent. The von Hippel-Lindau syndrome is inherited as an autosomal dominant trait and the gene has been localized to the short arm of chromosome 3 (97).

Clinically, angiomatosis retinae follows a typical sequence of events: 1) angiomatous dilatation and tumor formation; 2) retinal hemorrhages and exudates; 3) massive retinal detachment; and 4) glaucoma (93). The early lesions are small, red to gray, and not associated with abnormal vessels. These minute tumors may not leak fluorescein. Later, a pink or yellow retinal tumor of moderate size, located most commonly at the temporal periphery and supplied by a large artery and vein, becomes ophthalmoscopically apparent. If the lesion is predominately exophytic in relation to the peripapillary retina, the tumor may be difficult to visualize. The fluorescein angiographic pattern, however, is diagnostic. Bilateral retinal tumors occur in 30 to 50 percent of patients and unilateral multiple tumors occur in 30 percent (93).

Histopathologically, the tumor is composed of small vascular channels of different sizes, which have the appearance of capillaries. Among these are large foamy cells containing lipid within their cytoplasm (figs. 4-47, 4-48). The nature of these cells has been debated (92,96): they represent either histiocytes, endothelial cells, or astrocytes. Gliosis of the affected retina is a common finding, especially in the advanced stages of the disease. Larger tumors may have marked cystic degeneration within the tumor and surrounding retina. Marked exudation may also occur leading to retinal detachment. Frequently, by the time enucleation is performed, secondary changes have taken place, leading to phthisis bulbi. Hemorrhage, fibrosis, and reactive gliosis may obscure the fundamental vascular lesion, and the correct histopathologic diagnosis may not be made. Step sections through the eye may be required before the vascular tumor is found.

Endothelial cells, pericytes, and rarely, multilaminar pericyte-like cells with smooth muscle differentiation can be seen in the vessels of the retinal tumor by electron microscopy. The tumoral endothelium has fenestrations, which could explain the characteristic exudate of larger lesions (92,96).

Cavernous Hemangioma

Cavernous hemangioma is an extremely rare nonprogressive congenital malformation, with a probable autosomal dominant inheritance pattern with incomplete penetrance. It is not related to the Sturge-Weber syndrome. Patients with cavernous hemangiomas of both the retina and the brain have

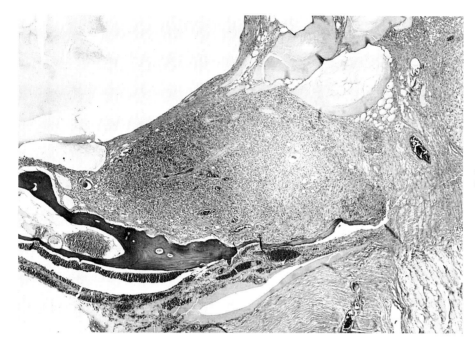

Figure 4-47
VON HIPPEL
ANGIOMATOSIS
Lesion located adjacent
to optic nerve head with os-
seous metaplasia.

Figure 4-48
VON HIPPEL
ANGIOMATOSIS
Higher power magnifica-
tion of tumor in figure 4-47
showing vascular proliferation with vacuolated stromal
cells.

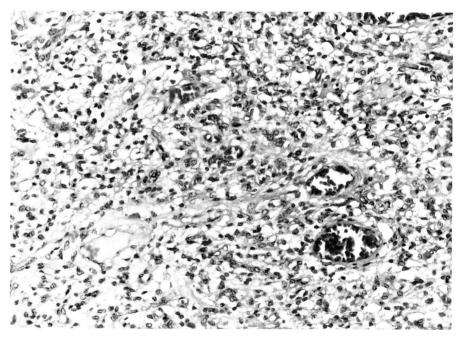

been reported. An association of seizures or cranial nerve palsies with retinal cavernous hemangioma has been described (94).

Clinically, the affected retina shows isolated clusters of dilated vessels. Fluorescein angiography displays a normal arterial supply, slowed transmission of dye, and slowed venous drainage. There is no arteriovenous shunting and no disturbance of per-meability. For these reasons, cavernous hemangiomas are rarely a source of bleeding.

Histopathologically, the retina is greatly thickened by large vascular channels with normal walls. The inner retinal layers are discontinuous in the area of the vascular lesions. Vitreous involvement may occur over the lesion, with posterior vitreous detachment. In the area of the hemangioma, traction of the retina may lead to retinal and vitreous hemorrhage (98).

TUMORS OF HEMATOPOIETIC AND LYMPHOID TISSUES

Malignant Lymphoma

Retinal involvement by a lymphoid neoplasm is usually a manifestation of a primary malignant lymphoma of the central nervous system; in older literature this was called microgliomatosis or reticulum cell sarcoma of the retina. Some ophthalmologists still use the term reticulum cell sarcoma. Retinal involvement may be the initial or only manifestation of the disease. The retinal neoplasm is frequently associated with brain lesions (99,101–103) but rarely is there involvement of the reticuloendothelial system. The initial site and intensity of the retinal involvement varies considerably. Modern immunohistochemical techniques have shown that these neoplasms are usually B-cell lymphomas. In comparison, lymphomas of the uveal tract are well differentiated and associated with systemic lymphoma, whereas retinal and vitreal lymphomas are poorly differentiated and associated with lymphoma of the central nervous system. Rarely, a cellular infiltrate in the vitreous may be the only manifestation of an intraocular lymphoma (100).

Clinical Features. The patients are typically over 40 years of age (range, 27 to 77 years) and usually have no history of malignant lymphoma (102). Most often, the disease presents initially with signs of uveitis: cells and flare in the anterior chamber and cells and debris in the vitreous. Extensive infiltration of the retina and optic nerve head may lead to coagulative necrosis (pl. IXA). Mound-like elevations of the RPE by lymphoma cells are highly characteristic (pl. IXB). A secondary glaucoma may be present. The intraocular manifestations usually precede the central nervous system symptoms. The mnemonic GUN (glaucoma, uveitis, neurologic signs) syndrome was coined for this condition (99). When the diagnosis is suspected, the work-up should include imaging studies of the central nervous system. The diagnosis may be microscopically confirmed by cytologic examination of cells from the cerebral spinal fluid, vitrectomy, or vitreous aspiration, (see pls. IB, C, IIA), or from biopsy of brain or retina.

Pathologic Findings. The gross findings include thickening of a detached retina, subretinal pigment epithelial tumors, and cloudiness of the vitreous. Occasionally, the thickened retina is focally hemorrhagic with a "pizza pie" appearance (pl. IXB). The subretinal pigment epithelial mounds are white on cross section. Vitreous infiltration varies markedly; with intense infiltration the vitreous is opaque with a dirty brown color.

The microscopic features include involvement of the retina, subretinal pigment epithelial space, and the vitreous by malignant neoplastic cells (pl. IXC, figs. 4-49–4-52). Extensive areas of hemorrhagic necrosis of tumor cells and retina are common. In many instances, the neoplastic cells accumulate on the inner surface of the Bruch membrane, producing irregular, nodular elevations of the RPE (pl. IXC, figs. 4-49–4-52). The neoplastic lymphocytes undergo necrosis at the apex of the mounds. Typically, in the retina the viable neoplastic cells are arranged around blood vessels (figs. 4-49, 4-50). The neoplastic cells are usually large B cells (pl. IXC) with discernible cytoplasm and large, round nuclei that are frequently indented with finger-like processes. The nuclear membrane is prominent. Most of the nuclei contain large single or multiple nucleoli. Mitotic figures may be numerous. The optic nerve may show neoplastic involvement (fig. 4-49). A reactive inflammatory infiltrate composed of mature T lymphocytes may be found in the choroid (pl. IXC, figs. 4-51, 4-52).

The differential diagnoses include leukemic infiltration, metastatic undifferentiated carcinoma, and any inflammatory process causing a chorioretinitis.

Treatment and Prognosis. Once the diagnosis is established, radiation therapy to the eyes and brain is the treatment of choice (102). Chemotherapy has also been used in some patients as an adjuvant therapy. Despite treatment, the prognosis is poor and most patients die as a result of central nervous system involvement.

Leukemia

Acute and chronic leukemias may involve the retina (104,105). The most severe retinal manifestations are seen in patients with acute myeloid leukemia that has a rapid onset and course. The retinal findings include retinal venous dilation

PLATE IX
PRIMARY INTRAOCULAR LYMPHOMA

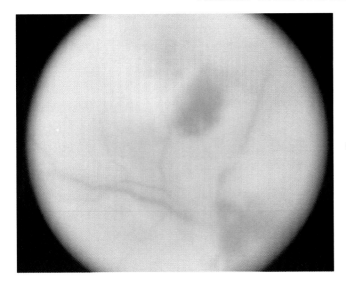

A. Fundus photograph of yellowish white hemorrhagic retinal infiltrates.

B. Focally hemorrhagic white infiltrates thicken the retina. A subretinal pigment epithelial infiltrate is present at the cut edge (arrow).

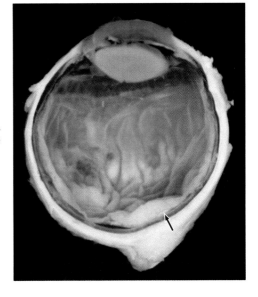

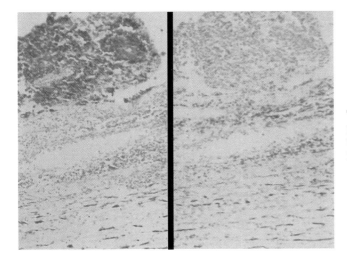

C. Immunohistochemistry for B cells (left) and T cells (right). Lymphocytes in the choroid are predominately reactive T cells, whereas those in the subretinal pigment epithelial space are neoplastic B cells.

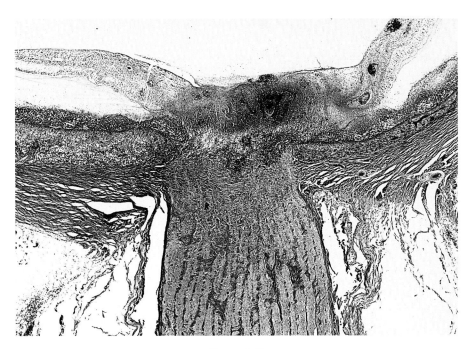

Figure 4-49
PRIMARY INTRAOCULAR LARGE CELL LYMPHOMA
Tumor involves the optic nerve head and peripapillary retina with extensive areas of necrosis.

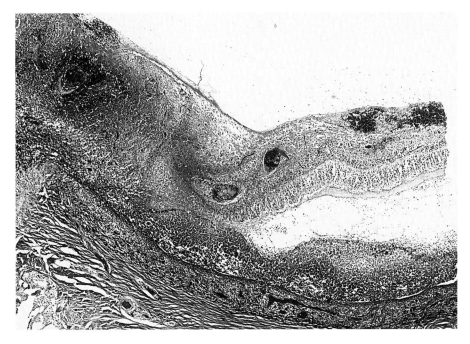

Figure 4-50
PRIMARY INTRAOCULAR LARGE CELL LYMPHOMA
Higher power magnification of tumor seen in previous figure showing retinal involvement and neoplastic cells typically located between detached retinal pigment epithelium and Bruch membrane.

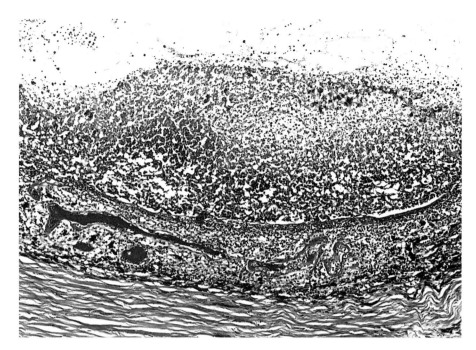

Figure 4-51
PRIMARY INTRAOCULAR
LARGE CELL LYMPHOMA

Higher power magnification of tumor in figure 4-49 showing viable and necrotic neoplastic cells located between detached retinal pigment epithelium and Bruch membrane and smaller benign reactive lymphocytes within the choroid.

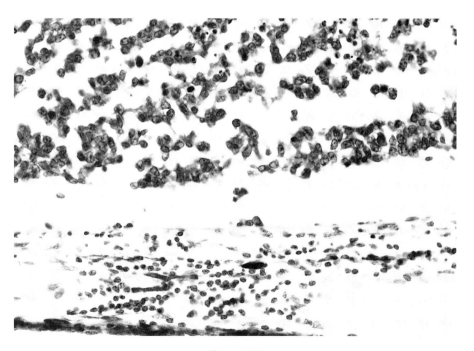

Figure 4-52
PRIMARY INTRAOCULAR
LARGE CELL LYMPHOMA

Large neoplastic lymphocytes located between detached retinal pigment epithelium and Bruch membrane and smaller benign reactive lymphocytes within the choroid.

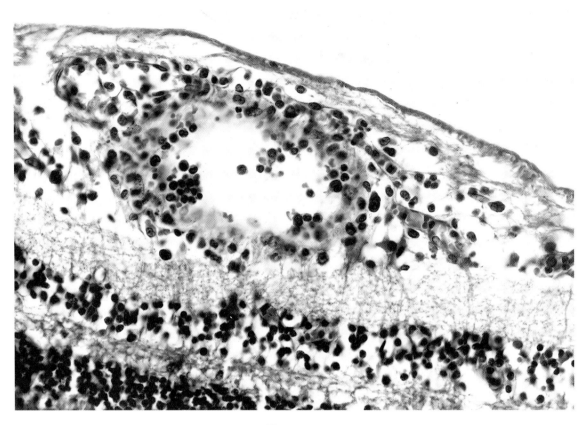

Figure 4-53
LYMPHOBLASTIC LEUKEMIA
Intravascular and perivascular retinal involvement.

and segmentation, vascular sheathing due to perivascular infiltration, and vascular occlusion (fig. 4-53). The vessel may become yellower because of the increase of leukemic cells and decrease of erythrocytes. Retinal hemorrhages are caused by the vascular occlusions. They are most frequent in the posterior pole, may involve all layers of the retina, and may break into the vitreous cavity.

Histopathologically, the retina is variably infiltrated with immature leukocytes. In some examples, the neoplastic cells accumulate at various levels of the retina, producing nodular masses. The retinal blood vessels may be packed with immature blood cells. Perivascular accumulation of neoplastic cells is common around the vessels (fig. 4-53). In the later stages, there is glial cell hyperplasia and neuronal degeneration of retinal tissues. Infiltrates in the choroid, vitreous, and anterior segment of the eye may also be present (104,105).

The differential diagnoses include retinal lymphoma and other undifferentiated neoplasms involving the retina.

NEUROEPITHELIAL TUMORS

Tumors of the neuroepithelium of the eye are rare (Table 4-5). Zimmerman proposed dividing these tumors, which usually occur in the ciliary body but can grow from neuroepithelium anywhere in the eye, into two classes: congenital and acquired. The congenital lesions are either choristomatous malformations or neoplasms composed of embryonic tissue. The acquired lesions occur after embryologic development. Although some authors refer to the acquired tumors as adult diktyomas or adult medulloepitheliomas, the World Health Organization prefers diagnosing these tumors as adenomas and carcinomas of ciliary epithelium. Congenital tumors include the rare glioneuroma and the less rare medulloepithelioma.

Tumors of the Retina

Table 4-5

NEUROEPITHELIAL TUMORS*

Type of Tumor	Number of Cases
Embryonic tumors	
Medulloepithelioma	
Benign	4
Malignant	9
Nonembryonic tumors	
Nonpigmented ciliary epithelium	
Adenoma	4
Carcinoma	8
Pigmented ciliary epithelium	
Adenoma	4
Carcinoma	1
Retinal pigment epithelium	
Adenoma	1
Adenocarcinoma	2

*Frequency distribution of 33 tumors in the AFIP Registry of Ophthalmic Pathology collected between 1984 and 1989.

Glioneuroma

This rare benign tumor is a choristomatous malformation of the ciliary body and iris. It is composed of well-differentiated tissue that resembles disorganized brain (fig. 4-54).

Medulloepithelioma (Diktyoma, Teratoneuroma)

This tumor arises from the medullary epithelium and contains elements resembling the optic vesicle during embryonic development. Since both benign and malignant forms of this tumor grow progressively, they are classified as neoplasms rather than as choristomas. In some, there is a network of neuroepithelial bands, which led Fuchs (110) to call them diktyomas. Verhoeff (110) observed structures resembling primitive retina and vitreous in some of these tumors and introduced the term teratoneuroma but he did not describe heteroplastic elements. Since both of these terms at best describe only a subset of these tumors, the name medulloepithelioma is now preferred.

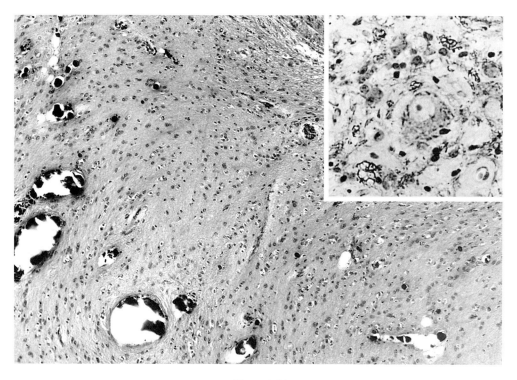

Figure 4-54
GLIONEUROMA
Tumor of ciliary body composed predominately of glial cells with scattered foci of calcification. Insert: Large neuron.

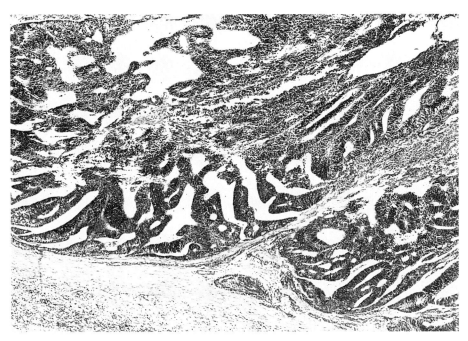

Figure 4-55
MALIGNANT
MEDULLOEPITHELIOMA
Tumor composed of a network of cords of neuroepithelial cells.

The neuroepithelium in medulloepithelioma may differentiate toward RPE, nonpigmented and pigmented ciliary epithelium, neurons, and neuroglia. Vitreous production is often observed. Medulloepitheliomas that contain heterologous tissues (cartilage, skeletal muscle, and brain) are classified as teratoid (107). If the medulloepithelioma contains totally undifferentiated cells resembling those of retinoblastoma or if the heteroplastic tissue is anaplastic with high mitotic activity, the tumor is classified as malignant.

Clinically, medulloepitheliomas usually present as tumors of the ciliary body; rarely, they arise in the optic nerve head or retina. Some ciliary body medulloepitheliomas are cystic. Occasionally, these cysts become detached from the ciliary body and are carried by aqueous flow through the pupil into the anterior chamber.

Histologically, the proliferating medullary epithelium is characteristically arranged in cords and sheets (figs. 4-55, 4-56). The cords vary from a single layer of columnar epithelium to a stratified multilayered structure that resembles embryonic retina. Along the apical side of the cords, there is a fenestrated membrane resembling the external limiting membrane of the retina. On the basal side, the medulloepithelial cells produce a basement membrane that separates the epithelium from a cystic space containing hyaluronic

acid. In some instances, spherical cysts containing hyaluronic acid become free floating in the aqueous humor. Small cords of pigmented neuroepithelial cells are often present but are usually enmeshed in nonpigmented tissue, so that the tumor appears white, gray, or yellow. In rare instances, the pigmented neuroepithelial cell component may be large enough to give the tumor a pigmented appearance on clinical examination.

With the possible exception of metastatic blastic tumors to the eye (neuroblastoma, Wilms tumor, leukemia), medulloepithelioma is the only primary ocular childhood neoplasm that can histologically mimic retinoblastoma and cause a diagnostic problem for the pathologist. Malignant medulloepitheliomas can have undifferentiated blastic areas that are indistinguishable from retinoblastoma. Structures resembling Flexner-Wintersteiner rosettes (fig. 4-56) may occasionally be observed in these blastic areas, indicating photoreceptor differentiation (110). Most of the rosettes in medulloepithelioma have a lumen surrounded by more than a single layer of cells.

Broughton and Zimmerman (107) studied 56 medulloepitheliomas from the ROP. The mean age of the patients was 5 years at the time of definitive diagnosis. There was histologic evidence of malignancy in 37 (66 percent) and extraocular extension in 10 of these. Follow-up was

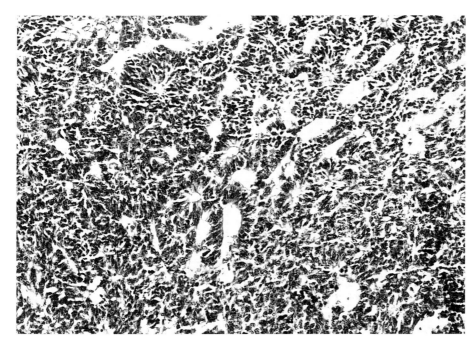

Figure 4-56
MALIGNANT
MEDULLOEPITHELIOMA
An area of the same
tumor as in previous figure
composed of less differentiated cells with structures
mimicking rosettes.

possible in 33 of the 56 cases. Four patients (12.1 percent) died of metastatic disease, and all 4 had extraocular extension. Heteroplastic elements (brain tissue, cartilage, or rhabdomyoblasts) were observed in 4 benign and 17 malignant tumors (figs. 4-57, 4-58). Possibly related to the teratoid medulloepithelioma is the rare primary rhabdomyosarcoma of the iris (109). Although neuroepithelial elements are not observed in iris rhabdomyosarcomas, they, like medulloepitheliomas, are believed to be of neuroepithelial origin.

Acquired Neuroepithelial Tumors of the Ciliary Body

These tumors have a wide spectrum of clinical and histopathologic features and biologic behavior. Most are rare, and most studies have consisted of single case reports. Classification is based on the presence or absence of pigmentation, the cellular pattern, and malignant behavior.

Fuchs Adenoma (Hyperplasia of the Nonpigmented Ciliary Epithelium, Pseudoadenomatous Hyperplasia, Coronal Adenoma)

In contrast to the other acquired tumors of the ciliary epithelium, Fuchs adenoma is relatively common. The adenoma consists of small age-related hyperplastic nodules. In a series of donor eyes from 59 patients, 12 had one or more Fuchs ade-

nomas (111). The median age of the 12 patients was 82. Rarely, Fuchs adenomas may be large enough to cause a sectoral cataract or simulate a malignant melanoma of the ciliary body.

Grossly, Fuchs adenomas are small white nodules that usually measure less than 1 mm in diameter and are located on the pars plicata. The maximum size is approximately 4 mm in diameter. Histologically, the lesion consists of a nodule of hyperplastic, nonpigmented ciliary epithelium arranged in sheets and tubules, embedded in a matrix of PAS-positive basement membrane-like material.

Adenomas of the Nonpigmented Ciliary Epithelium

These tumors are much rarer and larger than Fuchs adenomas. Histologically, they have a solid, papillary, tubular, or pleomorphic appearance. They are often confused clinically with malignant melanoma of the ciliary body (108).

Carcinomas of the Nonpigmented Ciliary Epithelium

These tumors span a spectrum from localized, low-grade, well-differentiated malignant neoplasms that resemble the ciliary epithelium to poorly differentiated pleomorphic tumors, some of which resemble sarcomas (figs. 4-59, 4-60). The poorly differentiated pleomorphic tumors usually

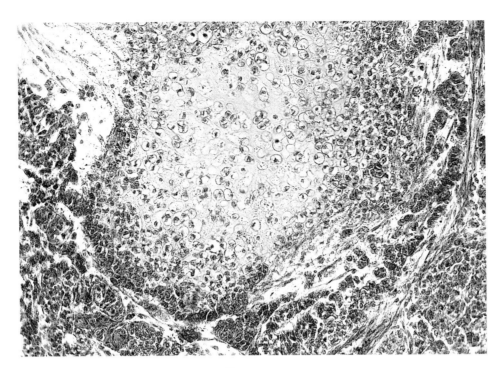

Figure 4-57
MALIGNANT TERATOID MEDULLOEPITHELIOMA
Malignant neuroepithelial cells surround an island of anaplastic cartilage.

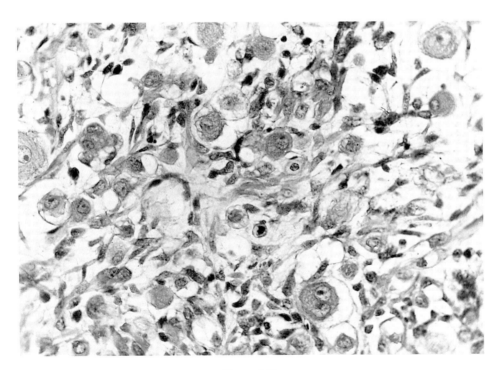

Figure 4-58
MALIGNANT TERATOID MEDULLOEPITHELIOMA
Rhabdomyoblastic differentiation in the same tumor as in figure 4-57.

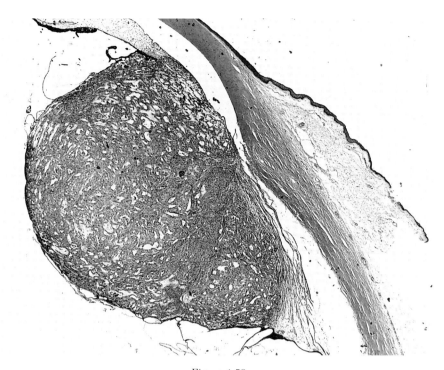

Figure 4-59
ADENOCARCINOMA: CILIARY EPITHELIUM
Nonpigmented tumor has invaded ciliary muscle and root of the iris.

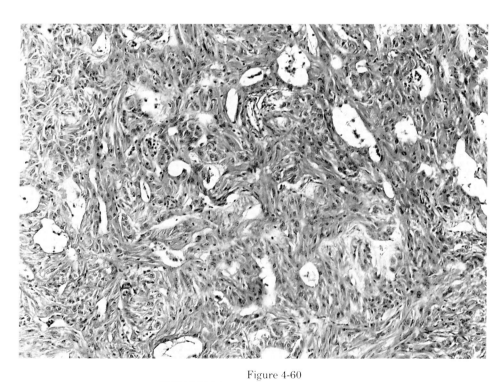

Figure 4-60
ADENOCARCINOMA: CILIARY EPITHELIUM
Higher power magnification of tumor in figure 4-59 showing a pleomorphic mixture of spindle- and epithelial-shaped neoplastic cells.

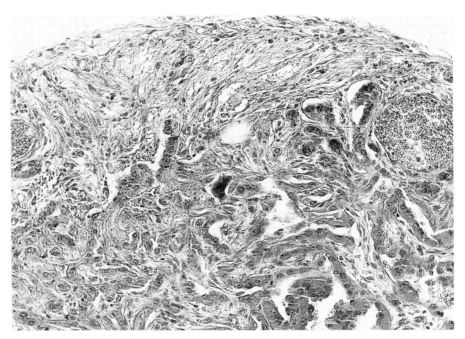

Figure 4-61
ADENOMA: CILIARY
EPITHELIUM
Partially pigmented tumor composed of a mixture of tubular and papillary patterns.

occur in eyes that were previously traumatized or had longstanding inflammatory disease. These tumors may be a form of "scar carcinoma" resulting from neoplastic transformation of reactive hyperplasia of the ciliary epithelium. Of 21 cases from the ROP, follow-up information was available for 16: 3 patients died of other causes, 5 died of disease, and 8 were alive and well after a median follow-up interval of 5.7 years. Two of these 8 patients had a recurrence. One was an intraocular recurrence treated by iridocyclectomy and the other was a metastasis to the parotid gland that was treated surgically. Of the five patients that died from tumor extension into the central nervous system or widespread metastasis, all had orbital involvement.

Adenomas and Carcinomas of the Pigmented Ciliary Epithelium

In a study of 30 adult ciliary body epithelial tumors (106), 7 were of pigment epithelial origin; all were considered benign, although most showed local infiltration. The diagnosis of this tumor is usually made only after histopathologic study, with most cases being confused clinically with malignant melanoma. Histologically, a variety of cellular patterns may be observed, including solid, tubular, papillary, and vacuolated (fig. 4-61). Some of the pigmented tumors have suffi-

ciently anaplastic features, mitotic activity, and invasiveness to be classified as adenocarcinoma but none have metastasized.

The vacuolated or cystic variety of adenoma of the pigmented ciliary epithelium appears to be quite characteristic, composed of large pigmented cells arranged in nodules, lobules, and sheets. Vacuoles containing small amounts of mucopolysaccharide that is not sensitive to hyaluronidase are scattered throughout the tumor. By electron microscopy, these vacuoles consist of intercommunicating intercellular spaces lined by cells with microvilli and occasional cilia.

Adenomas and Carcinomas of the Retinal Pigment Epithelium

True neoplasms of the RPE are uncommon. In contrast, reactive hyperplasia is frequent. It may be difficult to differentiate hyperplasia from true neoplasia, since both types of proliferation show variable histologic features and true neoplasms may develop from reactive hyperplasia (112).

Clinically, adenomas and adenocarcinomas of RPE are jet black and may be misinterpreted as malignant melanomas. Patients may present with visual loss or are asymptomatic.

The adenomas and adenocarcinomas of the RPE occur in middle-aged individuals (fifth or sixth decades) and have a variety of histologic patterns ranging from most differentiated to least differentiated: mosaic, tubular, papillary, vacuolated, and pleomorphic. The tumors often show different histologic patterns in different regions (figs. 4-62–4-66). All the characteristics of RPE cells can be seen by electron microscopy, including basement membrane production, junctional complexes, microvilli, and melanosomes.

The adenocarcinomas reveal anaplastic cells with variable-sized nuclei; some are large and hyperchromatic with prominent nucleoli. The most important criteria for malignancy is extensive invasion. Adenomas and hyperplasias are usually confined to the subretinal space, whereas adenocarcinomas invade into the choroid and retina. Adenocarcinomas have increased mitotic activity and more pleomorphism than benign tumors. Distant metastases have not been histologically demonstrated (112).

METASTATIC NEOPLASMS

Metastatic tumors to the retina are exceedingly rare (113–115). The most common primary sites, as with the metastasis to the uveal tract, are breast and lung. Malignant melanoma is the most common nonepithelial tumor.

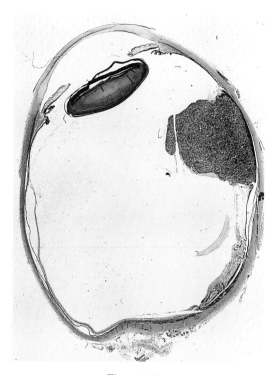

Figure 4-62
ADENOCARCINOMA:
RETINAL PIGMENT EPITHELIUM
Solid pigmented tumor has arisen in the periphery of the retina.

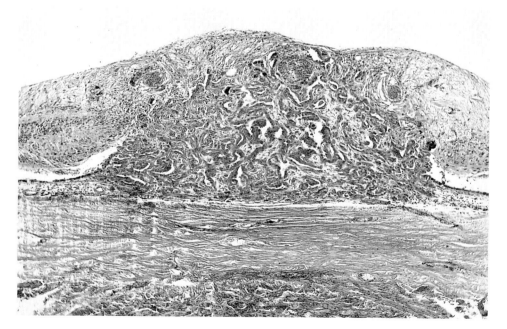

Figure 4-63
ADENOCARCINOMA: RETINAL PIGMENT EPITHELIUM
Pigmented tumor with tubular and papillary pattern has invaded the retina and choroid.

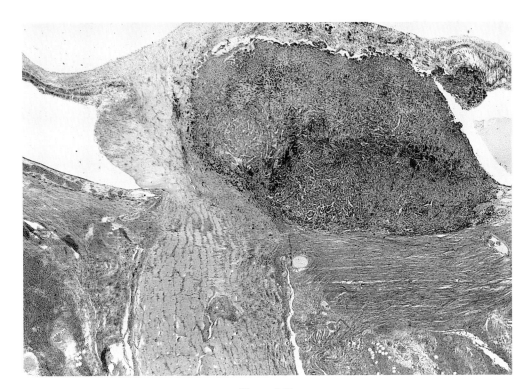

Figure 4-64
ADENOCARCINOMA: RETINAL PIGMENT EPITHELIUM
Adjacent to the optic nerve head a variably pigmented tumor has arisen and invaded the choroid.

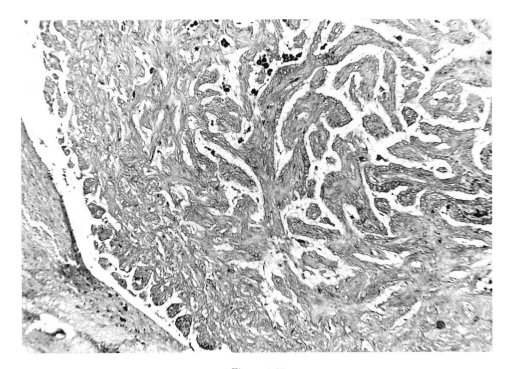

Figure 4-65
ADENOCARCINOMA: RETINAL PIGMENT EPITHELIUM
Higher power magnification of a less pigmented pleomorphic and papillary area of the tumor seen in figure 4-64.

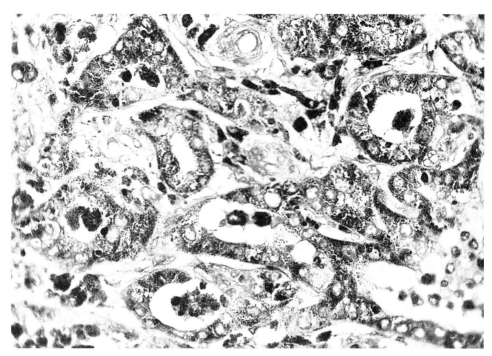

Figure 4-66
ADENOCARCINOMA: RETINAL PIGMENT EPITHELIUM
Higher power magnification of a heavily pigmented tubular area of the tumor seen in figure 4-64.

REFERENCES

General References

Fine BS, Yanoff M. Ocular histology. A text and atlas. 2nd ed. New York: Harper & Row, 1979:61–127.

Jakobiec FA. Ocular anatomy, embryology and teratology. Philadelphia: Harper & Row, 1982:441–552.

Mafee MF, Goldberg MF, Greenwald MJ, Schulman J, Malmed A, Flanders AE. Retinoblastoma and simulating lesions: role of CT and MR imaging. Radiol Clin North Am 1987;25:667–82.

Classification and Frequency

1. Burnier MN, Neves RA, Pereira MG, Alberti VN, Rigueiro MP. The use of the peroxidas-anti-peroxidas technique in ocular pathology. Arch I P B 1988;30:181–4.
2. Klauss V, Chana HS. Ocular tumors in Africa. Soc Sci Med 1983;17:1743–50.
3. Shields JA, Shields CL. Intraocular tumors. A text and atlas. Philadelphia: WB Saunders, 1992.
4. _____, Shields CL, Donoso LA, Lieb WE. Changing concepts in the management of retinoblastoma. Ophthalmic Surg 1990;21:72–6.

Retinoblastoma and Retinocytoma

5. Aaby AA, Price RL, Zakov ZN. Spontaneously regressing retinoblastomas, retinoma, or retinoblastoma group 0. Am J Ophthalmol 1983;96:315–20.

6. Abramson DH, Ellsworth RM, Zimmerman LE. Non-ocular cancer in retinoblastoma survivors. Trans Am Acad Ophthalmol Otolaryngol 1976;81(3 Pt 1):454–7.
7. _____, Greenfield DS, Ellsworth RM. Bilateral retinoblastoma. Correlations between age at diagnosis and time course for new intraocular tumors. Ophthalmic Paediatr Genet 1992;13:1–7.
8. _____, McCormick B, Fass D, et al. Retinoblastoma. The long-term appearance of radiated intraocular tumors. Cancer 1991;67:2753–5.
9. Albert DM. Historic review of retinoblastoma. Ophthalmology 1987;94:654–62.
10. Amendola BE, Markoe AM, Augsburger JJ, et al. Analysis of treatment results in 36 children with retinoblastoma treated by scleral plaque irradiation. Int J Radiat Oncol Biol Phys 1989;17:63–70.
11. Bader JL, Meadows AT, Zimmerman LE, et al. Bilateral retinoblastoma with ectopic intracranial retinoblastoma: trilateral retinoblastoma. Cancer Genet Cytogenet 1982;5:203–13.
12. Balmer A, Munier F, Gailloud C. Retinoma. Case studies. Ophthalmic Paediatr Genet 1991;12:131–7.
13. Benedict WF, Srivatsan ES, Mark C, Banerjee A, Sparkes RS, Murphree AL. Complete or partial homozygosity of chromosome 13 in primary retinoblastoma. Cancer Res 1987;47:4189–91.
14. _____, Xu HJ, Takahashi R. The retinoblastoma gene: its role in human malignancies. Cancer Invest 1990;8:535–40.

15. Boniuk M, Zimmerman LE. Spontaneous regression of retinoblastoma. Int Ophthalmol Clin 1962;2:525–42.

16. Bunt AH, Tso MO. Feulgen-positive deposits in retinoblastoma. Incidence, composition, and ultrastructure. Arch Ophthalmol 1981;99:144–50.

17. Burnier MN, McLean IW, Zimmerman LE, Rosenberg SH. Retinoblastoma. The relationship of proliferating cells to blood vessels. Invest Ophthalmol Vis Sci 1990;31:2037–40.

18. Canning S, Dryja TP. Short, direct repeats at the breakpoints of deletions of the retinoblastoma gene. Proc Natl Acad Sci USA 1989;86:5044–8.

19. Chader GJ. Multipotential differentiation of human Y-79 retinoblastoma cells in attachment culture. Cell Differ 1987;20:209–16.

20. Chang M, McLean IW, Merritt JC. Coats's disease. A study of 62 histological confirmed cases. J Pediatr Ophthalmol Strabis 1984;21:163–8.

21. Committee for the National Registry of Retinoblastoma, The. Survival rate and risk factors for patients with retinoblastoma in Japan. Jpn J Ophthalmol 1992;36:121–31.

22. Derkinderen DJ, Koten JW, Wolterbeek R, Beemer FA, Tan KE, Den Otter W. Non-ocular cancer in hereditary retinoblastoma survivors and relatives. Ophthalmic Paediatr Genet 1987;8:23–5.

23. Donoso LA, Shields CL, Lee EY. Immunohistochemistry of retinoblastoma. A review. Ophthalmic Paediatr Genet 1989;10:3–32.

24. Draper GJ, Sanders BM, Kingston JE. Second primary neoplasms in patients with retinoblastoma. Br J Cancer 1986;53:661–71.

25. Eagle RC Jr, Shields JA, Donoso L, Milner RS. Malignant transformation of spontaneously regressed retinoblastoma, retinoma/retinocytoma variant. Ophthalmology 1989;96:1389–95.

26. Erwenne CM, Franco EL. Age and lateness of referral as determinants of extra-ocular retinoblastoma. Ophthalmic Paediatr Genet 1989;10:179–84.

27. Friend SH, Bernards R, Rogelj S, et al. A human DNA segment with properties of the gene that predisposes to retinoblastoma an osteosarcoma. Nature 1986;323:643–6.

28. Gallie BL, Phillips RA, Ellsworth RM, Abramson DH. Significance of retinoma and phthisis bulbi for retinoblastoma. Ophthalmology 1982;89:1393–9.

29. Gamel JW, McLean IW, Rosenberg SH. Proportion cured and mean log survival time as functions of tumor size. Stat Med 1990;9:999–1006.

30. Grabowski EF, Abramson DH. Intraocular and extraocular retinoblastoma. Hematol Oncol Clin North Am 1987;1:721–35.

31. Haddad R, Font RL, Reeser F. Persistent hyperplastic primary vitreous. A clinicopathologic study of 62 cases and review of the literature. Surv Ophthalmol 1978;23:123–34.

32. Hungerford J, Kingston J, Plowman N. Orbital recurrence of retinoblastoma. Ophthalmic Paediatr Genet 1987;8:63–8.

33. John-Mikolajewski V, Messmer E, Sauerwein W, Freundlieb O. Orbital computed tomography. Does it help in diagnosing the infiltration of choroid, sclera and/or optic nerve in retinoblastoma? Ophthalmic Paediatr Genet 1987;8:101–4.

34. Keith CG. Chemotherapy in retinoblastoma management. Ophthalmic Paediatr Genet 1989;10:93–8.

35. Kingston JE, Hungerford JL, Plowman PN. Chemotherapy in metastatic retinoblastoma. Ophthalmic Paediatr Genet 1987;8:69–72.

36. Kivelä T. Glycoconjugates in retinoblastoma. A lectin histochemical study of ten formalin-fixed and paraffin-embedded tumours. Virchows Arch [A] 1987;410:471–9.

37. Knudson AG Jr. Mutation and cancer: a statistical study of retinoblastoma. Proc Natl Acad Sci USA 1971;68:820–8.

38. Kopelman JE, McLean IW, Rosenberg SH. Multivariate analysis of risk factors for metastasis in retinoblastoma treated by enucleation. Ophthalmology 1987; 94:371–7.

39. Lane JC, Klintworth GK. A study of astrocytes in retinoblastomas using the immunoperoxidase technique and antibodies to glial fibrillary acidic protein. Am J Ophthalmol 1983;95:197–207.

40. Lee WH. The molecular basis of cancer suppression by the retinoblastoma gene. Princess Takamatsu Symp 1989;20:159–70.

41. _____, Bookstein R, Hong F, Young LJ, Shew JY, Lee EY. Human retinoblastoma susceptibility gene: cloning, identification, and sequence. Science 1987; 235:1394–9.

42. Lueder GT, Judisch GF, O'Gorman TW. Second nonocular tumors in survivors of heritable retinoblastoma. Arch Ophthalmol 1986;104:372–3.

43. _____, Judisch GF, Wen BC. Heritable retinoblastoma and pinealoma. Arch Ophthalmol 1991; 109:1707–9.

44. Madreperla SA, Whittum-Hudson JA, Prendergast RA, Chen PL, Lee WH. Intraocular tumor suppression of retinoblastoma gene-reconstituted retinoblastoma cells. Cancer Res 1991;51(23 Pt 1):6381–4.

45. Magramm I, Abramson DH, Ellsworth RM. Optic nerve involvement in retinoblastoma. Ophthalmology 1989;96:217–22.

46. Mansour AM, Greenwald MJ, O'Grady R. Diffuse infiltrating retinoblastoma. J Pediatr Ophthalmol Strabismus 1989;26:152–4.

47. Margo C, Hidayat A, Kopelman J, Zimmerman LE. Retinocytoma: a benign variant of retinoblastoma. Arch Ophthalmol 1983;101:1519–31.

48. Margo CE, Zimmerman LE. Retinoblastoma: the accuracy of clinical diagnosis in children treated by enucleation. J Pediatr Ophthalmol Strabismus 1983;20:227–9.

49. McLean IW, Rosenberg SH, Messmer EP, et al. Prognostic factors in cases of retinoblastoma: analysis of 974 patients from Germany and the United States treated by enucleation. In: Bornfeld N, Gragoudas ES, Lommatzsch PK, eds. Tumors of the eye. Proceedings of the International Symposium on Tumors of the Eye. Amsterdam: Kugler Publications, 1991;69–72.

50. Meli FJ, Boccaleri CA, Manzitti J, Lylyk P. Meningeal dissemination of retinoblastoma: CT findings in eight patients. AJNR Am J Neuroradiol 1990;11:983–6.

51. Messmer EP, Font RL, Kirkpatrick JB, Höpping W. Immunohistochemical demonstration of neuronal and astrocytic differentiation in retinoblastoma. Ophthalmology 1985;92:167–73.

52. _____, Heinrich T, Höpping W, de Sutter E, Havers W, Saverwein W. Risk factors for metastases in patients with retinoblastoma. Ophthalmology 1991;98:136–41.

53. Morgan KS, McLean IW. Retinoblastoma and persistent hyperplastic vitreous occurring in the same patient. Ophthalmology 1981;88:1087–9.

54. Neafie RC, Connor DH. Viceral larva migrans. In: Binford CH, Connor DH, eds. Pathology of tropical and extraordinary diseases. An atlas. Vol 2. Washington, D.C.: Armed Forces Institute of Pathology, 1976:433–6.

55. Nicholson DH, Norton EW. Diffuse infiltrating retinoblastoma. Trans Am Ophthalmol Soc 1980;78:265–89.

56. Pratt CB, Meyer D, Chenaille P, Crom DB. The use of bone marrow aspirations and lumbar punctures at the time of diagnosis of retinoblastoma. J Clin Oncol 1989;7:140–3.

57. Roarty JD, McLean IW, Zimmerman LE. Incidence of second neoplasms in patients with bilateral retinoblastoma. Ophthalmology 1988;95:1583–7.

58. Robertson DM, Campbell RJ. Analysis of misdiagnosed retinoblastoma in a series of 726 enucleated eyes. Mod Probl Ophthalmol 1977;18:156–9.

59. Rubinstein LJ. Tumors of the central nervous system. Atlas of Tumor Pathology, 2nd Series, Fascicle 6 (Suppl). Washington, D.C.: Armed Forces Institute of Pathology, 1982:15–20.

60. Sanders BM, Draper GJ, Kingston JE. Retinoblastoma in Great Britain 1969-80: incidence, treatment, and survival. Br J Ophthalmol 1988;72:576–83.

61. Schipper J. Retinoblastoma: a medical and experimental study [Thesis]. Utrecht: Univ Utrecht, 1980:144.

62. Shields JA. Diagnosis and management of intraocular tumors. St. Louis: CV Mosby, 1983.

63. _____, Parsons H, Shields CL, Giblin ME. The role of cryotherapy in the management of retinoblastoma. Am J Ophthalmol 1989;108:260–4.

64. _____, Shields CL, Eagle RC, Blair CJ. Spontaneous pseudohypopyon secondary to diffuse infiltrating retinoblastoma. Arch Ophthalmol 1988;106:1301–2.

65. _____, Shields CL, Parsons H, Giblin ME. The role of photocoagulation in the management of retinoblastoma. Arch Ophthalmol 1990;108:205–8.

66. _____, Shields CL, Sivalingam V. Decreasing frequency of enucleation in patients with retinoblastoma. Am J Ophthalmol 1989;108:185–8.

67. _____, Shields CL, Suvarnamani C, Schroeder RP, DePotter P. Retinoblastoma manifesting as orbital cellulitis. Am J Ophthalmol 1991;112:442–9.

68. Smith JL. Histology and spontaneous regression of retinoblastoma. Tran Ophthalmol Soc UK 1974;94:953–67.

69. Stafford WR, Yanoff M, Parnell BL. Retinoblastoma initially misdiagnosed as primary ocular inflammations. Arch Ophthalmol 1969;82:771–3.

70. Stannard C, Lipper S, Sealy R, Sevel D. Retinoblastoma: correlation of invasion of the optic nerve and choroid with prognosis and metastases. Br J Ophthalmol 1979;63:560–70.

71. Tamboli A, Podgor MJ, Horm JW. The incidence of retinoblastoma in the United States: 1974 through 1985. Arch Ophthalmol 1990;108:128–32.

72. Tarlton JF, Easty DL. Immunohistological characterisation of retinoblastoma and related ocular tissue. Br J Ophthalmol 1990;74:144–9.

73. Tso MO, Fine BS, Zimmerman LE. The Flexner-Wintersteiner rosettes in retinoblastoma. Arch Pathol 1969;88:664–71.

74. _____, Fine BS, Zimmerman LE. The nature of retinoblastoma. II. Photoreceptor differentiation: an electron microscopic study. Am J Ophthalmol 1970;69:350–9.

75. _____, Fine BS, Zimmerman LE, et. Photoreceptor elements in retinoblastoma. A preliminary report. Arch Ophthalmol 1969;82:57–9.

76. _____, Zimmerman LE, Fine BS. The nature of retinoblastoma. I. Photoreceptor differentiation: a clinical and histopathologic study. Am J Ophthalmol 1970;69:339–49.

77. _____, Zimmerman LE, Fine BS, Ellsworth RM. A cause of radioresistance in retinoblastoma: photore-

ceptor differentiation. Tran Am Acad Ophthalmol Otolaryngol 1970;74:959–69.

78. Varley JM, Armour J, Swallow JE, et al. The retinoblastoma gene is frequently altered leading to loss of expression in primary breast tumours. Oncogene 1989;4:725–9.

79. Vrabec T, Arbizo V, Adamus G, McDowell JH, Hargrave PA, Donoso LA. Rod cell-specific antigens in retinoblastoma. Arch Ophthalmol 1989;107:1061–3.

80. Weichselbaum RR, Zakov ZN, Albert DM, Friedman AH, Nove J, Little JB. New findings in the chromosome 13 long-arm deletion syndrome and retinoblastoma. Trans Am Acad Ophthalmol Otolaryngol 1979;86:1191-8.

81. White L. Chemotherapy for retinoblastoma: where do we go from here? A review of published literature and meeting abstracts, including discussions during the Vth International Symposium on Retinoblastoma, October 1990. Ophthalmic Paediatr Genet 1991;12:115–30.

82. Wiggs J, Nordenskjold M, Yandell D, et al. Prediction of the risk of hereditary retinoblastoma, using DNA polymorphisms within the retinoblastoma gene. N Engl J Med 1988;318:151–7.

83. Yunis JJ, Ramsay N. Retinoblastoma and subband deletion of chromosome 13. Am J Dis Child 1978;132:161–3.

84. Zimmerman LE. Retinoblastoma and retinocytoma. In: Spencer WH, ed. Ophthalmic pathology. An atlas and textbook. 3rd ed. Philadelphia: WB Saunders, 1985:1292–1351.

85. _____, Burns RP, Wankum G, Tully R, Esterly JA. Trilateral retinoblastoma: ectopic intracranial retinoblastoma associated with bilateral retinoblastoma. J Pediatr Ophthalmol Strabismus 1982;19:320–5.

Glial Tumors and Tumor-like Conditions

86. Bornfeld N, Messmer EP, Theodossiadis G, Meyer-Schwickerath G, Wessing A. Giant cell astrocytoma of the retina. Clinicopathologic report of a case not associated with Bourneville's disease. Retina 1987;7:183–9.

87. Jakobiec FA, Brodie SE, Haik B, Iwamoto T. Giant cell astrocytoma of the retina. A tumor of possible Mueller cell origin. Ophthalmology 1983;90:1565–76.

88. Reeser FH, Aaberg TM, Van Horn DL. Astrocytic hamartoma of the retina not associated with tuberous sclerosis. Am J Ophthalmol 1978;86:688–98.

89. Robertson DM. Ophthalmic manifestations of tuberous sclerosis. Ann N Y Acad Sci 1991;615:17–25.

90. Ulbright TM, Fulling KH, Helveston EM. Astrocytic tumors of the retina. Differentiation of sporadic tumors from phakomatosis-associated tumors. Arch Pathol Lab Med 1984;108:160–3.

91. Yanoff M, Zimmerman LE, Davis RL. Massive gliosis of the retina. Int Ophthalmol Clin 1971;11:211–29.

Vascular Tumors and Tumor-like Conditions

92. Ehlers N, Jensen OA. Juxtapapillary retinal hemangioblastoma (angiomatosis retinae) in an infant: light microscopical and ultrastructural examination. Ultrastruct Pathol 1982;3:325–33.

93. Font RL, Ferry AP. The phakomatoses. Int Ophthalmol Clin 1972;12:1–50.

94. Goldberg RE, Pheasant TR, Shields JA. Cavernous hemangioma of the retina: a four-generation pedigree with neurocutaneous manifestations and an example of bilateral retinal involvement. Arch Ophthalmol 1979;97:2321–4.

95. Horton WA, Wong V, Eldridge R. Von Hippel-Lindau Disease. Clinical and pathological manifestations in nine families with 50 affected members. Arch Intern Med 1976;136:769–77.

96. Jakobiec FA, Font RL, Johnson FB. Angiomatosis retinae: an ultrastructural study and lipid analysis. Cancer 1976;38:2042–56.
97. Jordan DK, Patil SR, Divelbiss JE, et al. Cytogenetic abnormalities in tumors of patients with von Hippel-Lindau disease. Cancer Genet Cytogenet 1989;42:227–41.
98. Messmer E, Font RL, Laqua H, Höpping W, Naumann GO. Cavernous hemangioma of the retina. Immunohistochemical and ultrastructural observations. Arch Ophthalmol 1984;102:413–8.

Malignant Lymphoma

99. Kim EW, Zakov N, Albert DM, Smith TR, Craft JL. Intraocular reticulum cell sarcoma: a case report and literature review. Albrecht Von Graefes Arch Klin Exp Ophthalmol 1979;209:167–78.
100. Minckler DS, Font RL, Zimmerman LE. Uveitis and reticulum cell sarcoma of brain with bilateral neoplastic seeding of vitreous without retinal or uveal involvement. Am J Ophthalmol 1975;80(3 Pt 1):433–9.
101. Neault RW, Van Scoy RE, MacCarty CS. Uveitis associated with isolated reticulum cell sarcoma of the brain. Am J Ophthalmol 1972;73:431–6.
102. Siegel MJ, Dalton J, Friedman AH, Strauchen J, Watson C. Ten-year experience with primary ocular "reticulum cell sarcoma" (large cell non-Hodgkin's lymphoma). Br J Ophthalmol 1989;73:342–6.
103. Weiner JM, Ramsay RJ, Anand N, Cairns JD. Vitreous cytology in primary cerebroretinal malignant lymphoma. Aust J Ophthalmol 1984;12:33–7.

Leukemia

104. Kincaid MC, Green WR. Ocular and orbital involvement in leukemia. Surv Ophthalmol 1983;27:211–32.

105. Rosenthal AR. Ocular manifestations of leukemia. A review. Ophthalmology 1983;90:899–905.

Neuroepithelial Tumors

106. Anderson SR. Medulloepithelioma of the retina. Int Ophthalmol Clin 1962;2:483–506.
107. Broughton WL, Zimmerman LE. A clinicopathologic study of 56 cases of intraocular medulloepitheliomas. Am J Ophthalmol 1978;85:407–18.
108. Chang M, Shields JA, Wachtel DL. Adenoma of the pigment epithelium of the ciliary body simulating a malignant melanoma. Am J Ophthalmol 1979;88:40–4.
109. Font RL, Zimmerman LE. Electron microscopic verification of primary rhabdomyosarcoma of the iris. Am J Ophthalmol 1972;74:110–7.
110. Green WR. Retina. In: Spencer WH, ed. Ophthalmic pathology. An atlas and textbook. 3rd ed. Philadelphia: WB Saunders, 1985:589–1291.
111. Iliff WJ, Green WR. The incidence and histology of Fuchs' adenoma. Arch Ophthalmol 1972;88:249–54.
112. Tso MO, Albert DM. Pathologic conditions of the retinal pigment epithelium: neoplasms and nodular nonneoplastic lesions. Arch Ophthalmol 1972;889:27–38.

Metastatic Tumors

113. Klein R, Nicholson DH, Luxenberg MN. Retinal metastasis from squamous cell carcinoma of the lung. Am J Ophthalmol 1977;83:358–61.
114. Letson AD, Davidorf FH. Bilateral retinal metastases from cutaneous malignant melanoma. Arch Ophthalmol 1982;100:605–7.
115. Young SE, Cruciger M, Lukeman J. Metastatic carcinoma to the retina: case report. Trans Am Acad Ophthalmol Otolaryngol 1979;86:1350–4.

❖❖❖

5

TUMORS OF THE UVEAL TRACT

ANATOMY AND HISTOLOGY

The uveal tract is the pigmented vascular coat of the eye consisting of the iris, ciliary body, and choroid. It is composed of many blood vessels, a variable number of melanocytes, supporting connective tissue, and nerves.

The Iris

Anatomy. The iris is located in front of the crystalline lens, and divides the anterior aqueous-containing part of the eye into the anterior and posterior chambers (fig. 5-1). The iris forms a diaphragm, permitting light to enter the eye only through the pupil. The amount of light transmitted into the eye is controlled by changes in pupillary size. Contraction of the iris reduces the amount of light and increases the depth of focus of the eye.

The surface of the iris is coarsely ribbed with depressions and ridges. This trabeculated appearance is created by the iris vessels and fibrous bands in the stroma, coursing radially from the pupil toward the base of the iris. The iris collarette or minor vascular circle of the iris

is formed by a ring of vessels in the anterior stroma at the junction of the inner and middle thirds, dividing the iris into a narrow, thinner pupillary zone and a broad ciliary zone.

The crypts (of Fuchs) are excavations of varying size into the anterior surface of the iris. Clusters of pigmented cells, "iris freckles," may be present in the anterior iris stroma. Contraction furrows, concentric with the periphery of the iris, may be visualized when the pupil is dilated.

The color of the iris is determined by the content of pigmented cells in the stroma. Many irides appear blue at birth when the uveal tract is not fully pigmented. By 3 to 6 months of age, the iris reaches its maximum pigmentation. If the stroma of the iris lacks pigmented cells (melanocytes) but its double layer of pigment epithelium is normally pigmented, the iris appears blue. In contrast, the iris of some albino individuals is melanin deficient not only in the stromal cells but also in the pigment epithelium. In these individuals, the iris appears pink because the red glow of the illuminated fundus shows through the amelanotic iris.

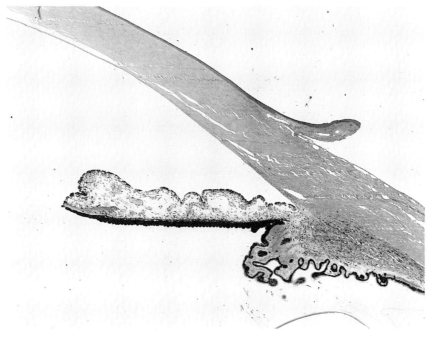

Figure 5-1
NORMAL ANTERIOR
SEGMENT
Iris and ciliary body with open anterior chamber angle.

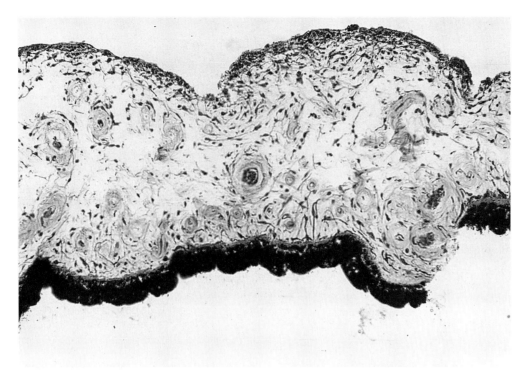

Figure 5-2
NORMAL IRIS
Lightly pigmented iris is organized into four layers.

Histology. The iris is composed of four layers: the anterior limiting or border layer, the stroma, the dilator muscle, and the posterior epithelium (fig. 5-2).

The anterior border layer is a condensation of stromal cells and melanocytes. It varies considerably in thickness and pigmentation in different eyes and in different areas of the same iris. This layer may also be extremely attenuated or even absent, particularly over the iris crypts where no cell processes cover the underlying iris stroma.

The stroma of the iris contains blood vessels, nerves, melanocytes, and the sphincter muscle of the pupil embedded in a loose connective tissue. The tissue characteristics of the stroma permit rapid expansion and contraction. The blood vessels, which are particularly numerous in the iris, run radially. They enter at the iris root and pass through the ciliary zone in several layers. At the junction of the ciliary and pupillary zones, they anastomose to form the minor circle of the iris, which consists of both arteries and veins. The iris vessels are characteristically thick walled with an endothelial lining and a collar of collagen fibrils. The nerve fibers are sensory, vasomotor, and motor; the latter supply the iris muscles. Some clump cells are observed within the iris stroma. Electron microscopic studies have shown two types of clump cells: type I (clump cells of Koganei) are macrophages with phagocytosed melanin; type II (neuroepithelial cells) are less common and possess a surrounding basement membrane and uniform cytoplasmic melanin granules. These rounded cells are probably pigment epithelial cells that have migrated into the stroma in the region of the sphincter.

The sphincter muscle of the iris is a smooth muscle located in the posterior iris stroma next to the pupil. Its attachments to the stromal collagen fibers permit some function even after removal of a segment of the pupillary portion of the iris. The dilator muscle of the iris is continuous with the anterior layer of the iris pigment epithelium and extends from the region of the sphincter muscle to the base of the iris. The dilator and sphincter muscles of the pupil are derived from the outer layer of the optic cup and, therefore, are of neuroectodermal derivation.

The epithelium of the iris consists of two layers of densely pigmented cells, distinguishable as separate layers after bleaching and by electron microscopy. This double layer of pigment epithelium covers the posterior iris surface and results from apposition of the two epithelial layers forming the anterior extremity of the embryonic optic cup.

The anterior layer of the iris epithelium is highly specialized. At their apices, these pigmented cells are cuboidal and form a single epithelial layer. However, at their bases the cytoplasm expands to form the overlapping plate-like smooth muscle cells that make up the dilator muscle, except in the region behind the sphincter muscle where the dilator muscle is lacking. The columnar cells of the posterior layer of pigment epithelium are arranged apex-to-apex with the cells of the anterior layer.

The Ciliary Body

Anatomy. The ciliary body is approximately 6 mm wide and extends from the base of the iris to become continuous posteriorly with the choroid, retinal pigment epithelium (RPE), and neurosensory retina at the ora serrata. On sagittal section, it looks like a triangle that has one corner at the scleral spur, the second corner at the apex of the first ciliary process, and the third corner at the ora serrata posteriorly (fig. 5-1). It is composed of two regions: the pars plicata and the pars plana. The pars plicata or corona ciliaris forms the anterior 2 mm of the ciliary body and contains the ciliary processes, which are irregular radial ridges 2 mm long, 0.8 mm high, and approximately 70 in number. The pars plana or orbicularis ciliaris is the posterior flat part of the ciliary body, about 4 mm in length.

Histology. The ciliary body can be divided histologically into seven layers:

1. The outermost lamina fusca or suprachoroidal tissue plane is a potential space between the sclera and the ciliary body.
2. The ciliary muscles are divided into three groups of fibers. The outermost Brücke muscle forms the longitudinal portion that attaches anteriorly to the scleral spur and trabecular meshwork. The innermost Müller muscle forms the circular portion. The radial portion is formed by some of the fibers of the longitudinal muscle (Brücke muscle) which run obliquely to become continuous with the circular fibers.

3. The vascular layer is a direct continuation of the vascular layer of the choroid.
4. The basement membrane of the pigmented ciliary epithelium (lamina vitrea) is a thick structure and has a reticular pattern.
5. The pigmented ciliary epithelium is the outermost layer of ciliary epithelium and is a continuation of the RPE. It is firmly attached at its apex to the apical surface of the nonpigmented ciliary epithelium.
6. The nonpigmented ciliary epithelium is the innermost layer of ciliary epithelium and is a continuation of the neurosensory retina. It acquires pigment as it approaches the iris root.
7. The basement membrane of the nonpigmented ciliary epithelium is a complex meshwork, to which the zonular fibers of the lens are attached.

The aging ciliary body frequently reveals hyalinization of the ciliary processes and the circular portions of the ciliary muscle, and nodular hyperplasia of the nonpigmented epithelium of the pars plicata.

One of the most important functions of the ciliary body is the production of aqueous. The production of vitreous hyaluronic acid is attributed to the nonpigmented ciliary epithelium of the pars plana.

The Choroid

Anatomy. The choroid is the vascular and pigmented tissue that forms the middle coat of the posterior part of the eye (fig. 5-3). It extends from the ora serrata to the optic nerve and is loosely attached to the sclera by connective tissue strands. Posteriorly, the ciliary blood vessels and nerves enter the choroid from the sclera, anchoring the choroid to the sclera at these points. The choroid varies in thickness from 0.1 mm anteriorly to 0.2 mm posteriorly. Small amounts of choroidal tissue, including melanocytes, extend into the scleral canals through which the ciliary vessels and nerves enter the eye (fig. 5-4). In darkly pigmented individuals, melanocytes may be observed in the inner layers of the sclera and in the lamina cribrosa of the optic nerve head.

Histology. The choroid has four layers:

1. The outermost lamina fusca consists of collagenous and elastic fibers and fibrocytes, and has a prominent number of melanocytes. It is a potential space between the sclera and choroid when the choroid is detached.

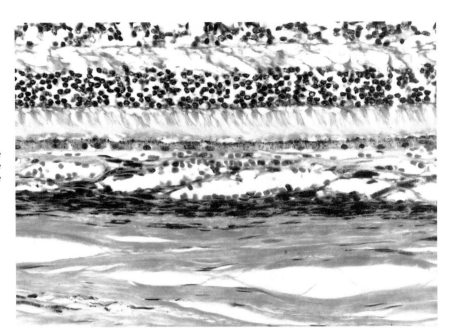

Figure 5-3
NORMAL CHOROID
The choroid consists of the vascularized pigmented tissue between the Bruch membrane and sclera.

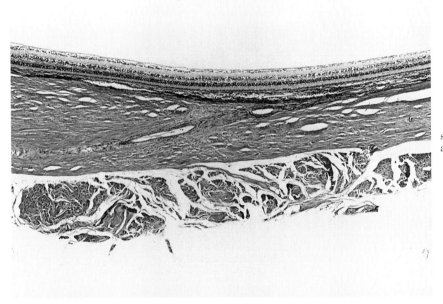

Figure 5-4
NORMAL CHOROID
Uveal tissue extends into the sclera within scleral canals around a long ciliary vessel.

2. The stroma contains arteries and veins embedded in a loose fibrous matrix that contains numerous melanocytes. The arteries decrease in caliber as they approach the choriocapillaris.

3. The choriocapillaris is the capillary layer of the choroid and provides sustenance for the RPE and the outer retinal layers, including the photoreceptor layer, outer plexiform layer, and the outer aspect of the inner nuclear layer. The choriocapillaris is arranged in lobules (1). The endothelial cells lining it are fenestrated and joined by gap junctions.

4. The Bruch membrane is formed by five components: the basement membrane of the RPE, an inner collagenous band, an elastic layer, an outer collagenous zone, and the basement membrane of the endothelium of choriocapillaris. Some authors consider the basement membrane of the RPE to be part of the retina.

CLASSIFICATION AND FREQUENCY

Uveal malignant melanoma is the most common primary intraocular tumor in white people. In the experience of the Armed Forces Institute of Pathology (AFIP) Registry of Ophthalmic Pathology (ROP), the prevalence of uveal malignant melanoma is 3.5 times that of retinoblastoma (Tables 4-1, 5-1). This ratio is lower than the 6.6 reported in the National Cancer Institute's SEER study (3) and probably reflects the referral of cases from Africa and Asia to the AFIP ROP. More heavily pigmented or younger populations have a lower incidence of uveal melanoma. Data from the Brazilian Registry (2) indicating an almost equal frequency of retinoblastoma and uveal malignant melanoma reflects the greater pigmentation in that population. Our experience suggests that retinoblastoma is at least 10 times more common than uveal malignant melanoma in black African patients. Primary uveal tumors other than nevi and malignant melanoma are exceedingly rare (Table 5-1).

MELANOCYTIC NEVI

Melanocytic nevi of the uvea are common small benign tumors. Between 5 and 10 percent of eyes enucleated at autopsy have uveal nevi (35). Nevi of the choroid are the most common and tend to be larger than nevi of the ciliary body and iris. Most choroidal nevi are flat lesions less than 5 mm in diameter. Rarely, they attain a diameter greater than 10 mm and a thickness greater than 1.5 mm. Patients with choroidal nevi are usually asymptomatic, but careful perimetry can detect visual field defects in many (35). The frequency of visual field defects increases with the size of the nevus.

Histologic examination may reveal degenerative changes in the tissues overlying the nevus that could result in a visual field defect. The earliest changes are compression and obliteration of the choriocapillaris, followed by drusen formation by the RPE, serous detachment of the RPE and neurosensory retina, and degeneration of the RPE and photoreceptor cells (fig. 5-5) (60).

Uveal nevi are composed of four histologic types of melanocytes (61). Polyhedral nevus cells have small ovoid nuclei with fine chromatin and small nucleoli. The amount of cytoplasm is variable. When the nevus is composed entirely of

Table 5-1

PRIMARY TUMORS OF THE UVEAL TRACT*

Type of Tumor	Number of Cases
Melanocytic	
Nevi	69
Malignant melanoma	656
Nonmelanocytic	
Hemangioma	4
Leiomyoma	3
Neurofibroma (neurofibromatosis)	1
Osteoma	1
Lymphoma	3

*Frequency distribution of 737 tumors in the AFIP Registry of Ophthalmic Pathology collected between 1984 and 1989.

heavily pigmented, plump polyhedral cells it is referred to as a *melanocytoma* (96). Spindle nevus cells have smaller, less hyperchromatic nuclei with a lower nuclear-cytoplasmic ratio than Callender spindle A type melanoma cells (58). Dendritic nevus cells have long branching processes and larger, rounder nuclei with more prominent nucleoli than the spindle type nevus cells. The balloon nevus cells are polyhedral, with vacuolated or clear cytoplasm. Except for melanocytoma cells, which are always heavily pigmented, and balloon cells, which are always lightly pigmented, the other types of nevus cells vary dramatically in their degree of pigmentation. Many uveal nevi are composed of a mixture of these different types of cells (figs. 5-5, 5-6).

Nevi of the iris differ from nevi of the choroid and ciliary body in at least three ways. First, the anterior border layer of the iris does not provide a barrier to the spread of iris nevus cells and they can grow onto the anterior surface of the iris. In unusual cases, the nevus cells extend beyond the iris and grow onto the surface of the trabecular meshwork, causing glaucoma (64). This behavior is much more common with melanomas than nevi (77). Second, nevi of the iris often have irregular nuclear membranes, with cytoplasm prolapsed into the nuclei. These intranuclear cytoplasmic inclusions are rare in nevi of the choroid and

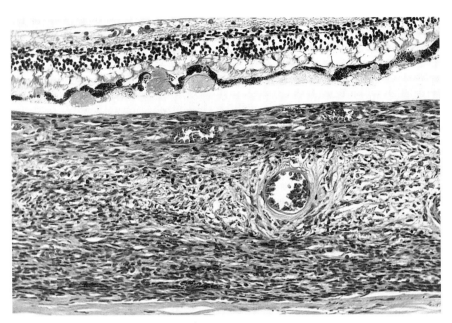

Figure 5-5
CHOROIDAL NEVUS
The choroid is doubled in thickness by a proliferation of benign melanocytes with drusen of the overlying retinal pigment epithelium and mild disruption of photoreceptors.

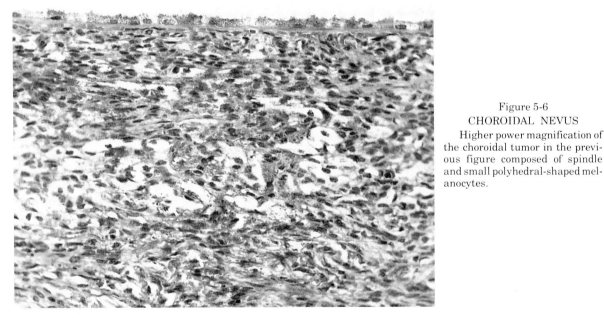

Figure 5-6
CHOROIDAL NEVUS
Higher power magnification of the choroidal tumor in the previous figure composed of spindle and small polyhedral-shaped melanocytes.

ciliary body. Third, iris nevi may contain large, sometimes multinucleated epithelioid nevus cells (41), similar to the epithelioid cells of the Spitz nevus. Epithelioid cells are not seen in nevi of the posterior uvea.

Clinically, it is difficult to differentiate between large nevi and small melanomas of the uveal tract. Shields and Shields (80) recommend using the term "suspicious nevi" for tumors in this grey zone. About 10 percent of suspicious nevi grow, whereas growth of nonsuspicious nevi is uncommon. Growth of a suspicious nevus does not necessarily mean that the lesion is a malignant melanoma, since growth has been documented in a benign choroidal nevus (49). Gass (33) pointed out that because the incidence of choroidal nevi increases with age, they must grow. Also, orange lipofuscin pigment, a pigment associated with tumors that grow, can be seen on the surface of some suspicious nevi (26).

MALIGNANT MELANOMA
OF THE UVEAL TRACT

Historical Aspects and Terminology.
Uveal malignant melanoma has had a variety of descriptive names: *melanosarcoma* for tumors of spindle cell type; *melanocarcinoma* for tumors of epithelioid cell type; *leukosarcoma* for amelanotic varieties; *angiosarcoma* for highly vascular tumors; and *giant cell sarcoma* for anaplastic tumors containing bizarre, often multinucleated, giant cells. In the last few decades the term *uveal malignant melanoma* has gained popularity and is recommended by the World Health Organization. We do not recommend a diagnosis of uveal melanoma without an indication of malignancy because some pathologists define "melanoma" to include both benign and malignant melanocytic tumors. We designate the former as nevi and the latter as malignant melanomas to avoid confusion.

Virchow (95) recognized that malignant melanoma is a tumor of melanocytes and that these tumors are not always pigmented. Both benign and malignant melanocytic tumors of the uvea vary greatly in pigmentation. While the amelanotic tumors cause the greatest problems in diagnosis, there is a special problem with heavily pigmented intraocular tumors as well. The eye contains two types of melanocytic cells: uveal melanocytes and the pigment epithelial cells of the retina, ciliary body, and iris. Tumors of these two different origins have very different prognoses and must be differentiated. The tumors of the pigmented epithelia are referred to as adenomas and carcinomas to distinguish them from nevi and malignant melanomas of uveal melanocytic origin. The pigmented neuroepithelial tumors are described in the chapter on tumors of the retina.

Etiology.
The cause of uveal malignant melanoma is unknown but several risk factors for the development of this tumor have been identified. These include age, race, sex, predisposing lesions, genetic factors, and possibly, environmental factors (27).

Age. The incidence increases with age (16). The median age at diagnosis in the cases on file in the AFIP ROP is 53. Barr and associates (8) found that only 1.6 percent of 6358 cases in the ROP were in patients under 20 years of age. They noted that this

prevalence was probably inflated since some cases were submitted to the Registry only because the patient was so young. Congenital uveal malignant melanoma is exceedingly rare (10).

Racial Pigmentation. Because the racial make-up of the population of patients whose cases are referred to the ROP is not known, the relative risk of uveal melanoma in blacks and whites cannot be calculated from ROP data. Still, the prevalence in blacks appears to be very low. Margo and McLean (52) reviewed 3876 cases of uveal malignant melanoma in which the race of the patient was known from the ROP; only 39 (1 percent) of these patients were black. Scotto et al. (73) found that the incidence in whites (six per million per year) is 8.5 times greater than in blacks, which is consistent with Margo and McLean's data, assuming that blacks make up 13 percent of the referral population. Margo and McLean also found that the tumors in blacks were larger, more heavily pigmented, and more extensively necrotic than the tumors in whites; however, there was no difference in survival between black and white patients.

In black Africans there is suggestive evidence that the incidence of uveal malignant melanoma is even lower than in black Americans, who often have some white ancestors. Asians have an incidence intermediate between American blacks and whites. Among whites, blue-eyed blonds have the highest incidence. These findings indicate an inverse relationship between racial pigmentation and incidence.

Sex. Uveal malignant melanoma is more common in men than women. In the AFIP ROP there are 2764 men and 2231 women with choroidal and ciliary body melanomas. A similar male predominance was reported from Canada (27) and in the Third National Cancer Survey (16) from the United States. The reason for the higher rate in men is unknown.

Geographic Factors. There is great variation in the incidence of uveal malignant melanoma around the world but these variations appear to reflect the dominant racial groups in the different regions. The incidence is the lowest in Africa, where the most heavily pigmented individuals predominate and highest in the Scandinavian countries, where blond, blue-eyed people predominate. There is suggestive data that actinic exposure is a pathogenetic factor in uveal malignant

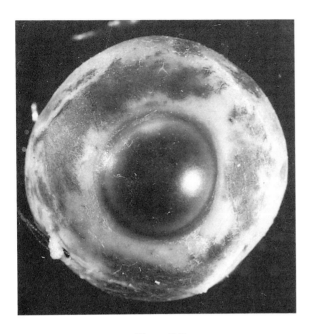

Figure 5-7
MELANOSIS OCULI
Congenital diffuse anterior scleral pigmentation. (Figures 5-7–5-10 are from the same patient.)

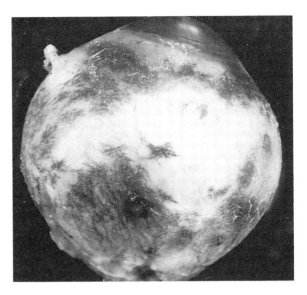

Figure 5-8
MELANOSIS OCULI
Congenital diffuse posterior scleral pigmentation that was not seen clinically.

melanoma but the relative risk is much lower than it is with cutaneous malignant melanoma (40,75). This is not surprising since most of the ultraviolet light is absorbed before it reaches the uveal melanocytes.

Predisposing Lesions. Congenital melanosis (36,37) and nevi (33,61,93) are the best documented lesions that predispose to the development of uveal malignant melanoma. Both ocular melanocytosis and oculodermal melanocytosis have been frequently observed to precede the development of the tumor. Almost without exception, malignant melanoma occurs in the more heavily pigmented eye (figs. 5-7–5-11). Congenital oculodermal melanocytosis (nevus of Ota) is more common in blacks and Asians than whites. Patients of all races develop uveal malignant melanoma in the eye with congenital melanosis (65) but progression to uveal malignant melanoma is most often observed in whites.

Uveal nevi progress to malignant melanoma less frequently than congenital melanosis. The rate of transformation of nevi has been estimated to be 1 per 10,000 to 15,000 per year. Another reason for considering nevi a precursor

of uveal malignant melanoma is that nevoid-appearing cells are observed at the periphery or along the scleral edge in about 75 percent of tumors (93). This frequency is considered too high by some investigators who believe that the nevoid appearance of cells along the sclera represents a compression artifact.

Genetic Factors. Although rare, familial occurrence has been recorded (48,89). Among the patients whose data are on file in the ROP, we have observed two families with uveal malignant melanoma in successive generations. The rarity of these cases suggests that family members of patients with uveal malignant melanoma have at most a low risk of developing this tumor but this risk is probably far greater than that of the general population.

The role of specific gene alterations in the pathogenesis of uveal melanoma is less well defined than it is in retinoblastoma. Chromosomal analysis has demonstrated that abnormalities of chromosomes 3 and 8 are most frequently observed (67,83,92): mostly a loss of chromosome 3 alleles and multiplication of chromosome 8 alleles. These findings suggest that there is a tumor-suppressor gene (antioncogene) on chromosome 3 that is deleted and an oncogene on

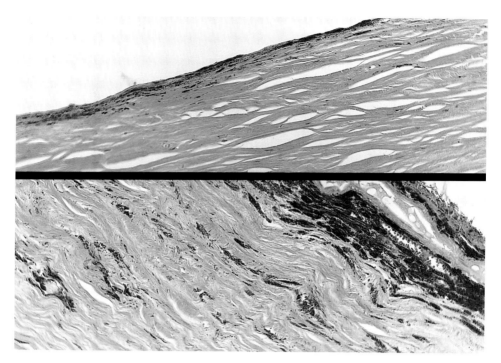

Figure 5-9
MELANOSIS OCULI
Diffuse uveal and scleral pigmentation.

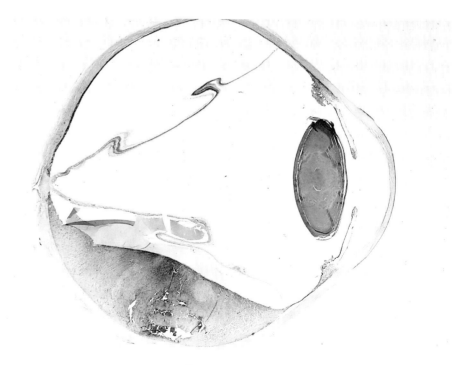

Figure 5-10
MELANOSIS OCULI WITH MALIGNANT MELANOMA
Medium-sized choroidal tumor with retinal detachment.

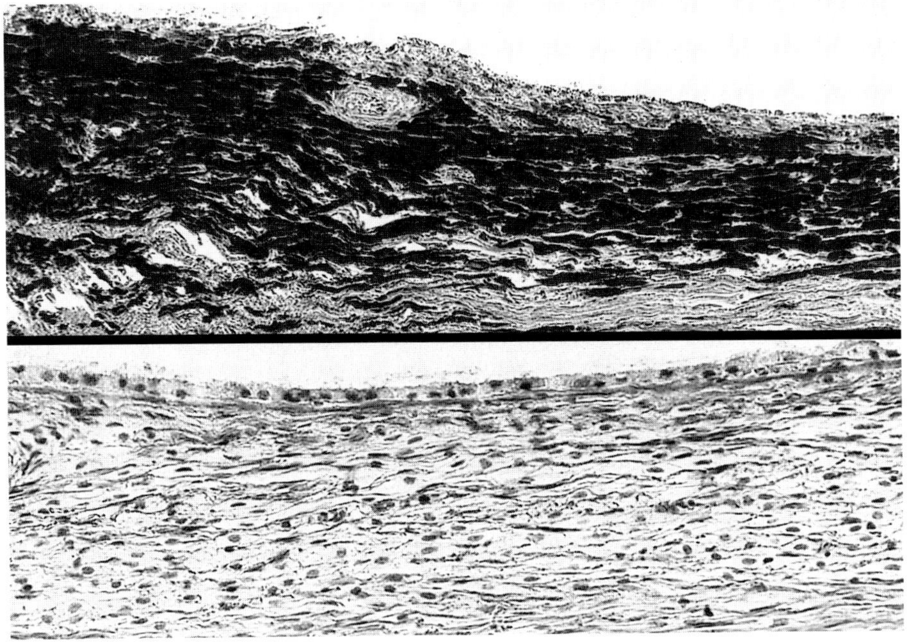

Figure 5-11
MELANOSIS OCULI
Diffuse proliferation of benign, heavily pigmented, polyhedral melanocytes (regular and bleached sections).

chromosome 8 that is amplified in uveal melanoma. Neither of these genes has been identified. Detectable deletions of the long arm of chromosome 6 are less frequent than in cutaneous melanoma (67,83,92), which suggests that the putative melanoma tumor-suppressor gene in this location (15) is less frequently altered in uveal melanoma than in cutaneous melanoma.

The tumor-suppressor gene p53 located on the short arm of chromosome 17 is mutated in a variety of cancers. It may also play a role in the pathogenesis of uveal melanomas. This gene, like the retinoblastoma gene, codes for a nucleoprotein that is involved in regulating the cell cycle. Point mutations in the p53 gene alter the tumor-suppressor function of the protein product and increase its stability, so that it accumulates in cells to levels that can be detected immunohistochemically. Thus, immunohistochemical detection of p53 protein in cells can be used to screen for point mutations. In 12 of 18 uveal melanomas, Tobal et al. (86) measured increased expression of p53 protein. Polymerase chain reaction and sequencing of the p53 gene in 2 of the 12 tumors revealed point mutations in both tumors. Interestingly, neither of these mutations were the cytosine to thymidine conversions characteristic of ultraviolet light injury (94).

Jay and McCartney (43) demonstrated mutant p53 gene product in a uveal malignant melanoma from an 150-year-old ocular specimen. This tumor was from a member of a family in which four generations had uveal melanoma associated with breast cancer. Parsons first described this family in 1905 (43).

Associated Tumors. Although several authors have commented on the high rate of death due to other neoplasms in the follow-up of patients with uveal malignant melanoma, these authors failed to consider the expected cancer mortality for these patients. United States Life Tables indicate that approximately one fourth of deaths in 55- to 75-year-old people are due to cancer. Using cases from the ROP, we compared the mortality due to cancers other than metastatic melanoma for patients treated for uveal melanoma with the expected mortality due to cancer of matched people and found no difference. Holly et al. (39) found no increased risk of prior cancer in patients with uveal melanoma. These data suggest that there is not a strong association between uveal melanoma and other malignancies.

Ten cases of uveal malignant melanoma have been reported in patients with dysplastic nevus syndrome (87). We observed one case from the ROP in which a choroidal spindle cell nevus was

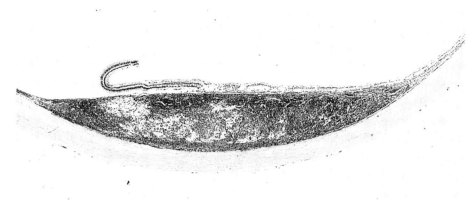

Figure 5-12
DYSPLASTIC
NEVUS SYNDROME
Spindle cell nevus of the
choroid. (Figures 5-12–5-16
are from the same patient.)

Figure 5-13
DYSPLASTIC
NEVUS SYNDROME
High-power magnifica-
tion of spindle cell nevus of
the choroid showing hypo-
cellular and hypercellular
areas.

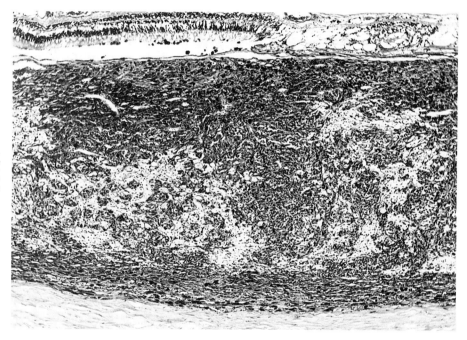

associated with multiple cutaneous malignant melanomas (figs. 5-12–5-16). This association appears to be weak: Taylor et al. (85) found the same prevalence of dysplastic nevi in patients with uveal melanoma as observed in the general population.

Bilaterality and multicentricity in one eye are rare in uveal melanoma whereas in retinoblastoma multiple tumors are common and indicative of a genetic predisposition. There is a strong association with other cancers in a small subgroup of patients with bilateral uveal melanoma (9). This subgroup has a unique constellation of findings: rapid bilateral loss of vision in older patients (57 to 78 years) who eventually die with carcinoma of bowel, ovary, gallbladder, pancreas, or lung; a confusing clinical appearance that gives the impression of multiple choroidal tumors suggesting metastatic carcinoma or metastatic melanoma; and bilateral diffuse melanocytic tumors in which the majority of the cells are cytologically benign.

Clinical Features. Uveal malignant melanomas may arise in the iris, ciliary body, or choroid. Those in the iris are visible and usually noticed by the patient when relatively small. Choroidal and ciliary body malignant melanomas are divided

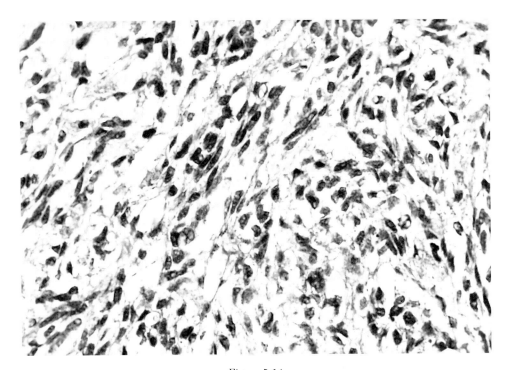

Figure 5-14
DYSPLASTIC NEVUS SYNDROME
High-power magnification of spindle cell nevus of the choroid showing benign cytologic features.

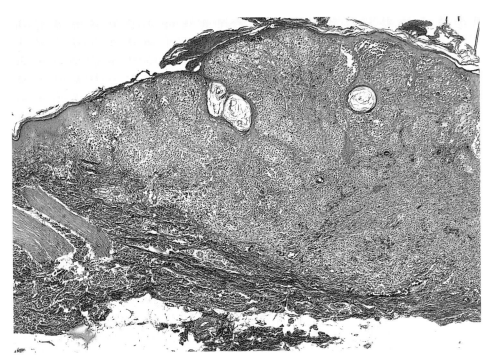

Figure 5-15
DYSPLASTIC NEVUS SYNDROME
Malignant melanoma of the skin.

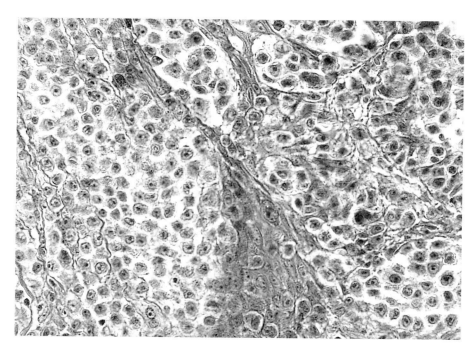

Figure 5-16
DYSPLASTIC NEVUS SYNDROME
Higher power magnification of malignant melanoma of the skin.

into stages based on clinical presentation. The first stage is asymptomatic and represents those tumors discovered on a routine ophthalmoscopic examination. Use of the indirect ophthalmoscope has greatly improved the ability of ophthalmologists to detect and diagnose small choroidal tumors (14). These tumors tend to be small lesions confined to the uvea without associated retinal detachment or involvement of the macular area. In the second stage, there is either a field defect or loss of vision, which is usually due to associated retinal detachment. In the third stage, the patient develops ocular pain from glaucoma or inflammation. In the fourth stage, there are symptoms of extraocular extension, either proptosis or a visible subconjunctival mass. Of 2627 cases of uveal melanoma obtained between 1936 and 1975 from the ROP, 2.8 percent were stage 1, 64 percent stage 2, 32 percent stage 3, and 1.4 percent stage 4 (97). Over the 40-year period in which these cases were collected, the proportion of patients that were stage 1 and 2 increased and the proportion with more advanced disease decreased by 23 percent. Despite treatment at earlier stages, there was no significant improvement in survival rates (97).

Pathologic Findings. The gross pathologic features of uveal malignant melanoma depend on the size and location of the tumor. Choroidal tumors are the most common. Although ophthalmologists use both the diameter and height of the tumor to determine size, most pathologists use a simpler classification based only on the largest dimension of the tumor (pl. XIA). Uveal malignant melanomas are divided into three groups: small, if the largest dimension is 10 mm or less; medium, if the largest dimension is 11 to 15 mm; and large, if the largest dimension is greater than 15 mm. Most small tumors are discoid and confined to the choroid (pls. XA, XIIA, figs. 5-17, 5-18). The tough fibrous sclera prevents expansion of the tumor externally but internally the Bruch membrane is relatively weak. As these tumors grow and produce a larger discoid mass (pl. XB) the Bruch membrane is stretched over the tumor and eventually ruptures. The tumor herniates through the rupture and grows into the subretinal space, giving the tumor a "collar button" configuration. The growth in the subretinal space is often greater than the growth in the choroid and as the mass in the subretinal space becomes larger, the

PLATE X
MALIGNANT MELANOMA

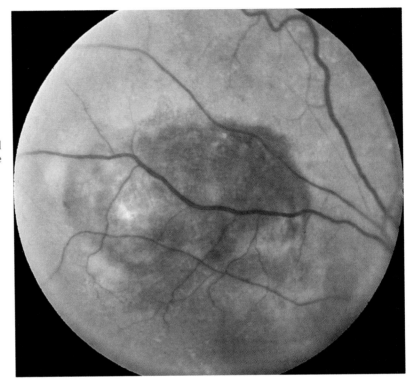

A. Fundus photograph of a small tumor with orange pigment on the surface.

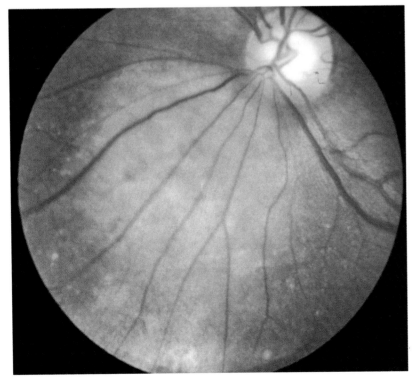

B. Fundus photograph of a medium-sized tumor. Vessels over the dome of the tumor are out of focus due to the elevation of the mass.

PLATE XI

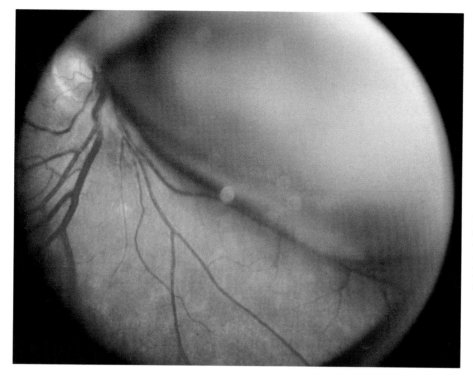

A. MALIGNANT MELANOMA
Fundus photograph of a choroidal tumor. The dome of the tumor is out of focus due to the elevation of the mass. Because of the elevation this tumor would be classified as large clinically and medium-sized pathologically.

B. Large transillumination defect produced by a pigmented tumor of the ciliary body and choroid.

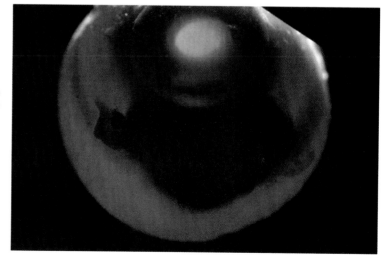

PLATE XII
MALIGNANT MELANOMA

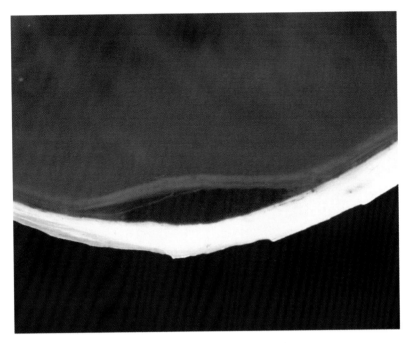

A. Small, heavily pigmented choroidal tumor.

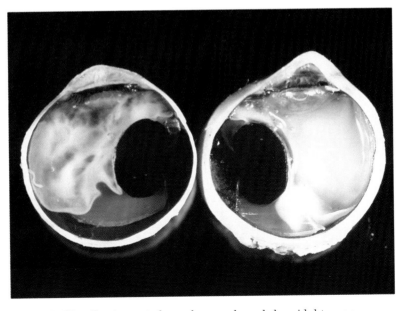

B. Heavily pigmented, mushroom-shaped choroidal tumor.

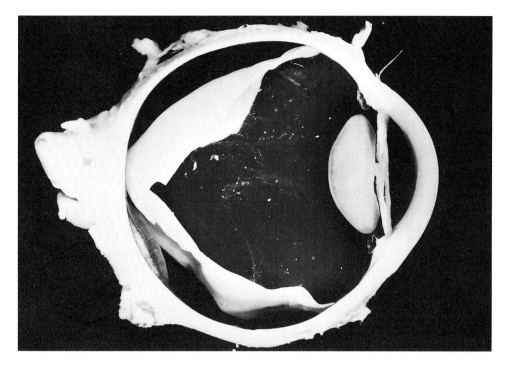

Figure 5-17
MALIGNANT MELANOMA
Small pigmented tumor confined to the choroid.

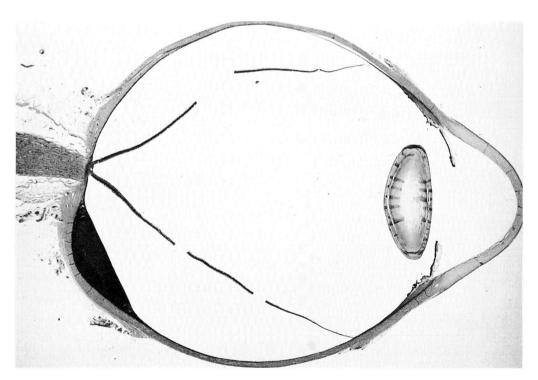

Figure 5-18
MALIGNANT MELANOMA
Tumor seen in previous figure is composed of tightly packed melanoma cells.

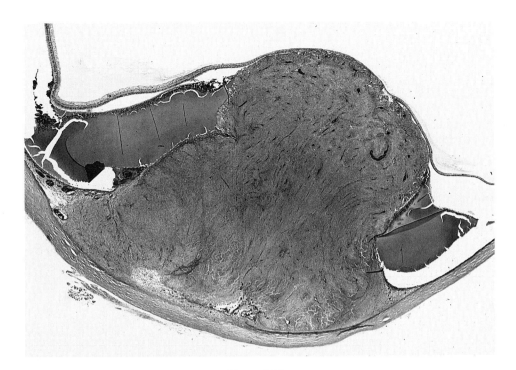

Figure 5-19
MALIGNANT MELANOMA
Mushroom-shaped choroidal tumor with exudative retinal detachment.

tumor develops a mushroom-like appearance. The collar button and mushroom configurations are typically seen in medium-sized tumors (pls. XIA, XIIB–XIVA, figs. 5-19, 5-20). The retina overlying a uveal melanoma undergoes atrophy or cystoid degeneration while the retina surrounding the tumor is detached by the accumulation of serous exudate between the retina and the RPE. As the tumors become even larger, they invade and destroy the ocular tissues, eventually completely filling the globe. Some tumors invade posteriorly through the sclera, usually along the course of perforating nerves and vessels into the orbit or anteriorly into the conjunctiva (4,81).

The diffuse infiltrating type of choroidal melanoma is an uncommon variant (25). These tumors grow laterally in the choroid without producing much thickness (pl. XIVB, figs. 5-21–5-26). They are more likely to invade through the sclera than discoid uveal malignant melanomas and may produce an orbital mass larger than the intraocular tumor (pl. XIVB).

Malignant melanomas that arise in the ciliary body are less common, smaller, and have a more spherical shape than choroidal tumors (pls. XIB,

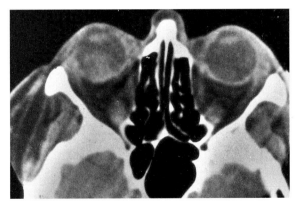

Figure 5-20
MALIGNANT MELANOMA
Computed tomograph of a mushroom-shaped choroidal tumor.

XIVC, D, figs. 5-27, 5-28). Anterior invasion to involve the iris root, angle structures, and anterior chamber is common. Clinically, the anterior extension may be noticed by the patient and what is thought to be a small iris tumor may represent only the tip of the iceberg (figs. 5-27, 5-28). Bruch membrane does not exist in the ciliary body and

PLATE XIII
MALIGNANT MELANOMA

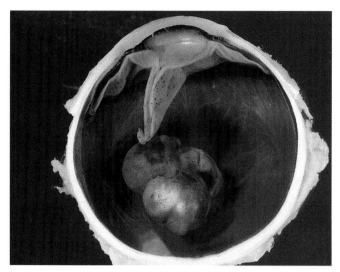

A. Variably pigmented, mushroom-shaped choroidal tumor has ruptured the Bruch membrane and grown into the subretinal space.

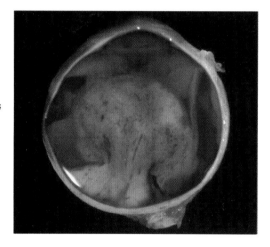

B. Slightly pigmented, mushroom-shaped choroidal tumor has caused a subretinal hemorrhage and a total retinal detachment.

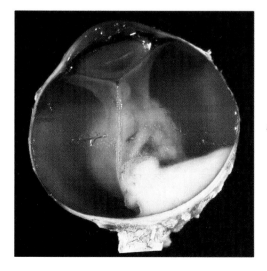

C. Amelanotic, mushroom-shaped choroidal tumor has caused a total retinal detachment.

PLATE XIV
MALIGNANT MELANOMA

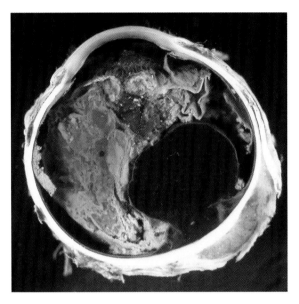

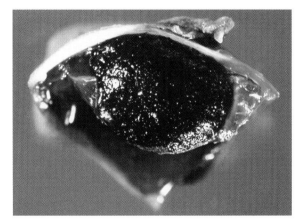

C. Heavily pigmented ciliary body tumor excised by iridocyclectomy.

A. Heavily pigmented, mushroom-shaped choroidal tumor has caused a large, partially organized subretinal hemorrhage and a total retinal detachment.

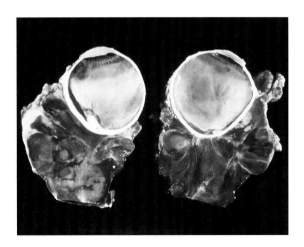

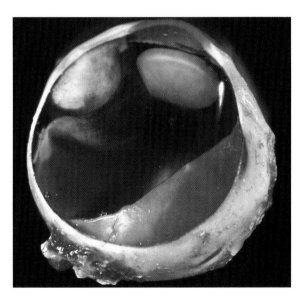

B. Diffuse pigmented choroidal tumor with massive extraocular extension.

D. Lightly pigmented tumor of the ciliary body.

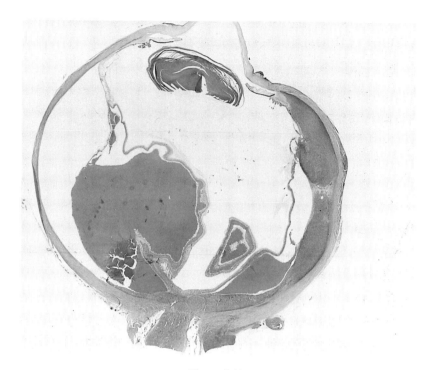

Figure 5-21
DIFFUSE MALIGNANT MELANOMA
Tumor extends from ciliary body to optic nerve and has produced an exudative retinal detachment.

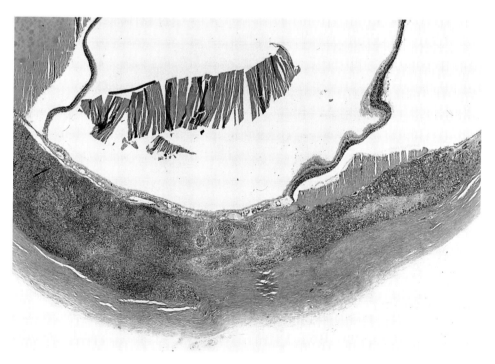

Figure 5-22
DIFFUSE MALIGNANT MELANOMA
Focal areas of necrosis and scleral invasion.

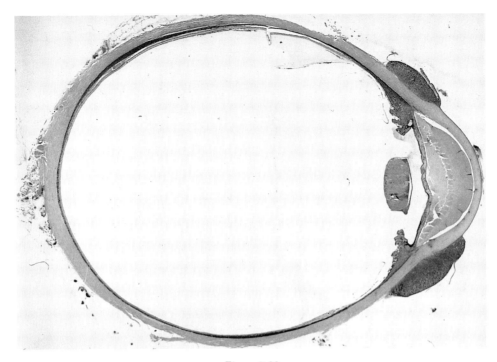

Figure 5-23
DIFFUSE MALIGNANT MELANOMA
An unusually diffuse tumor involving the entire uveal tract, with extraocular extension anteriorly in a ring configuration. (Figures 5-23–5-26 are from the same patient.)

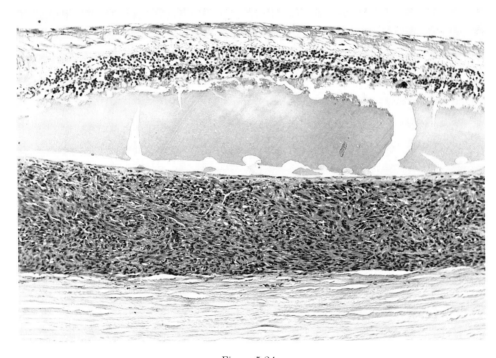

Figure 5-24
DIFFUSE MALIGNANT MELANOMA
Higher power magnification of the choroidal portion of the tumor in the previous figure showing spindle-shaped melanocytes.

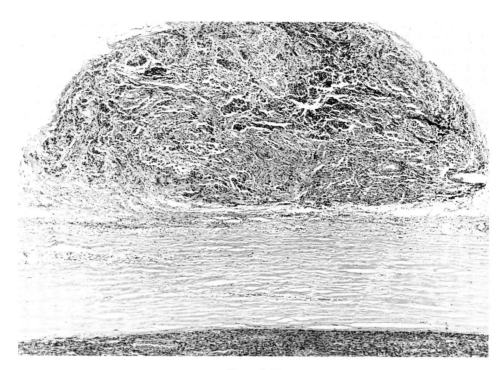

Figure 5-25
DIFFUSE MALIGNANT MELANOMA
Another area of the same tumor with a nodular area of extraocular extension.

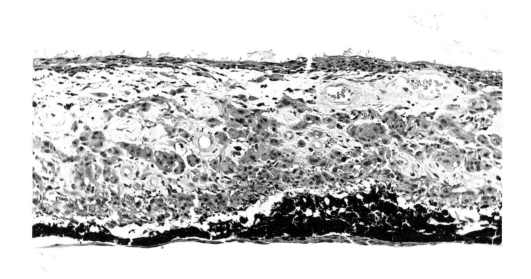

Figure 5-26
DIFFUSE MALIGNANT MELANOMA
Iris involvement by small epithelioid cells.

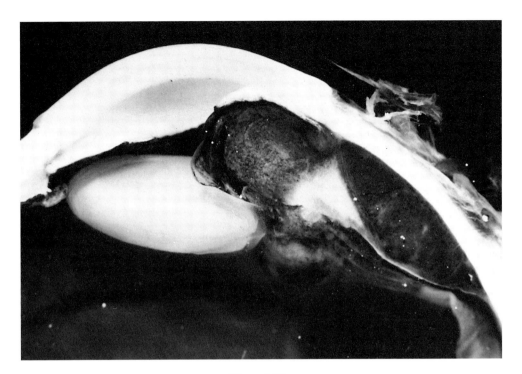

Figure 5-27
MALIGNANT MELANOMA
Large iris and ciliary body tumor with subluxation of the lens.

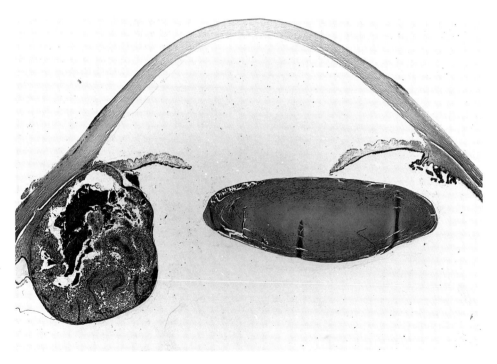

Figure 5-28
MALIGNANT MELANOMA
Ciliary body tumor with areas of necrosis and hemorrhage.

the ciliary epithelium does not provide an effective barrier to inward growth. Commonly, ciliary body malignant melanomas invade into the posterior chamber and indent the lens, creating a lenticular notch, cataract, or subluxation (fig. 5-27). The diffuse type of malignant melanoma also occurs in the ciliary body (fig. 5-23) where the tumor tends to grow in a ring configuration (50). Like diffuse tumors of the choroid, these tumors frequently invade outside of the eye. The extraocular extension is usually along the aqueous outflow channels from the trabecular meshwork and Schlemm canal. This extension may be mistaken for a primary malignant melanoma of the conjunctiva (fig. 5-29).

Tumors of the iris are the least common of the uveal malignant melanomas. Because the iris is visible, these tumors tend to be detected when relatively small (figs. 5-30–5-33) and in patients who are significantly younger. Tumors of the choroid measuring up to 10 mm are considered small but a 10-mm tumor would completely fill the anterior chamber of the eye. Because of early detectability and surgical accessibility, iris tumors are usually treated by local excision (iridectomy or iridocyclectomy). If the tumor is confined to the iris, a simple iridectomy is adequate (figs. 5-30–5-32); when the tumor extends into the ciliary body (fig. 5-33), a more extensive iridocyclectomy is required (pl. XIVC) (59). These procedures enable the ophthalmologist to remove the tumor and preserve the eye, usually with useful vision. Because iris tumors are excised when relatively small, a large percentage of lesions removed for suspected malignant melanoma of the iris prove to be benign nevi (42).

Iris melanomas may be associated with large dilated blood vessels (figs. 5-30, 5-31). In some, the tortuous enlarged blood vessels may be more prominent than the melanocytic component. These tumors have been misdiagnosed both clinically and pathologically as hemangioma of the iris. A true hemangioma of the iris is an uncommon lesion that may not even exist (22).

In the iris there is no barrier between the stroma and the anterior chamber and growth onto the anterior surface of the iris is often seen with nevi and melanomas. Melanomas of epithelioid cell type are composed of cells that lack cohesion. With this type tumor, it is not uncommon for malignant cells to be shed from the

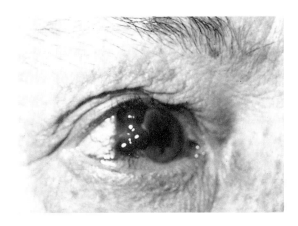

Figure 5-29
MALIGNANT MELANOMA
Tumor of ciliary body with extraocular extension mimicking a primary conjunctival neoplasm.

surface of the iris tumor and seed throughout the anterior chamber, clog the trabecular meshwork, and elevate intraocular pressure (figs. 5-34–5-36). There is also a diffuse variant of malignant melanoma of the iris. These tumors spread through the iris stroma and along the surface of the iris causing heterochromia but no mass. They tend to be of epithelioid cell type and usually seed the anterior chamber (figs. 5-26, 5-34–5-36).

Extraocular Extension. The sclera provides a barrier to egress of uveal malignant melanomas. Invasion outside of the eye is usually along the emissaries of the vortex veins and the ciliary arteries and nerves (figs. 5-37, 5-38). Occasionally, neoplastic cells invade into the lumen of the vortex veins (fig. 5-39), but vascular invasion within the tumor is a more common source of hematogenous metastasis. Peripapillary uveal malignant melanomas frequently invade the optic nerve head but unlike retinoblastomas, uveal malignant melanomas only rarely extend retrolaminarly within the optic nerve. Seeding of the cerebral spinal fluid has been reported (72) but we have not observed this as a cause of death.

Cytology and Histopathologic Findings. In 1931, Callender (12) classified uveal malignant melanomas based on cytologic and histopathologic features. He (13), his co-workers (90), his successors at the AFIP (29,54,55,66), and other investigators (38,44,68,69,76) demonstrated the prognostic value of this classification. The cells of uveal malignant melanoma are divided into

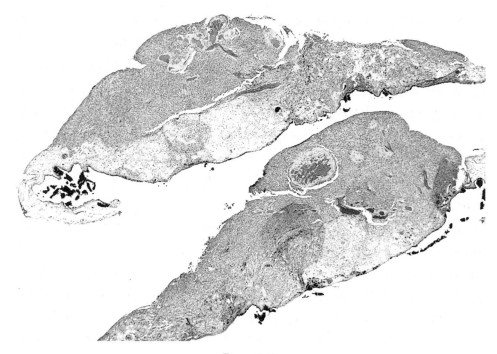

Figure 5-30
MALIGNANT MELANOMA
Iridectomy specimen containing a spindle cell iris tumor. (Figures 5-30–5-32 are from the same patient.)

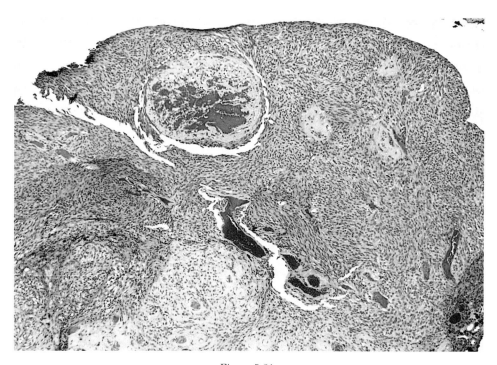

Figure 5-31
MALIGNANT MELANOMA
Higher power magnification of previous tumor showing an area composed of nevus cells, an area with spindle-shaped melanoma cells, and a large thrombosed blood vessel.

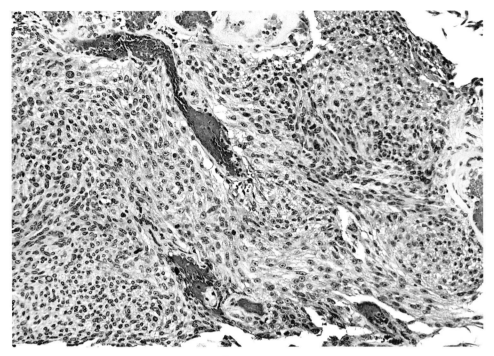

Figure 5-32
MALIGNANT MELANOMA
Higher power magnification of an area composed of spindle A and B type cells.

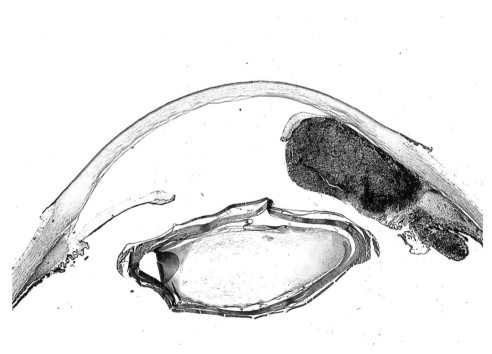

Figure 5-33
MALIGNANT MELANOMA
A large iris tumor has extended to the ciliary body.

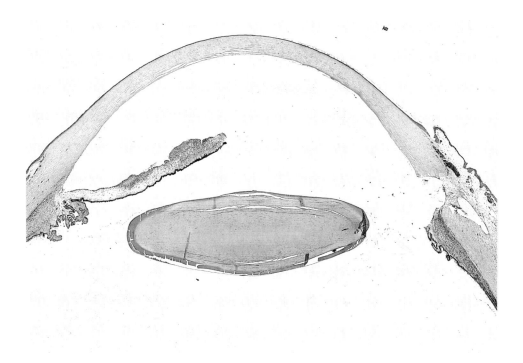

Figure 5-34
MALIGNANT MELANOMA
Recurrent diffuse tumor of the iris following iridectomy. (Figures 5-34–5-36 are from the same patient.)

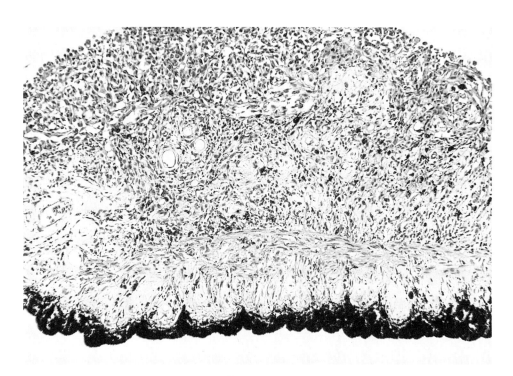

Figure 5-35
MALIGNANT MELANOMA
Higher power magnification of tumor in the previous figure showing a mixture of spindle and epithelioid type cells.

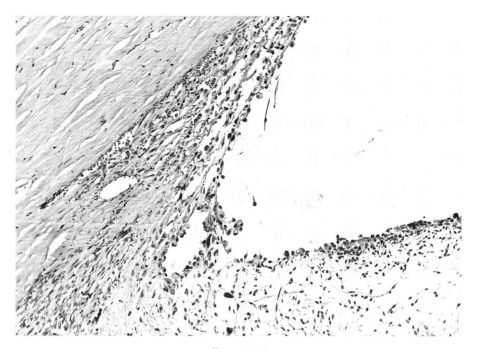

Figure 5-36
MALIGNANT MELANOMA
Seeding of anterior chamber angle by small epithelioid cells.

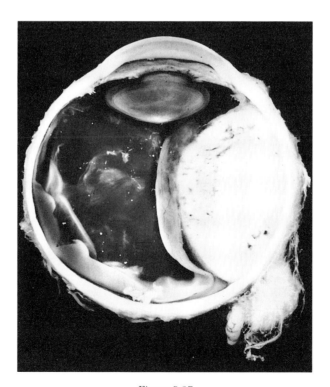

Figure 5-37
MALIGNANT MELANOMA
Amelanotic large choroidal tumor with extraocular extension.

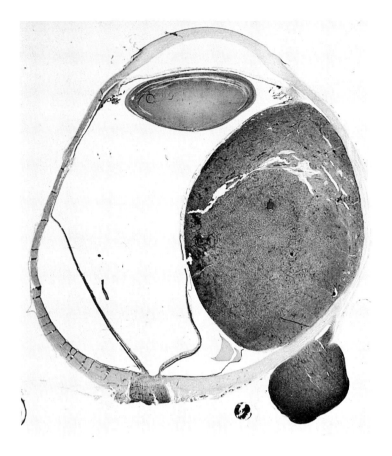

Figure 5-38
MALIGNANT MELANOMA
Same tumor as in previous figure.

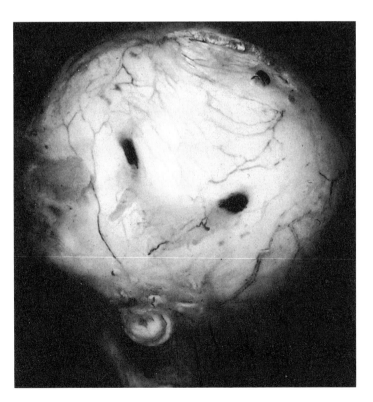

Figure 5-39
MALIGNANT MELANOMA
Vortex vein invasion.

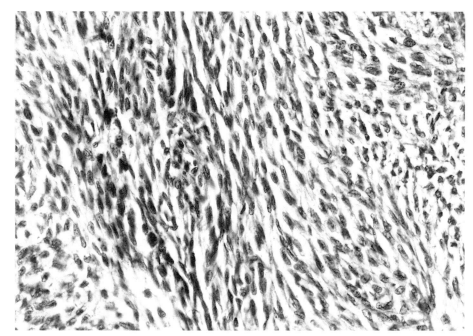

Figure 5-40
MALIGNANT
MELANOMA
Tumor composed almost
exclusively of spindle A type
cells.

two main cytologic types: spindle and epithelioid. Spindle type cells are fusiform and usually arranged in tightly cohesive bundles. By light microscopy, the plasma membranes of the cells within the bundles are indistinct, giving the appearance of a syncytium. The cytoplasm has a fibrillar or finely granular character. Callender identified two subtypes of spindle cells based on nuclear features. Subtype A has a slender nucleus with fine chromatin and an indistinct nucleolus (figs. 5-40, 5-41); there is often a longitudinal fold in the nuclear envelope that gives the appearance of a chromatin streak. Subtype B has a plumper nucleus, coarser chromatin, and a more prominent and eosinophilic nucleolus (figs. 5-42, 5-43). Mitotic activity is rare in spindle A type cells and infrequent in most spindle B type cells.

The epithelioid type cells are larger and more pleomorphic than the spindle type cells (figs. 5-44, 5-45). They usually have abundant glassy cytoplasm, giving the cell a polyhedral shape. The cells have a distinct cell border, often with extracellular space between adjacent cells. This loss of cohesion is characteristic of epithelioid type cells and is one of the main features that distinguishes them from the spindle type (figs. 5-42–5-45). Other distinguishing features are a larger and rounder nucleus and a more angular nuclear envelope with irregular indentations and outpouchings. The chromatin is very coarse and marginated. A very large eosinophilic nucleolus is usually present within the center of a nucleus that is often cleared of chromatin. Occasional bizarre and multinucleated epithelioid cells may be seen. Mitotic activity is usually greater in epithelioid type cells than in spindle type cells.

Callender et al. (13) classified uveal malignant melanomas into six groups: four were based on the cytologic make-up of the tumor and two were based on histologic features. The four groups based on cytology were: tumors composed of spindle A type cells, tumors composed of spindle B type cells, tumors composed of epithelioid type cells, and tumors composed of a mixture of epithelioid and spindle type cells. The fifth group consisted of tumors with a fascicular pattern. Two fascicular patterns exist in uveal melanomas, vasocentric and Verocay-like. In tumors with the vasocentric pattern (fig. 5-46), the cells are predominately of the spindle B type, with nuclei arranged in columns perpendicular to a central blood vessel. In tumors with the Verocay-like pattern (fig. 5-47), the cells, usually of the spindle A type, are arranged in bundles with palisaded nuclei forming stripes across the bundle. The sixth group was composed of tumors too necrotic to classify into one of the other groups.

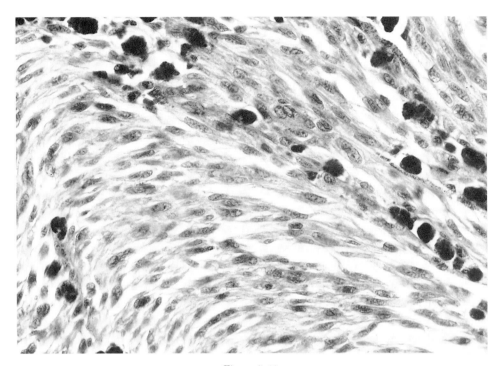

Figure 5-41
MALIGNANT MELANOMA
Tumor composed predominantly of spindle A type cells.

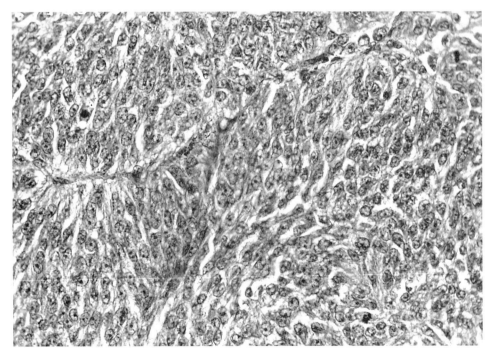

Figure 5-42
MALIGNANT MELANOMA
Spindle B type cells arranged in bundles.

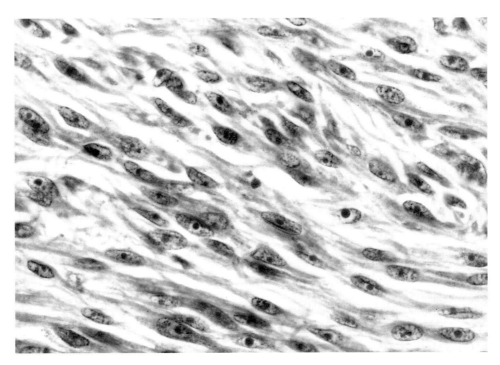

Figure 5-43
MALIGNANT MELANOMA
Spindle B type cells with prominent nucleoli.

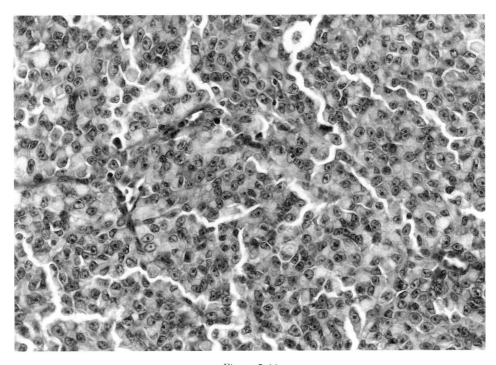

Figure 5-44
MALIGNANT MELANOMA
An area of a tumor composed of small epithelioid type cells.

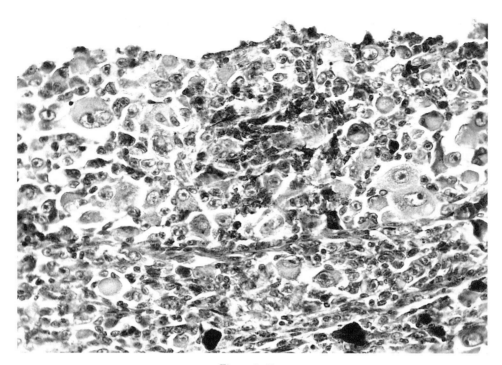

Figure 5-45
MALIGNANT MELANOMA
Large epithelioid cells with large nucleoli and lack of cohesion.

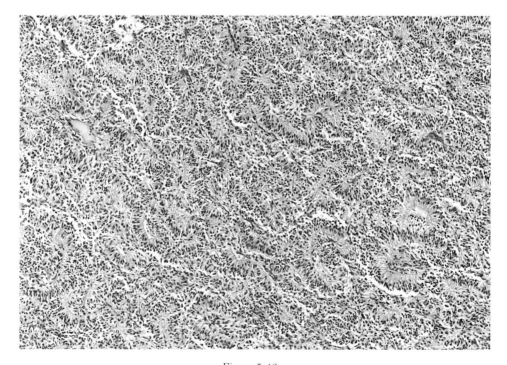

Figure 5-46
MALIGNANT MELANOMA
Fascicular type tumor with neoplastic cells palisading around blood vessels (vasocentric pattern).

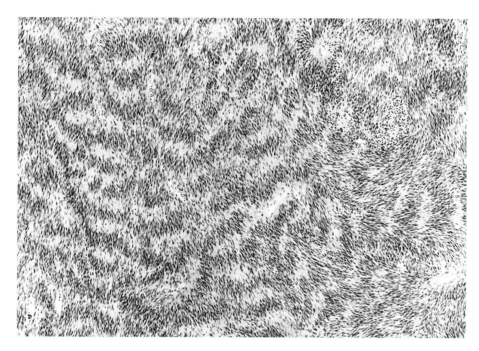

Figure 5-47
MALIGNANT MELANOMA
Within bundles of this fascicular type tumor the nuclei of the neoplastic cells are arranged in stripes (Verocay-like pattern).

Several authors documented the frequency and prognostic significance of the six classes of uveal melanoma. By 1951, Wilder and Paul (90) had studied 1064 cases of uveal melanoma with at least a 5-year follow-up from the ROP. Approximately half (48 percent) were mixed cell type tumors and one third (32 percent) were tumors of spindle B cell type. The percentages of necrotic, spindle A, fascicular, and epithelioid cell type tumors were 8, 6, 5, and 2, respectively. There were two prognostic groups. The group with a better prognosis consisted of tumors of spindle A, spindle B, and fascicular cell types; patients with tumors of these types had a 22 percent death rate due to metastasis. The group with a poorer prognosis consisted of tumors of necrotic, mixed, or epithelioid cell types; patients with these types of tumors had a 62 percent death rate due to metastasis.

Callender's classification has been criticized both because it is too complicated and because it is an oversimplification. Investigators at the AFIP have simplified Callender's classification by deleting the fascicular class and combining the spindle A and B types of tumors. In 1962, Paul and co-workers (66) argued that the prognosis for patients with fascicular and spindle B

types of tumors was similar and combined them for statistical analysis. Since 1962, fascicular tumors have been classified at the AFIP by their cytologic composition. Although most fascicular tumors are composed of a mixture of spindle A and B type cells, some contain only bland spindle A cells while others are of mixed cell type.

In 1972, McLean and co-workers (58) reexamined 105 tumors classified as spindle A type by their predecessors at the AFIP. The purpose of this study was to investigate two problems with Callender's classification. First, Callender provided no criteria for distinguishing spindle A type malignant melanomas from nevi. Second, there was no clear criteria for classifying tumors composed of a mixture of spindle A and B cells. In their study, McLean et al. found that 15 of the 105 tumors originally classified as spindle A type were cytologically benign. These tumors were composed of spindle-shaped cells that had a lower nuclear-cytoplasmic ratio and finer, less hyperchromatic chromatin than the cytologically malignant spindle A type cells. Because none of the 15 patients with these tumors died, McLean et al. reclassified these tumors as spindle cell nevi. They documented several examples of tumors composed of cytologically malignant spindle A type cells, without the spindle B or epithelioid types of cells, which killed by metastasis. In one case, examination of foci of metastatic melanoma in the liver revealed that the metastases were composed of a pure population of spindle A type cells. Thus, tumors classified by Callender as spindle A type included both benign and malignant neoplasms. Since the prognosis of cytologically malignant spindle A type tumors is similar to that of spindle B type tumors, McLean et al. (58) recommended that Callender's spindle A and B types be combined and designated spindle cell type melanomas. This designation also eliminates the problem of classifying tumors composed of a mixture of spindle A and B type cells.

The major problem with Callender's classification is that it represents an oversimplification. Callender recognized only three types of cells in uveal malignant melanomas, but the cells actually exist in a spectrum ranging from bland spindle A type to anaplastic bizarre epithelioid cells. Within this spectrum are spindle-shaped cells that lack cohesion. These cells may have the relatively large eosinophilic nucleolus characteristic of epithelioid cells. There are also polyhedral cells that are cohesive, with fibrillar cytoplasm and relatively small eosinophilic nucleoli characteristic of spindle B type cells. Should these cells be classified purely on the basis of shape or by their other features?

Callender's mixed cell type causes additional problems. There is no agreement as to what percentage of the cells have to be epithelioid to classify a tumor as mixed cell type. Are fewer epithelioid cells required if they are large and anaplastic than if they deviate only minimally from spindle B type cells? Because of these complexities, there is poor agreement among pathologists when using the Callender classification. When five ophthalmic pathologists from different countries reviewed uveal melanomas for the World Health Organization, at least two of the five disagreed with the other pathologists' classification of cell type 60 percent of the time.

Immunohistochemical Findings. Since uveal melanocytic cells are of neural crest derivation, the tumors derived from them would be expected to contain S-100 protein (45). HMB-45 is a monoclonal antibody against a protein obtained from cutaneous malignant melanoma and

Table 5-2

COMPARISON OF DEGREE OF POSITIVITY FOR HMB-45, S-100 PROTEIN, AND NEURON-SPECIFIC ENOLASE IN UVEAL NEVI AND MELANOMAS*

Antibody	Grade[†]	Nevi	Malignant Melanomas
HMB-45	0	0	0
	1	6	0
	2	4	1
	3	3	19
S-100	0	5	2
	1	3	10
	2	3	4
	3	2	4
NSE**	0	5	1
	1	8	8
	2	0	7
	3	0	4

*From reference 11.
**Neuron-specific enolase.
[†]Grade 0 = negative, grade 3 = strongly positive.

is a marker for cells derived from uveal melanocytes as well as from cutaneous melanocytes (fig. 5-48). Neuron-specific enolase (NSE) is an enzyme found in neurons, but a variety of nonneuronal cells express NSE to varying degrees. Burnier et al. (11) compared the immunohistochemical reactivity of 13 uveal nevi and 20 uveal melanomas for HMB-45, S-100 protein, and NSE in formalin-fixed paraffin-embedded sections (Table 5-2). All 33 lesions were positive for HMB-45 (see fig. 5-48). The false-negative rates for S-100 protein and NSE were 21 percent and 18 percent, respectively. If only strongly positive reactions were considered, more than half of the tumors would be interpreted as negative for S-100 protein and NSE. Nevi stained with less intensity than melanomas with all three antibodies. The expression of HMB-45 appeared to be greater in active nevi than in inactive nevi.

Differential Diagnosis. The ability of ophthalmologists to correctly diagnose uveal malignant melanoma and the pseudomelanomas has dramatically improved in the past two decades (14, 17,20,21,70,78,79,82). The most important reason for this has been better education of ophthalmologists and use of the indirect ophthalmoscope. For

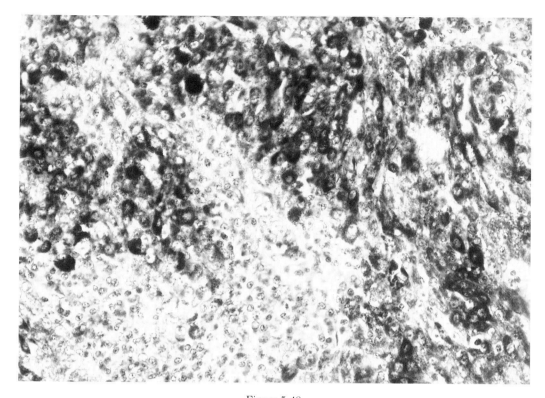

Figure 5-48
MALIGNANT MELANOMA
HMB-45 positive immunoperoxidase staining in a mixed cell type tumor.

medium and large melanomas, the diagnostic error rate for experienced ocular oncologists is less than 1 percent. For very small melanomas, there is no certain way to clinically differentiate these tumors from large nevi. In the United States and Europe many small tumors are treated with photocoagulation or radiotherapy without a histopathologic confirmation of the diagnosis (80) and for these tumors the diagnostic error rate remains unknown.

Diagnostic errors by pathologists are uncommon with uveal melanoma and pseudomelanoma. Tumors that may be confused with uveal malignant melanoma are nevi, leiomyomas, schwannomas, carcinomas of the pigmented neuroepithelia of the eye, and metastatic neoplasms. Immunohistochemistry can aid in correctly diagnosing many of these tumors. An additional diagnostic problem for the inexperienced ocular pathologist is the uveal melanoma that is totally necrotic. These tumors can be overlooked when mixed with other necrotic or degenerated tissues in a phthisical eye.

Prognostic Features. Callender's classification of cell types, as modified at the AFIP, remains one of the most reliable prognosticators despite its lack of reproducibility. Gamel and co-workers (30–32,53,56) searched for more reliable and reproducible techniques by measuring cytologic features. They measured the area, circumference, width, and length of nuclei and nucleoli of cells in 50 uveal malignant melanomas and computed the mean and standard deviation of these measurements. These statistics were compared with Callender's cell types for discriminating between fatal and nonfatal patient outcomes. They found that measurement of nucleolar size was a better predictor of outcome than measurement of nuclear size and that the standard deviation was a better predictor than the mean. The standard deviation of the area, circumference, length, and width of the nucleolus were all better predictors of patient outcome than Callender's cell type. This indicated that the most important prognostic feature in uveal malignant melanoma is not the shape of the cell but the size and variability in size of the nucleolus. They suggested that pathologists should place greater emphasis on nucleolar size and variability than on other cytologic features when using Callender's classification in order to better predict patient outcome (56).

Although the measurement of cytologic features is a more reproducible indicator of prognosis than Callender's classification, it is also more time consuming. Gamel and co-workers (28,29) used a semiautomated image analysis system to measure the standard deviation of the area of 200 nucleoli. An optical drawing tube permitted a technician to trace the outline of the nucleoli of the melanoma cells onto a digitizer. The problem with this methodology is that it took a well-trained technician approximately 30 minutes to trace 200 nucleoli. Two approaches to improving this method are the development of computer-assisted morphometry to the point that manual tracing is obsolete and simplification of the measurements. Both approaches are being explored, however, more progress has occurred in simplifying nucleolar measurement. Measuring the diameter of the 10 largest nucleoli in a uveal malignant melanoma with a Filar micrometer can be done more easily and quickly than measuring the standard deviation of nucleolar area; these two parameters are equally associated with patient outcome (29,53).

The size of the uveal malignant melanoma is as important a predictor of patient outcome as the cytologic features. The problem with using size as a prognostic feature, however, is related to the difficulty in measuring the size of an irregularly shaped object. Flocks et al. (23) suggested using the volume of a cube equal to the length times the width of the base of the tumor times the maximum height. This volume obviously exaggerates the true volume of the tumor but was strongly associated with patient outcome. Of 210 tumors, those larger than the median volume of 1344 mm^3 were associated with a 54 percent mortality rate while the smaller tumors were associated with a 15 percent mortality rate. Surprisingly, when these tumors were divided into quartiles based on volume, there was no difference in mortality between the first and second quartiles and between the third and fourth quartiles. This finding gave rise to the popular notion that a dramatic transition occurs in uveal malignant melanomas at a volume of 1345 mm^3 that results in increased mortality.

McLean et al. (54) analyzed 217 cases of uveal malignant melanoma in which the tumor measured less than 1400 mm3 (length times width times height). This sample included the 105 small uveal malignant melanomas in which Flocks et al. (23) reported no association between volume and patient outcome. In this larger series of small tumors, there was a weak association between volume and outcome, but more important, the largest tumor dimension was a much better prognosticator than volume. There are probably several reasons why largest dimension has a better association with patient outcome than does volume. Most important is that diffuse type malignant melanomas, which have a poor prognosis, typically have a very large linear size but a small volume. Another reason is the difficulty in measuring the volume of uveal malignant melanomas. It is possible that more accurate methods of measuring volume than those employed by Flocks and McLean would result in better prediction.

In 1977, McLean et al. (54) introduced the use of multivariate analysis in the study of prognostic factors for uveal malignant melanoma. This type of analysis determines which factors among a group of predictors are most directly associated with patient outcome. In multivariate analysis, the degree of the association between a prognostic factor and outcome that is due to its association with other factors can be determined. For example, by univariate analysis McLean found that pigmentation was strongly associated with a fatal outcome but pigmentation was not a significant predictor when the largest dimension and cell type of the tumors were taken into consideration. By multivariate analysis, the variables that were the best predictors of patient outcome were cell type and largest dimension of the tumor. Weaker associations with patient outcome, which were still significant by multivariate analysis, were found for invasion into the sclera and mitotic activity.

Univariate and multivariate analyses have been employed in a variety of studies investigating prognostic factors in uveal melanomas. Almost invariably, these studies reconfirmed the importance of tumor size and cytology as significant prognostic factors (29,38,54,55,76). Invasion into the sclera, tumor location within the

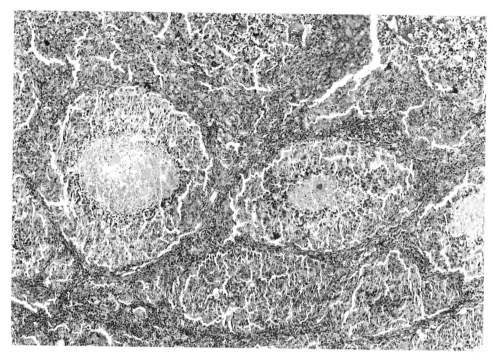

Figure 5-49
MALIGNANT MELANOMA
Partially necrotic tumor.

eye, mitotic activity, necrosis (fig. 5-49), DNA aneuploidy, and neovascularization characterized by the presence of closed vascular loops were significant factors in most studies (4,6,18,24,29, 57). All these studies were based on malignant melanomas of the choroid and ciliary body. Because iris tumors are smaller, less likely to contain epithelioid type cells, and less likely to metastasize than choroidal tumors, size and cell type are believed to be prognostic factors. Because of the rarity of metastasis of iris tumors, this belief has not been confirmed by direct analysis (5,42,71,84).

Most studies of prognostic factors in cases of uveal malignant melanoma have not examined host factors. McLean et al. (54) observed that even when multiple features were predictive of a fatal outcome, some patients survived for many years without developing metastasis. They suggested that a major reason for failure of predictions based on the features of the tumor was variation in host defenses. The majority of infiltrating lymphocytes in tumors including uveal malignant melanoma are cytotoxic/suppressor T lymphocytes (19). These lymphocytes are believed to represent an important component in the host's immune re-

sponse to tumors (63). Contrary to what has been found in many tumors, two studies of the prognostic significance of infiltrating lymphocytes in uveal melanomas (fig. 5-50) found that lymphocytic infiltration was associated with a worse prognosis (18,88). Kranda et al. (46) observed that an abnormal ganglioside profile on the surface of melanoma cells was related to both mixed cell type and lymphocytic infiltration, suggesting that more malignant uveal melanomas may be more antigenic.

Recurrence and Metastasis. The relationship between extension outside of the eye, orbital recurrence, and metastasis is not as important in uveal malignant melanoma as it is in retinoblastoma (81). In retinoblastoma, extraocular extension is the most important prognostic feature; in uveal malignant melanoma, this is of minor prognostic value. Most of the significance of extraocular extension results from association with other features of the tumor. Tumors that are large and contain epithelioid cells are more likely to have extraocular extension. For most fatal cases with extraocular extension, the cause of death is hematogenous metastasis to the liver.

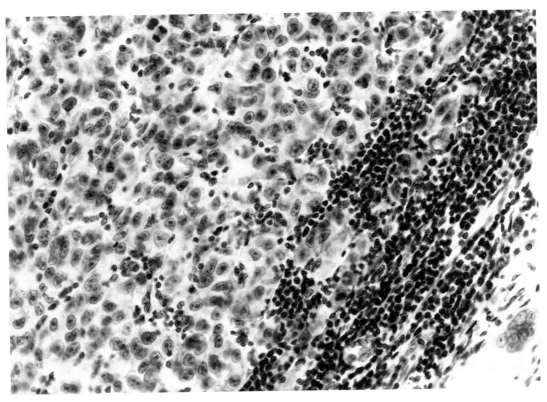

Figure 5-50
MALIGNANT MELANOMA
Tumor-infiltrating lymphocytes are present in small clusters and scattered throughout the mixed cell type neoplasm.

Detection of metastasis is uncommon at the time of enucleation, but with long-term follow-up metastases will develop in most patients. Lorigan et al. (47) studied the location of metastases using imaging in 110 patients with metastatic uveal melanoma. Hepatic metastasis developed in 101 patients (92 percent). The liver was involved initially in 94 patients (85 percent) and it was the only initial metastatic site in 60 patients (55 percent). Only one patient initially had isolated lymph node metastasis in the mediastinum. Abdominal and axillary lymph nodes were involved secondary to hepatic and pulmonary metastases in 13 patients (12 percent). We are aware of only a few cases of uveal malignant melanoma that spread to regional lymph nodes and in none of these cases did the patient die of local extension. This suggests that the biology of metastases of uveal melanoma is different from cutaneous melanoma and retinoblastoma, which are more likely to invade locally and spread to regional lymph nodes. The high prevalence of hepatic metastasis with uveal mela-

noma cannot be explained by venous drainage and indicates a selection process by the disseminated tumor cells.

Treatment. Most uveal melanomas are treated promptly after discovery. Gallagher et al. (28) found that in 47 percent of patients, treatment was initiated 4 or more months after presentation but in half of these cases the delay was intentional, occurring with patients whose small tumors were observed for growth to support the diagnosis of malignant melanoma. Unlike retinoblastoma, delays in treatment of uveal melanoma do not worsen survival (34). Some investigators have questioned the efficacy of enucleation (55,98) and some have postulated that enucleation may cause or stimulate metastasis (62,91). Radiation therapy seems as effective as enucleation (7,74) and is now being evaluated as an alternative to enucleation in a randomized clinical trial. Others argue that treatment other than enucleation can rarely be justified for uveal malignant melanoma (51).

HEMANGIOMA

Choroidal hemangiomas may be either localized or diffuse vascular hamartomas. The diffuse type involves most of the choroid and is associated with the Sturge-Weber syndrome (figs. 5-51, 5-52). The localized form involves only a small portion of the choroid, has no association with systemic abnormalities, and may be confused clinically with uveal melanoma.

In the series of Witschel and Font (100), the two types of choroidal hemangioma differed in their clinical presentation. The age at onset of ocular symptoms with solitary hemangioma (range, 8 to 66 years; median, 38.7 years) was slightly lower but similar to that of uveal melanoma. With the diffuse type, the age at onset of symptoms was usually in childhood but some lesions presented in adults (range, 0 to 52 years; median, 7.6 years). While most of the affected eyes in patients with localized hemangioma were enucleated because of a suspected uveal melanoma, the patients with the diffuse type were enucleated because of blind painful eyes

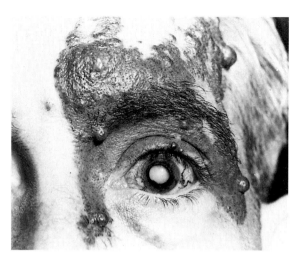

Figure 5-51
STURGE-WEBER SYNDROME
Nevus flammeus of the skin and conjunctiva, with glaucoma and secondary cataract.

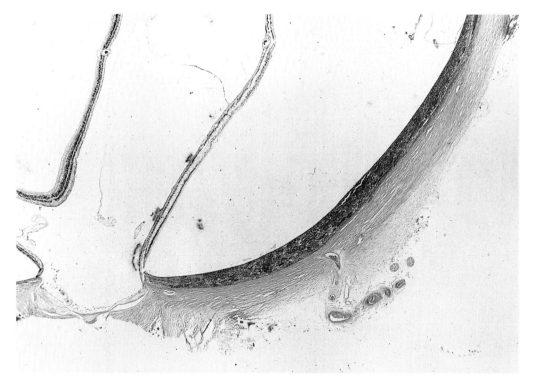

Figure 5-52
STURGE-WEBER SYNDROME
Diffuse hemangioma of the choroid.

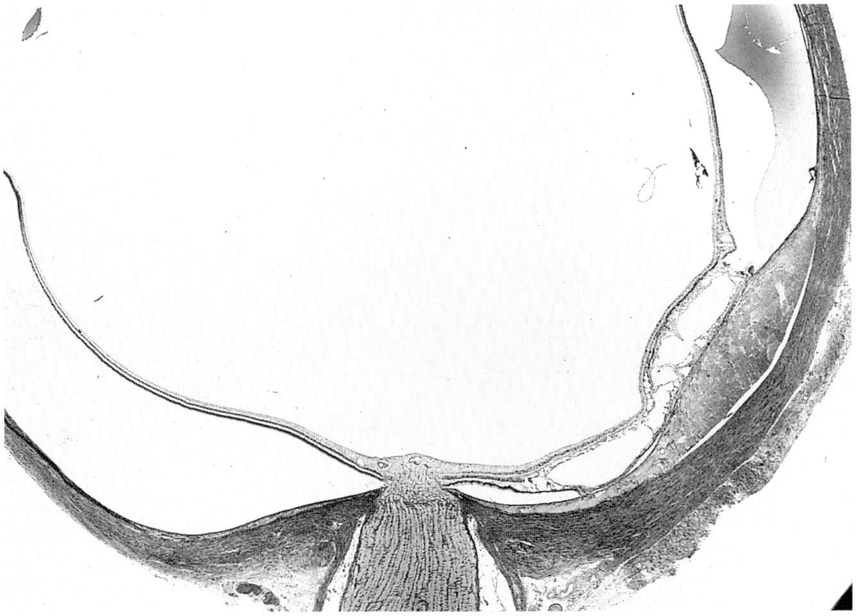

Figure 5-53
CAVERNOUS HEMANGIOMA
Localized choroid tumor with cystoid degeneration of the overlying retina and serous retinal detachment.

usually due to refractory glaucoma. The diffuse type occurred more commonly in males.

Histopathologically, all of the localized hemangiomas had clearly demarcated borders, frequently with compression of choroidal tissue adjacent to the lesion (figs. 5-53, 5-54). In the diffuse lesions, there was a gradual transition at the edge with progressively less engorgement of vessels. The size of the blood vessels in these tumors varied. Witschel and Font found that of 45 localized tumors, 3 were capillary, 20 were cavernous, and 22 were mixed capillary and cavernous. All 17 cases of diffuse hemangioma were mixed. The choroidal hemangiomas induced changes in the overlying RPE and retina (fig. 5-55). These changes, in part, were responsible for visual impairment and ophthalmoscopic abnormalities. The RPE changes ranged from mild atrophy and drusen formation to marked fibrous metaplasia. Focal chorioretinal adhesions, retinal detachment, and severe cystic degeneration with gliosis of the retina were common (fig. 5-53).

Glaucoma is frequently associated with choroidal hemangiomas. In Witschel and Font's series, 18 of 45 (40 percent) eyes with localized tumors had angle closure glaucoma caused by iris neovascularization. Of 17 eyes with diffuse hemangioma, 13 (76 percent) were glaucomatous. Nine had neovascular glaucoma, 3 had glaucoma attributed to incomplete development

of the anterior chamber angle, and 1 had an episcleral vascular hamartoma that presumably elevated the episcleral venous pressure.

Treatment with argon laser over the area of tumor may be effective in reducing or eliminating associated retinal detachment. Sanborn, Augsburger, and Shields (99) treated 40 choroidal hemangiomas with secondary nonrhegmatogenous retinal detachment involving the macula in an effort to bring about resolution of the retinal detachment and not destroy the tumor. Of the 40 eyes treated, 33 (83 percent) exhibited resolution of the detachment but in 17 of these 33 eyes the retinal detachment recurred.

CHOROIDAL OSTEOMA

Choroidal osteoma is a rare choristoma that is usually found in young white women; however some men, children, older adults, and nonwhites are also affected (101). The lesions are located in the posterior pole and may surround the optic disc. Ophthalmoscopically, there is an orange to yellow, discrete, geographic choroidal mass with a scalloped border. Clinical evidence of enlargement has been noted in many cases (101).

Histopathologically, the lesion is composed of normal-appearing cancellous bone located within the peripapillary choroid (figs. 5-56, 5-57). The intratrabecular spaces are filled with a loose

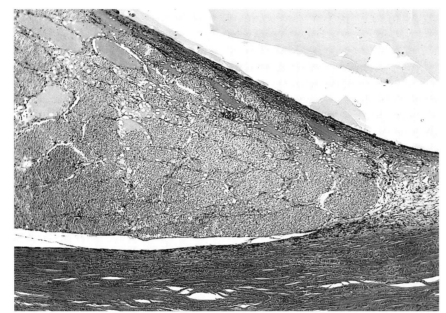

Figure 5-54
CAVERNOUS HEMANGIOMA
Higher power magnification of tumor in previous figure showing blood filled, dilated, thin-walled vessels.

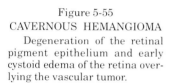

Figure 5-55
CAVERNOUS HEMANGIOMA
Degeneration of the retinal pigment epithelium and early cystoid edema of the retina overlying the vascular tumor.

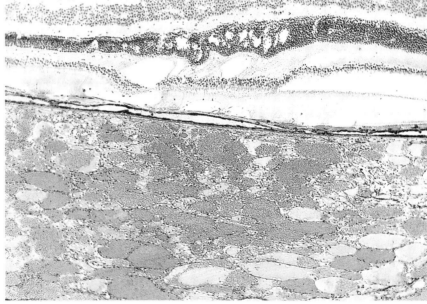

connective tissue containing large and small blood vessels and vacuolated mesenchymal cells (102).

A much more common lesion that must be distinguished from the choroidal osteoma is osseous metaplasia of the RPE. These lesions consist of masses of bone formed by metaplasia of large calcified drusen between the sensory retina and choroid, not within the choroid where osteomas develop. Osseous metaplasia most often occurs in phthisical eyes.

LEIOMYOMA AND MESECTODERMAL LEIOMYOMA

Most uveal leiomyomas occur in the ciliary body where they usually arise from the ciliary muscle, but elsewhere in the uvea they probably arise from vascular smooth muscle. Many of the leiomyomas that have been described in the iris without electron microscopic or immunohisto-chemical confirmation probably represent

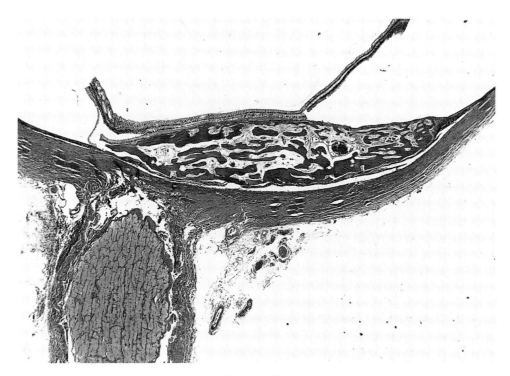

Figure 5-56
OSTEOMA
Choroidal tumor composed of mature bone located at the posterior pole.

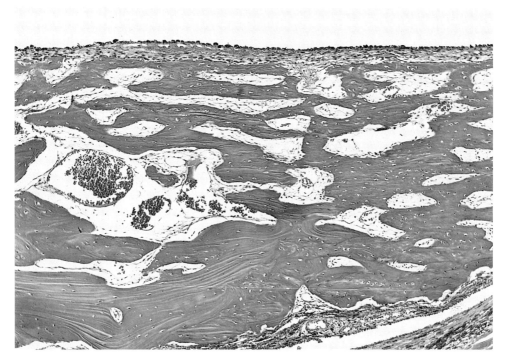

Figure 5-57
OSTEOMA
Higher power magnification of the tumor in the previous figure.

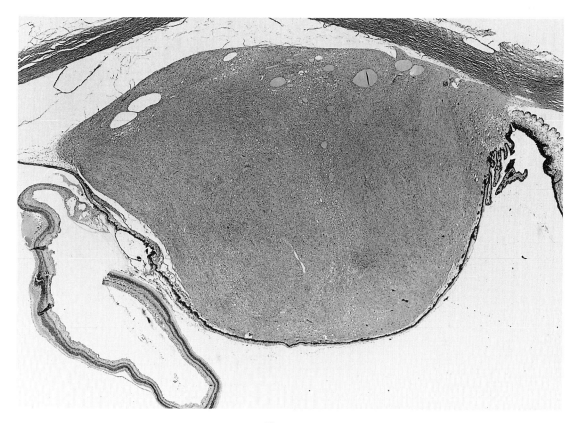

Figure 5-58
MESECTODERMAL LEIOMYOMA
Large, amelanotic tumor of the ciliary body.

melanocytic tumors of spindle cell type. In 1950, Blodi (103) conducted a critical review of the literature of leiomyomas of the ciliary body. He found 10 previously reported cases but none of these cases fulfilled his criteria for diagnosis.

Well-documented cases of ciliary body leiomyoma (figs. 5-58–5-63) have been reported since 1950 (104–107). Meyer and co-workers (106) noted that typical smooth muscle cells have several distinctive ultrastructural characteristics: numerous intracytoplasmic bundles of parallel filaments, fusiform densities in association with the cytoplasmic filaments, subplasmalemmal densities, small vesicular indentations of the plasmalemma (caveolae) between the subplasmalemmal densities, and a basement membrane that completely envelops the cell except for areas of cell attachment or close approximation to adjacent cells (fig. 5-63).

Immunohistochemistry has been helpful in the diagnosis of leiomyoma of the uvea. At the AFIP, we found that most of the tumors stain for muscle-specific actin (HHF-35) but only some stain for desmin. Some pleomorphic carcinomas of the ciliary epithelium may also be weakly reactive for muscle-specific actin. Positive staining for S-100 protein may help distinguish tumors of ciliary epithelial or Schwann cell origin from leiomyomas, which are S-100 negative.

Jakobiec et al. (104) studied two benign ciliary body tumors composed of cells that by light and electron microscopy had both myogenic and neurogenic features (figs. 5-58–5-60). Their first case was interpreted by light microscopy as being a ganglionic tumor or a glial tumor because of prominent cytoplasmic filaments. The second tumor had a prominent fibrillar background and the cystic degeneration suggestive of a schwannoma or neurofibroma, but since the cytoplasmic filaments were positive with phosphotungstic acid hematoxylin (PTAH), a glial or smooth muscle tumor was likely. Subsequent similar cases

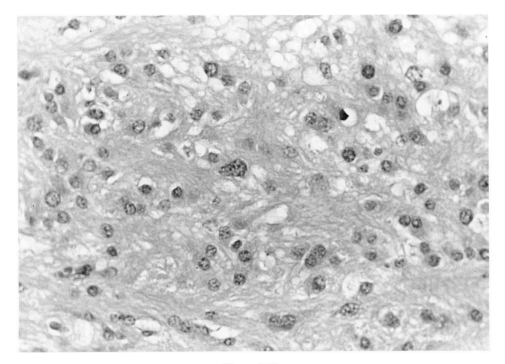

Figure 5-59
MESECTODERMAL LEIOMYOMA
Higher power magnification of tumor in figure 5-58 showing benign cells with round nuclei containing fine chromatin and interlacing fibrillar cytoplasmic processes resembling glial tissue.

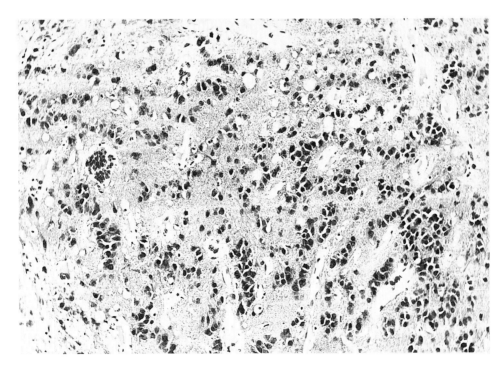

Figure 5-60
MESECTODERMAL LEIOMYOMA
Benign neoplastic cells with nuclei forming clusters separated by fibrillar cytoplasmic processes resembling neural tissue.

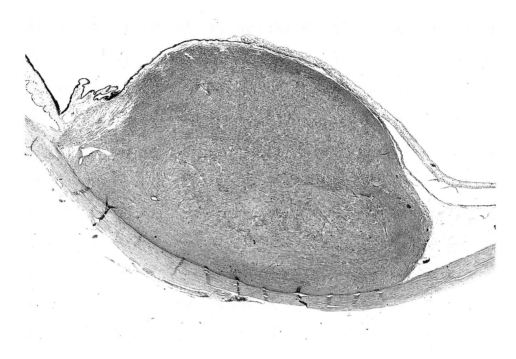

Figure 5-61
LEIOMYOMA
Amelanotic tumor of the ciliary body.

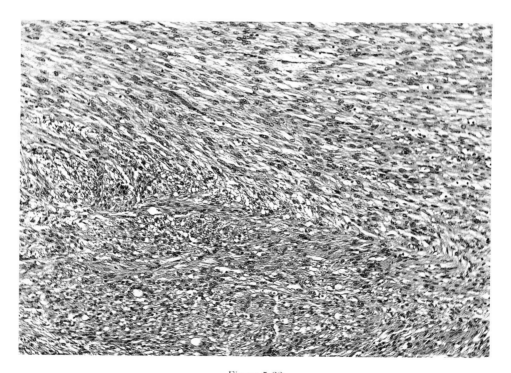

Figure 5-62
LEIOMYOMA
Higher power magnification of tumor seen in previous figure illustrating spindle-shaped neoplastic cells with cigar-shaped nuclei arranged in irregular bundles.

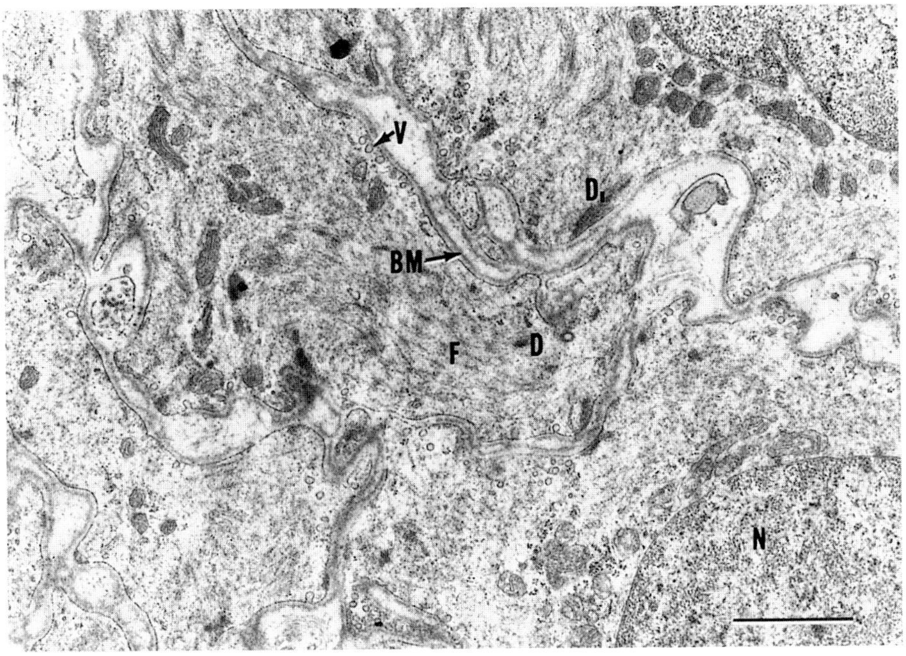

Figure 5-63
LEIOMYOMA
Electron micrograph of the previous tumor showing cells with basement membrane (BM), subplasmalemmal vesicles (V), and intracytoplasmic filaments (F) with fusiform densities (D).

studied at the AFIP have shown strong reactivity for muscle-specific actin and negative staining for S-100 protein and glial fibrillary acidic protein (GFAP).

Embryologic experiments in chicks have demonstrated that the ocular and orbital supporting tissues are of neural crest origin. The cells of the neural crest that contribute to the formation of bone, cartilage, connective tissue, and smooth muscle in the head and neck have been called mesectoderm. Jakobiec suggested that the neuroglial appearance of these tumors reflects their origin from mesectoderm, hence the name mesectodermal leiomyoma.

LEUKEMIA

Ocular involvement in the course of leukemia is very common. Clinically, the retina is most often involved but histopathologic studies indicate a higher rate of uveal involvement, which is often not detected clinically (108). The most common finding in eyes obtained at autopsy from patients with acute leukemia is dilated blood vessels stuffed with atypical blastic cells. Variable amounts of perivascular infiltration may be present with the formation of a choroidal tumor (figs. 5-64–5-66).

JUVENILE XANTHOGRANULOMA

This benign dermatologic disorder is characterized by yellowish pink nodules on the skin of children and young adults. The skin lesions typically involute spontaneously within a year leaving a small scar. In a few cases (109–112) there was ocular involvement and, rarely, ocular disease without cutaneous involvement. The anterior uvea is most frequently involved but other sites including the conjunctiva, optic nerve, and orbit may be affected (112). Clinically, the iris is thickened by a cellular infiltrate that can mimic a diffuse melanoma of the iris (fig. 5-67). There is usually neovascularization and hemorrhage into the anterior chamber. The iris lesions slowly resolve but, frequently, anterior synechia form, occluding the anterior chamber angle and leading to chronic glaucoma. Histologically, the iris and ciliary body are infiltrated by mildly atypical histiocytes (figs. 5-68–5-71). Mitotic activity is variable but xanthogranulomas with one or more mitotic figures per high-power field may be seen. A characteristic feature of the tumor is the presence of Touton giant cells (fig. 5-71); however, these can be rare. Frozen sections stained for fat usually show lipid droplets within the histiocytes and giant cells.

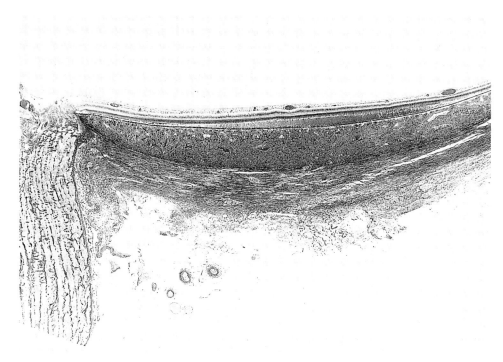

Figure 5-64
GRANULOCYTIC LEUKEMIA
Diffuse choroidal infiltration.

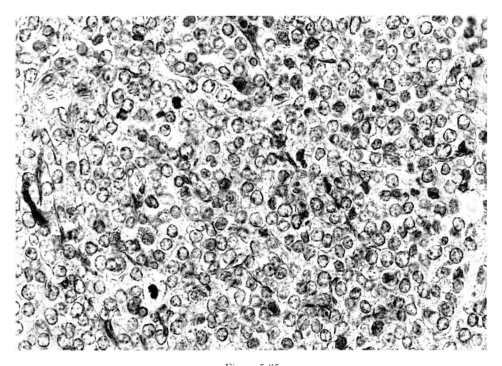

Figure 5-65
GRANULOCYTIC LEUKEMIA
Higher power magnification of the tumor in previous figure showing round malignant cells with mitotic activity.

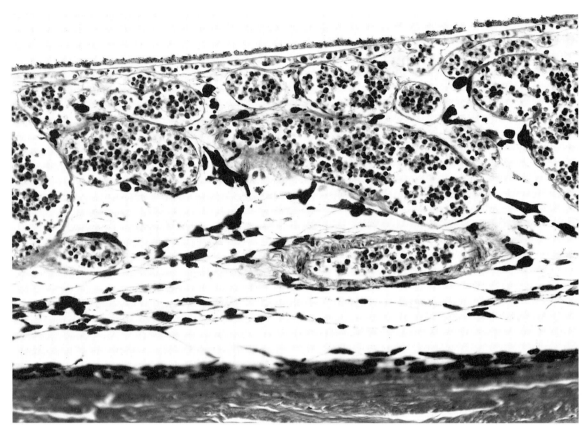

Figure 5-66
LYMPHOBLASTIC LEUKEMIA
Choroidal blood vessels filled with round neoplastic cells.

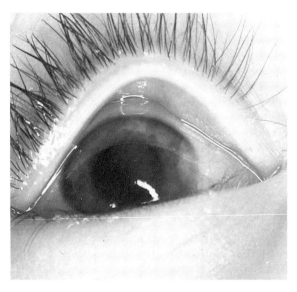

Figure 5-67
JUVENILE XANTHOGRANULOMA
Whitish tumor masses on the surface of the iris.

WELL-DIFFERENTIATED SMALL LYMPHOCYTIC OR LYMPHOPLASMACYTIC LYMPHOMA AND SECONDARY LYMPHOMAS OF THE UVEA

Clinical Features. These entities are difficult to diagnose clinically because the extensive thickening of the uvea may lead to the false impression of a diffuse uveal melanoma (113). Most of these lesions have been diagnosed only after enucleation.

Pathologic Findings. These tumors were originally classified as reactive lymphoid hyperplasias (113,115) but using modern immunohistochemistry, most of them display a monoclonal immunologic staining pattern indicative of a well-differentiated B-cell lymphoma. The uveal tract is diffusely thickened by an infiltrate of small mature lymphocytes. Germinal centers

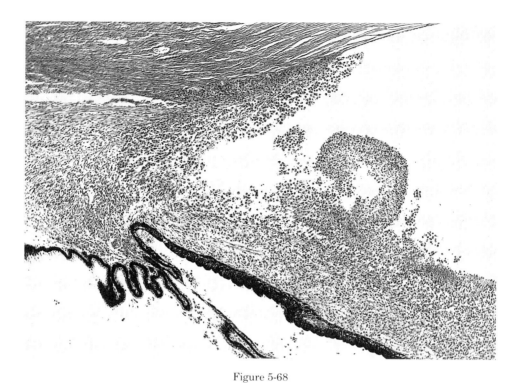

Figure 5-68
JUVENILE XANTHOGRANULOMA
Infiltrative histiocytic cells involving the iris and anterior chamber angle structures. (Figures 5-68–5-70 are from the same patient.)

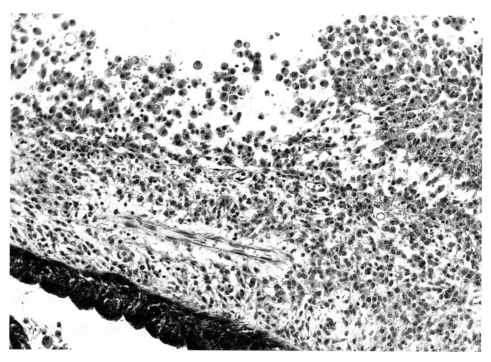

Figure 5-69
JUVENILE XANTHOGRANULOMA
Higher power magnification of tumor showing an iris stroma and anterior chamber.

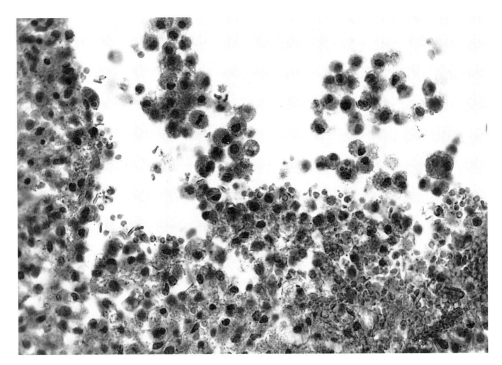

Figure 5-70
JUVENILE XANTHOGRANULOMA
Higher power magnification illustrating histiocytic cells with mitotic activity.

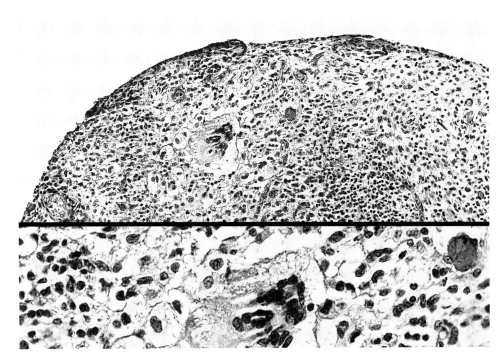

Figure 5-71
JUVENILE XANTHOGRANULOMA
Foamy histiocytic proliferation with Touton giant cells.

may be scattered throughout the uveal infiltrate, and there may be abundant plasma cells as well as lymphoplasmacytoid cells with periodic acid–Schiff (PAS)-positive intranuclear inclusions (Dutcher bodies) (115). Orbital involvement is seen in many of the cases (see fig. 7-50), but is usually not sufficiently exuberant to cause proptosis. Most of these patients present with localized disease but the work-up should include staging for systemic lymphoma and serum immunoelectrophoresis for Waldenström macroglobulinemia or other dysproteinemias when the tumors are lymphoplasmacytic. If the lesion can be accurately diagnosed clinically, systemically administered corticosteroids and low doses of radiotherapy to the globe itself can bring about a dramatic resolution of uveal tumefaction.

It is important to distinguish malignant lymphoma of the retina from malignant lymphoma of the uvea (see chapter, Tumors of the Retina). Malignant lymphoma of the retina is typically a high-grade, large cell lymphoma that affects the central nervous system. These patients usually die from involvement of the brain and rarely have systemic disease. Uveal lymphoma is usually a well-differentiated low-grade tumor with an indolent course. Some patients develop systemic lymphoma only after many years and central nervous system involvement is rare. The uvea may be involved secondarily by higher grade lymphomas but this usually occurs in patients with orbital involvement long after nodal or other visceral lesions have been recognized. Burkitt lymphoma of the orbit may also involve the uvea (114).

METASTATIC TUMORS

The incidence of cancer metastatic to the eye is unknown, but it is estimated to be greater than the incidence of primary uveal melanoma. Most ocular metastases occur in terminally ill patients whose eyes are not studied postmortem. In a 5-year period, we found metastases to the eye in 23 cases in the ROP (Table 5-3) and 18 cases in the Brazilian Registry (116). Only 22 cases of metastatic carcinoma to the eye and orbit were encountered in Denmark from 1944 to 1968 (121).

Ferry and Font (117,118) studied 227 metastatic tumors to the eye and orbit on file in the AFIP ROP. The eye was predominantly involved

Table 5-3

**METASTATIC TUMORS
OF THE UVEAL TRACT***

Type of Tumor	Number of Cases
Carcinoid	1
Melanoma	2
Carcinoma	20
Sarcoma	0

*Frequency distribution of 23 tumors in the AFIP Registry of Ophthalmic Pathology collected between 1984 and 1989.

in 196 cases, the orbit in 28, and the optic nerve in 3. The anterior segment of the eye was the only site of metastasis in 26 (11.4 percent) and the posterior segment in 112 (49.3 percent) patients. Stephens and Shields (123) observed the site of metastases in 83 eyes to be: choroid, 77 (93 percent); iris, 3 (4 percent); ciliary body, 1 (1 percent); iris and choroid, 1 (1 percent); and ciliary body and choroid, 1 (1 percent). Multiple foci were present in 30 of 227 eyes (13 percent) of the Ferry and Font series. Multiple foci of tumor in one eye or bilateral metastases were observed in 15 of the 70 cases (21 percent) reported by Stephens and Shields.

Ocular metastases are seen in all ages but are most common between 40 and 70 years of age. The presenting ocular signs and symptoms vary, depending on the size, location, and secondary effects of the tumor. Blurred vision and pain are the most common. There is a slight female predominance in most series, because breast carcinoma metastasizes most frequently. In the data combined from several reported series (117, 118,123), the sites of primary tumors were breast in 47 percent; lung in 25 percent; kidney and gastrointestinal tract in 3 percent each; testes in 2 percent; and prostate, pancreas, thyroid, and melanoma of skin in 1 percent each. Other sites of primary tumors (ovary and cervix) occurred as single cases. In 15 percent of the cases the primary site was unknown.

The diagnoses of the referring ophthalmologists in 56 patients of the Stephens and Shields series were metastatic tumor, 21 (38 percent);

retinal detachment, 17 (30 percent); mass lesion, 11 (20 percent); choroidal melanoma, 4 (7 percent); central serous chorioretinopathy, 1 (2 percent); choroidal hemangioma, 1 (2 percent); and endophthalmitis, 1 (2 percent).

Ocular metastasis may be the first sign of an asymptomatic primary tumor. In the Ferry and Font series, eye symptoms preceded the detection of the primary neoplasm in 105 of the 227 cases (46.3 percent). In 7 cases the detection of the primary and the onset of eye symptoms occurred at about the same time. In the study of Stephens and Shields, the ocular lesions preceded the detection of the primary in 22 of the 70 cases (31 percent). There was a striking difference in this feature with the two most common metastatic tumors. Only 9 of the 45 cases (12.8 percent) of ocular metastases of breast carcinoma preceded the detection of the primary tumor. Of the 10 cases of lung carcinoma, the ocular metastases preceded the detection of the primary in 7 (70 percent).

Generally, the development of ocular metastases is a bad prognostic sign. Of the 227 patients in the series of Ferry and Font, 192 died of metastatic tumor. In the study by Stephens and Shields, patients with primary lesions of the breast showed considerable variability, with a mean survival of 13.4 months and a median survival of 8 months. Patients with primary lung tumors had a mean survival of 5.2 months and a median survival of 3.3 months.

An exception to this dismal outlook is metastasis from a carcinoid tumor. A number of case reports have described uneventful follow-up 1 to 8 years after diagnosis of metastatic carcinoid tumor. Riddle et al. (122) reported the features of 15 cases of metastatic carcinoid. The site of the metastasis was the orbit in 7 cases, the choroid in 7 cases, and the iris in 1 case. The primary site of origin was determined in 12 cases: bronchus in 7, trachea in 1, and ileum in 4 cases.

Certain features are characteristic of metastatic tumors. Multiple tumors are more apt to occur with metastatic disease. The metastatic tumor is more likely to have a flat and diffuse configuration (fig. 5-72). Occasionally, metastatic lesions have a dome-shaped configuration similar to that seen with some primary choroidal melanomas. Mushroom-shaped configurations,

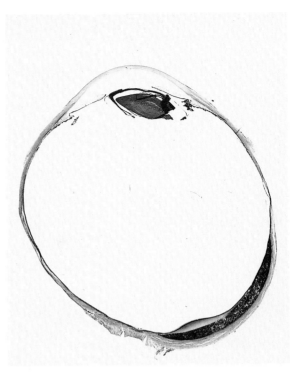

Figure 5-72
METASTATIC ADENOCARCINOMA
Flat choroidal tumor.

so typical of melanomas, are rarely seen with metastatic tumors.

The histopathologic features generally reflect those of the primary tumor (figs. 5-73–5-75). In many instances, the metastatic lesions are composed of undifferentiated cells and do not allow for identification of the probable primary. In such cases the history of a documented primary tumor becomes most important.

Differentiating among primary sites for carcinomas metastatic to the eye is usually difficult. Breast carcinoma metastases are usually moderately or well differentiated, maintaining features of an adenocarcinoma, with cells arranged in ducts surrounded by a desmoplastic stroma. Some show mucin production with the Alcian blue, colloidal iron, and mucicarmine stains. A single file or histiocytoid pattern is not seen in the uvea as often as it is in metastases to the lid and orbit. Metastases from bronchogenic carcinomas are often undifferentiated but may rarely have a squamoid appearance. Oat cell carcinoma

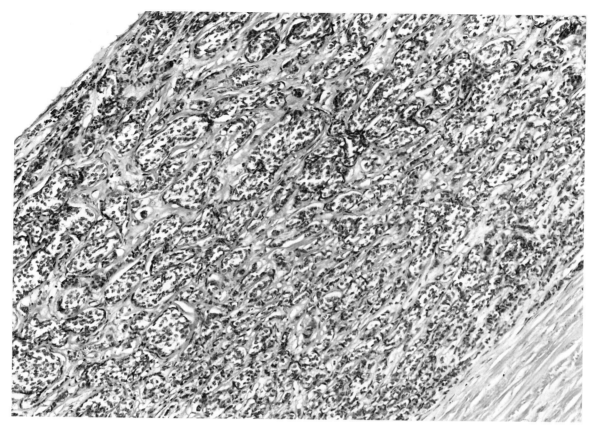

Figure 5-73
METASTATIC ADENOCARCINOMA
Choroidal infiltration by poorly differentiated neoplastic epithelial cells with desmoplastic reaction.

metastases of the lung consist of small cells that are often undifferentiated. Occasionally, a biphasic pattern of large and small cells may be observed. Metastatic tumors from the gastrointestinal tract usually demonstrate mucin production. Metastatic prostatic carcinoma often maintains an adenoid or glandular pattern. The tumor cells have round, vesicular nuclei, prominent nucleoli, and abundant eosinophilic cytoplasm. Metastatic thyroid carcinoma is usually of the follicular type.

Metastatic melanoma, although often not pigmented, usually shows microscopic histochemical evidence of melanin production (119). Differentiating between primary and metastatic melanoma may be difficult. Font and co-workers (120) noted the following helpful points: metastatic tumors are typically multiple and flat in the uveal tract; tumor emboli are observed in choroid, ciliary body, or retinal vessels; associated nevus cells at the base of the tumor are lacking; and epithelioid cell types are consistently present.

By light microscopy, carcinoid tumors are seen to be composed of round, polygonal, or spindle-shaped cells arranged in nests, strands, or cords that are separated by connective tissue. Carcinoid tumor cells may show a positive argyrophilic reaction, reduce ferric ferricyanide, and display the azocoupling reaction. By electron microscopy, membrane-bound neurosecretory granules are observed in the cytoplasm.

Immunohistochemistry is very helpful in the differential diagnosis of metastatic tumors to the eye. Cytokeratin and HMB-45 can be used to distinguish carcinomas from primary and metastatic melanomas. NSE, chromogranin, and synaptophysin can be used to identify carcinoid tumors. Staining for prostate-specific antigen (124) and thyroglobulin are useful for identifying metastatic prostate and thyroid tumors.

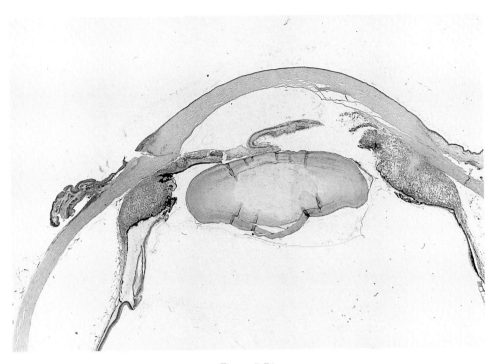

Figure 5-74
METASTATIC ADENOCARCINOMA
Iris and ciliary body involvement by an epithelial neoplasm. Specimen from an autopsy of a patient with a previous surgical wound from the iridectomy.

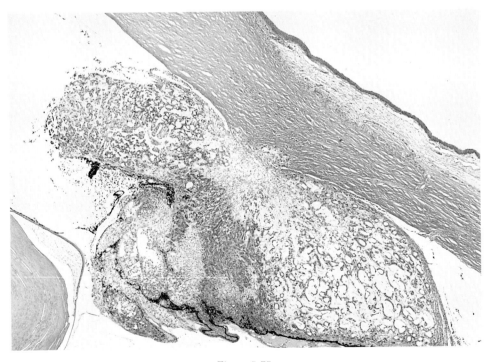

Figure 5-75
METASTATIC ADENOCARCINOMA
Higher power magnification of tumor in the previous figure showing a glandular pattern of the neoplastic epithelial cells.

REFERENCES

General References

Fine BS, Yanoff M. Ocular histology. A text and atlas. 2nd ed. Harper & Row: New York, 1979:195–248.

Jakobiec FA. Ocular anatomy, embryology and teratology. Philadelphia: Harper & Row, 1982:441–552.

Anatomy and Histology

1. Torczynski E, Tso MO. The architecture of the choriocapillaris at the posterior pole. Am J Ophthalmol 1976;81:428–40.

Classification and Frequency

2. Burnier MN Jr, Neves RA, Pereira MG, Alberti VN, Rigueiro MP. The use of the peroxidase-anti-peroxidase technique in ocular pathology. Arch I P B 1988;30:181–4.
3. Young JL, Percy CL, Asira AJ, et al. Surveillance, epidemiology, and end results: incidence and mortality data, 1973-77. NCI Monograph 57. Bethesda: National Institutes of Health, 1981.

Nevi and Malignant Melanoma

4. Affeldt JC, Minckler DS, Azen SP, Yeh L. Prognosis in uveal melanoma with extrascleral extension. Arch Ophthalmol 1980;98:1975–9.
5. Arentsen JJ, Green WR. Melanoma of the iris: report of 72 cases treated surgically. Ophthalmic Surg 1975;6:23–37.
6. Augsburger JJ, Gamel JW. Clinical prognostic factors in patients with posterior uveal malignant melanoma. Cancer 1990;66:1596–600.
7. _____, Gamel JW, Lauritzen K, Brady LW. Cobalt-60 plaque radiotherapy vs enucleation for posterior uveal melanoma. Am J Ophthalmol 1990;109:585–92.
8. Barr CC, McLean IW, Zimmerman LE. Uveal melanoma in children and adolescents. Arch Ophthalmol 1981;99:2133–6.
9. _____, Zimmerman LE, Curtin VT, Font RL. Bilateral diffuse melanocytic uveal tumors associated with systemic malignant neoplasms: a recently recognized syndrome. Arch Ophthalmol 1982;100:249–55.
10. Broadway D, Lang S, Harper J, et al. Congenital malignant melanoma of the eye. Cancer 1991;67:2642–52.
11. Burnier MN Jr, McLean IW, Gamel JW. Immunohistochemical evaluation of uveal melanocytic tumors. Expression of HMB-45, S-100 protein, and neuron-specific enolase. Cancer 1991;68:809–14.
12. Callender GR. Malignant melanotic tumors of the eye: a study of histologic types in 111 cases. Trans Am Acad Ophthalmol Otolaryngol 1931;36:131–42.
13. _____, Wilder HC, Ash JE. Five hundred melanomas of the choroid and ciliary body: followed five years or longer. Am J Ophthalmol 1942;25:562–7.
14. Chang M, Zimmerman LE, McLean IW. The persisting pseudomelanoma problem. Arch Ophthalmol 1984; 102:726–7.
15. Copeman MC. The putative melanoma tumor-suppressor gene on human chromosome 6q. Pathology 1992;24:307–9.
16. Cutler SJ, Young JL. Third National Cancer Survey. Incidence data. NCI Monograph, Vol 41. Bethesda: National Institutes of Health, 1975:1–9.
17. Davidorf FH, Letson AD, Weiss ET, Levine E. Incidence of misdiagnosed and unsuspected choroidal melano-

mas: a 50-year experience. Arch Ophthalmol 1983;101:410–2.
18. de la Cruz PO Jr, Specht CS, McLean IW. Lymphocytic infiltration in uveal malignant melanoma. Cancer 1990;65:112–5.
19. Durie FH, George WD, Campbell AM, Damato BE. Analysis of clonality of tumour infiltrating lymphocytes in breast cancer and uveal melanoma. Immunol Lett 1992;33:263–9.
20. Ferry AP. Hemangiomas of the iris and ciliary body. Do they exist? A search for a histologically proved case. Int Ophthalmol Clin 1972;12:177–94.
21. _____. Lesions mistaken for malignant melanoma of the iris. Arch Ophthalmol 1965;74:9–18.
22. _____. Lesions mistaken for malignant melanoma of the posterior uvea: a clinicopathologic analysis of 100 cases with ophthalmoscopically visible lesions. Arch Ophthalmol 1964;72:463–9.
23. Flocks M, Gerende JH, Zimmerman LE. The size and shape of malignant melanoma of the choroid and ciliary body in relation to prognosis and histologic characteristics. A statistical study of 210 tumors. Trans Am Acad Ophthalmol Otolaryngol 1955;59:740–56.
24. Folberg R, Pe'er J, Gruman LM, et al. The morphologic characteristics of tumor blood vessels as a marker of tumor progression in primary human uveal melanoma: a matched case-control study. Hum Pathol 1992;23:1298–305.
25. Font RL, Spaulding AG, Zimmerman LE. Diffuse malignant melanoma of the uveal tract. A clinicopathologic report of 54 cases. Trans Am Acad Ophthalmol Otolaryngol 1968;72:877–94.
26. _____, Zimmerman LE, Armaly MF. The nature of the orange pigment over a choroidal melanoma. Histochemical and electron microscopical observations. Arch Ophthalmol 1974;91:359–62.
27. Gallagher RP, Elwood JM, Rootman J. Epidemiologic aspects of intraocular malignant melanoma. Cancer Treat Res 1988;43:73–84.
28. _____, Elwood JM, Rootman J, Threlfall WJ, Davis J. Symptoms and time to presentation and treatment in ocular melanoma: the Western Canada Melanoma Study. Can J Ophthalmol 1988;23:11–3.
29. Gamel JW, McCurdy JB, McLean IW. A comparison of prognostic covariates for uveal melanoma. Invest Ophthalmol Vis Sci 1992;33:1919–22.
30. _____, McLean IW. Computerized histopathologic assessment of malignant potential. II. A practical method for predicting survival following enucleation for uveal melanoma. Cancer 1983;52:1032–8.
31. _____, McLean IW, Foster WD, Zimmerman LE. Uveal melanomas: correlation of cytologic features with prognosis. Cancer 1978;41:1897–901.
32. _____, McLean IW, Greenberg RA, Zimmerman LE, Lichtenstein SJ. Computerized histologic assessment of malignant potential: a method for determining the prognosis of uveal melanomas. Hum Pathol 1982;13:893–7.
33. Gass JD. Observation of suspected choroidal and ciliary body melanomas for evidence of growth prior to enucleation. Ophthalmology 1980;87:523–8.
34. _____. Problems in the differential diagnosis of choroidal nevi and malignant melanomas. The XXXIII Edward Jackson Memorial Lecture. Am J Ophthalmol 1977;83:299–323.

35. Green WR. Uveal tract. In: Spencer WH, ed. Ophthalmic pathology. An atlas and textbook. 3rd ed. WB Saunders: Philadelphia, 1985:1522–684.

36. Gonder JR, Ezell PC, Shields JA, Augsburger JJ. Ocular melanocytosis. A study to determine the prevalence rate of ocular melanocytosis. Ophthalmology 1982;89:950–2.

37. _____, Shields JA, Albert DM. Malignant melanoma of the choroid associated with oculodermal melanocytosis. Ophthalmology 1981;88:372–6.

38. Hayton S, Lafreniere R, Jerry LM, Temple WJ, Ashley P. Ocular melanoma in Alberta: a 38 year review pointing to the importance of tumor size and tumor histology as predictors of survival. J Surg Oncol 1989;42:215–8.

39. Holly EA, Aston DA, Ahn DK, Kristiansen JJ, Char DH. No excess prior cancer in patients with uveal melanoma. Ophthalmology 1991;98:608–11.

40. _____, Aston DA, Char DH, Kristiansen JJ, Ahn DK. Uveal melanoma in relation to ultraviolet light exposure and host factors. Cancer Res 1990;50:5773–7.

41. Jakobiec FA, Moorman LT, Jones IS. Benign epithelioid cell nevi of the iris. Arch Ophthalmol 1979;97:917–21.

42. _____, Silbert G. Are most iris "melanomas" really nevi? A clinicopathologic study of 189 lesions. Arch Ophthalmol 1981;99:2117–32.

43. Jay M, McCartney AC. Familial malignant melanoma of the uvea and p53: a Victorian detective story. Surv Ophthalmol 1993;37:457–62.

44. Jensen OA. Malignant melanomas of the human uvea. Recent follow-up of cases in Denmark, 1943-1952. Acta Ophthalmol (Copenh) 1970;48:1113–28.

45. Kan-Mitchell J, Rao N, Albert DM, Van Eldik LJ, Taylor CR. S100 immunophenotypes of uveal melanomas. Invest Ophthalmol Vis Sci 1990;31:1492–6.

46. Kanda S, Cochran AJ, Lee WR, Morton DL, Irie RF. Variations in the ganglioside profile of uveal melanoma correlate with cytologic heterogeneity. Int J Cancer 1992;52:682–7.

47. Lorigan JG, Wallace S, Mavligit GM. The prevalence and location of metastases from ocular melanoma: imaging study in 110 patients. AJR Am J Roentgenol 1991;157:1279–81.

48. Lynch HT, Anderson DE, Krush AJ. Heredity and intraocular malignant melanoma. Cancer 1968;21:119–25.

49. MacIlwaine WA, Anderson B, Klintworth GK. Enlargement of a histologically documented choroidal nevus. Am J Ophthalmol 1979;87:480–6.

50. Manschot WA. Ring melanoma. Arch Ophthalmol 1964;71:625–32.

51. _____, van Strik R. Uveal melanoma: therapeutic consequences of doubling times and irradiation results; a review. Int Ophthalmol 1992;16:91–9.

52. Margo CE, McLean IW. Malignant melanoma of the choroid and ciliary body in black patients. Arch Ophthalmol 1984;102:77–9.

53. McCurdy J, Gamel J, McLean I. A simple, efficient, and reproducible method for estimating the malignant potential of uveal melanoma from routine H&E slides. Pathol Res Pract 1991;187:1025–7.

54. McLean IW, Foster WD, Zimmerman LE. Prognostic factors in small malignant melanomas of choroid and ciliary body. Arch Ophthalmol 1977;95:48–58.

55. _____, Foster WD, Zimmerman LE. Uveal melanoma: location, size, cell type, and enucleation as risk factors in metastasis. Hum Pathol 1982;13:123–32.

56. _____, Foster WD, Zimmerman LE, Gamel JW. Modifications of Callender's classification of uveal melanoma at the Armed Forces Institute of Pathology. Am J Ophthalmol 1983;96:502–9.

57. _____, Gamel JW. Prediction of metastasis of uveal melanoma: comparison of morphometric determination of nucleolar size and spectrophotometric determination of DNA. Invest Ophthalmol Vis Sci 1988;29:507–11.

58. _____, Zimmerman LE, Evans RM. Reappraisal of Callender's spindle A type of malignant melanoma of choroid and ciliary body. Am J Ophthalmol 1978;86:557–64.

59. Memmen JE, McLean IW. The long-term outcome of patients undergoing iridocyclectomy. Ophthalmology 1990;97:429–32.

60. Naumann GOH, Hellner K, Naumann LR. Pigmented nevi of the choroid: clinical study of secondary changes in the overlying tissue. Trans Am Acad Ophthalmol Otolaryngol 1971;75:110–23.

61. Naumann G, Yanoff M, Zimmerman LE. Histiogenesis of malignant melanomas of the uvea. I. Histopathologic characteristics of nevi of the choroid and ciliary body. Arch Ophthalmol 1966;76:784–96.

62. Niederkorn JY. Enucleation-induced metastasis of intraocular melanoma in mice. Ophthalmology 1984;91:692–700.

63. _____. T cell subsets involved in the rejection of metastases arising from intraocular melanomas in mice. Invest Ophthalmol Vis Sci 1987;28:1397–403.

64. Nik NA, Hidayat A, Zimmerman LE, Fine BS. Diffuse iris nevus manifested by unilateral open angle glaucoma. Arch Ophthalmol 1981;99:125–7.

65. Nik ND, Glew WB, Zimmerman LE. Malignant melanoma of the choroid in the nevus of Ota of a black patient. Arch Ophthalmol 1982;100:1641–3.

66. Paul EV, Parnell BL, Fraker M. Prognosis of malignant melanomas of the choroid and ciliary body. Int Ophthalmol Clin 1962;2:387–402.

67. Prescher G, Bornfeld N, Becher R. Nonrandom chromosomal abnormalities in primary uveal melanoma. JNCI 1990;82:1765–9.

68. Rahi AH, Agrawal PK. Prognostic parameters in choroidal melanomata. Trans Ophthalmol Soc UK 1977; 97:368–72.

69. Raivio I. Uveal melanoma in Finland: an epidemiological, clinical, histological, and prognostic study. Acta Ophthalmol (Copenh) 1977;133(Suppl):1–64.

70. Robertson DM, Campbell RJ. Errors in the diagnosis of malignant melanoma of the choroid. Am J Ophthalmol 1979;87:269–75.

71. Rones B, Zimmerman LE. The prognosis of primary tumors of the iris treated by iridectomy. Arch Ophthalmol 1958;60:193–205.

72. Sassani JW, Weinstein JM, Graham WP. Massively invasive diffuse choroidal melanoma [clinical conference]. Arch Ophthalmol 1985;103:945–8.

73. Scotto J, Fraumenti JF Jr, Lee JA. Melanomas of the eye and other noncutaneous sites: epidemiologic aspects. JNCI 1976;56:489–91.

74. Seddon JM, Gragoudas ES, Egan KM, et al. Relative survival rates after alternative therapies for uveal melanoma. Ophthalmology 1990;97:769–77.

75. _____, Gragoudas ES, Glynn RJ, Egan KM, Albert DM, Blitzer PH. Host factors, UV radiation, and risk of uveal melanoma. A case-control study. Arch Ophthalmol 1990;108:1274–80.

76. Shammas HF, Blodi FC. Prognostic factors in choroidal and ciliary body melanomas. Arch Ophthalmol 1977; 95:63–9.

77. Shields CL, Shields JA, Shields MB, Augsburger JJ. Prevalence and mechanisms of secondary intraocular pressure elevation in eyes with intraocular tumors. Ophthalmology 1987;94:839–46.

78. Shields JA, McDonald PR. Improvements in the diagnosis of posterior uveal melanomas. Arch Ophthalmol 1974;91:259–64.

79. _____, Sanborn GE, Augsburger JJ. The differential diagnosis of malignant melanoma of the iris. A clinical study of 200 patients. Ophthalmology 1983;90:716–20.

80. Shields JA, Shields CL. Intraocular tumors. A text and atlas. Philadelphia: WB Saunders, 1992.

81. _____, Shields CL. Massive orbital extension of posterior uveal melanomas. Ophthal Plast Reconstr Surg 1991;7:238–51.

82. _____, Zimmerman LE. Lesions stimulating malignant melanoma of the posterior uvea. Arch Ophthalmol 1973;89:466–71.

83. Sisley K, Cottam DW, Rennie IG, et al. Non-random abnormalities of chromosomes 3, 6, and 8 associated with posterior uveal melanoma. Genes Chromosom Cancer 1992;5:197–200.

84. Sunba MS, Rahi AHS, Morgan G. Tumors of the anterior uvea. I. Metastasizing malignant melanoma of the iris. Arch Ophthalmol 1980;98:82–5.

85. Taylor MR, Guerry D IV, Bondi EE, et al. Lack of association between intraocular melanomas and cutaneous dysplastic nevi. Am J Ophthalmol 1984;98:478–82.

86. Tobal K, Warren W, Cooper CS, McCartney A, Hungerford J, Lightman S. Increased expression and mutation of p53 in choroidal melanoma. Br J Cancer 1992;66:900–4.

87. Vink J, Crijns MB, Mooy CM, Bergman W, Oosterhuis JA, Went LN. Ocular melanoma in families with dysplastic nevus syndrome. J Am Acad Dermatol 1990;23(5 Pt 1):858–62.

88. Vit VV. Prognostic role of morphologic characteristics of the immune response in uveal melanoblastomas of various cellular types [in Russian]. Arkh Patol 1983; 45:25–30.

89. Walker JP, Weiter JJ, Albert DM, Osborn EL, Weichselbaum RR. Uveal malignant melanoma in three generations of the same family. Am J Ophthalmol 1979;88:723–6.

90. Wilder HC, Paul EV. Malignant melanoma of the choroid and ciliary body: a study of 2,535 cases. Mil Surg 1951;109:370–8.

91. Wilson RS, Fraunfelder FT. "No-touch" cryosurgical enucleation: a minimal trauma technique for eyes harboring intraocular malignancy. Trans Am Acad Ophthalmol 1978;85:1170–5.

92. Wiltshire RN, Elner VM, Dennis T, Vine AK, Trent JM. Cytogenetic analysis of posterior uveal melanoma. Cancer Genet Cytogenet 1993;66:47–53.

93. Yanoff M, Zimmerman LE. Histogenesis of malignant melanomas of the uvea. II. Relationship of uveal nevi to malignant melanomas. Cancer 1967;20:493–507.

94. Ziegler A, Leffell DJ, Kunala S, et al. Mutation hotspots due to sunlight in the p53 gene of nonmelanoma skin cancers. Proc Natl Acad Sci U S A 1993;90:4216–20.

95. Zimmerman LE. Malignant melanoma. In: Spencer WH, ed. Ophthalmic pathology. An atlas and textbook. 3rd ed. Philadelphia: WB Saunders, 1985:2072–141.

96. _____. Melanocytes, melanocytic nevi and melanocytomas. Invest Ophthalmol 1965;4:11–41.

97. _____, McLean IW. Do growth and onset of symptoms of uveal melanomas indicate subclinical metastasis? Ophthalmology 1984;91:685–91.

98. _____, McLean IW, Foster WD. Does enucleation of the eye containing a malignant melanoma prevent or accelerate the dissemination of tumour cells? Br J Ophthalmol 1978;62:420–5.

Hemangioma

99. Sanborn GE, Augsburger JJ, Shields JA. Treatment of cumscribed choroidal hemangiomas. Ophthalmology 1982;89:1374–80.

100. Witschel H, Font RL. Hemangioma of the choroid. A clinicopathologic study of 71 cases and a review of the literature. Surv Ophthalmol 1976;20:415–31.

Choroidal Osteoma

101. Shields CL, Shields JA, Augsburger JJ. Choroidal osteoma. Surv Ophthalmol 1988;33:17–27.

102. Williams AT, Font RL, van Dyk HJ, Riehkof FT. Osseous choristoma of the choroid simulating a choroidal melanoma. Association with a positive 32P test. Arch Ophthalmol 1978;96:1874–7.

Leiomyoma

103. Blodi FC. Leiomyoma of the ciliary body. Am J Ophthalmol 1950;33:939–42.

104. Jakobiec FA, Font RL, Tso MO, Zimmerman LE. Mesectodermal leiomyoma of the ciliary body. A tumor of presumed neural crest origin. Cancer 1977;39:2102–13.

105. _____, Witschel H, Zimmerman LE. Choroidal leiomyoma of vascular origin. Am J Ophthalmol 1976;82:205–12.

106. Meyer SL, Fine BS, Font RL, Zimmerman LE. Leiomyoma of the ciliary body. Electron microscopic verification. Am J Ophthalmol 1968;66:1061–8.

107. Shields JA, Shields CL. Observations on intraocular leiomyomas. Trans Pa Acad Ophthalmol Otolaryngol 1990;42:945–50.

Leukemia

108. Green WR. Uveal tract. In: Spencer WH, ed. Ophthalmic pathology. An atlas and textbook. 3rd ed. WB Saunders: Philadelphia, 1985:1522–684.

Juvenile Xanthogranuloma

109. Cleasby GW. Nevoxanthogranuloma (juvenile xanthogranuloma of the iris). Arch Ophthalmol 1961;66:26–8.

110. Hadden OB. Bilateral juvenile xanthogranuloma of the iris. Br J Ophthalmol 1975;59:699–702.

111. Sanders TE. Intraocular juvenile xanthogranuloma (nevoxanthogranuloma): a survey of 20 cases. Trans Am Ophthalmol Soc 1960;58:59–74.

112. Wertz FD, Zimmerman LE, McKeown CA, Croxatto JO, Whitmore PV, LaPiana FG. Juvenile xanthogranuloma of the optic nerve, disc, retina and choroid. Ophthalmology 1982;89:1331–5.

Lymphoid Neoplasms

113. Desroches G, Abrams GW, Gass JD. Reactive lymphoid hyperplasia of the uvea. A case with ultrasonographic and computed tomographic studies. Arch Ophthalmol 1983;101:725–8.

114. Payne T, Karp LA, Zimmerman LE. Intraocular involvement in Burkitt's lymphoma. Arch Ophthalmol 1971;85:295–8.

115. Ryan SJ, Zimmerman LE, King FM. Reactive lymphoid hyperplasia. An unusual form of intraocular pseudotumor. Trans Am Acad Ophthalmol Otolaryngol 1972;76:652–71.

Metastatic Tumors

116. Burnier MN Jr, Neves RA, Pereira MG, Alberti VN, Rigueiro MP. The use of the peroxidase-anti-peroxidase technique in ocular pathology. Arch I P B 1988;30:181–4.
117. Ferry AP, Font RL. Carcinoma metastatic to the eye and orbit. I. A clinicopathologic study of 227 cases. Arch Ophthalmol 1974;92:276–86.
118. _____, Font RL. Carcinoma metastatic to the eye and orbit. II. A clinicopathologic study of 26 patients with carcinoma metastatic to the anterior segment of the eye. Arch Ophthalmol 1975;93:472–582.
119. Fishman ML, Tomaszewski MM, Kuwabara T. Malignant melanoma of the skin metastatic to the eye. Frequency in autopsy series. Arch Ophthalmol 1976; 94:1309–11.

120. Font RL, Naumann G, Zimmerman LE. Primary malignant melanoma of the skin metastatic to the eye and orbit. Report of ten cases and review of the literature. Am J Ophthalmol 1967;63:738–54.
121. Jensen OA. Metastatic tumors of the eye and orbit. A histopathological analysis of a Danish series. Acta Pathol Microbiol Scand 1970;212(Suppl):201–14.
122. Riddle PJ, Font RL, Zimmerman LE. Carcinoid tumors of the eye and orbit: a clinicopathologic study of 15 cases, with histochemical and electron microscopic observations. Hum Pathol 1982;13:459–69.
123. Stephens RF, Shields JA. Diagnosis and management of cancer metastatic to the uvea: a study of 70 cases. Ophthalmology 1979;86:1336–49.
124. Winkler CF, Goodman GK, Eiferman RA, Yam LT. Orbital metastasis from prostatic carcinoma. Identification by an immunoperoxidase technique. Arch Ophthalmol 1981;99:1406–8.

✧ ✧ ✧

6
TUMORS OF THE LACRIMAL GLAND AND SAC

ANATOMY AND HISTOLOGY

The lacrimal gland develops as epithelial buds that evaginate from the basal cells of the conjunctiva in the superotemporal portion of the embryonic fornix. Initially, solid cords are formed but by 3 months' gestation the central cells begin to vacuolate and lumina appear. The lateral portion of the aponeurosis of the levator palpebrae muscle divides the lacrimal gland into a superficial palpebral and a deeper orbital lobe at the fifth month of gestation. The full development of the lacrimal gland is not achieved until the third or fourth year of life.

In the normal fully developed orbit, the lacrimal gland is clinically impalpable and is situated in a small fossa behind the superotemporal orbital rim. It is not truly encapsulated and is composed of a collection of lobules of secretory tissue aggregated in the superotemporal orbital fat (figs. 6-1, 6-2). Accessory lacrimal glands with histologic features identical to those seen in the main lacrimal gland are often found in the substantia propria of the conjunctiva.

Many interlobular ducts converge into the main excretory ducts in the superotemporal fornix. The secretory acini are composed of an inner layer of columnar to cuboidal zymogen-bearing cells and an outer layer of contractile myoepithelial cells. The myoepithelial cells are not present in the terminal intralobular ductules or in the interlobular ducts.

The lacrimal drainage system is composed of the puncta, the lacrimal canaliculi, the lacrimal sac, and the nasolacrimal duct. The puncta are the openings for the drainage of tears into the canaliculi and lacrimal sac. They are located at the medial ends of the lid margins. The upper punctum is in a sulcus between the caruncle and the plica, whereas the lower is situated in a groove between the globe and the plica. Each punctum is a small oval aperture, measuring about 0.33 mm, and surrounded by an avascular ring of connective and elastic tissue, as well as skeletal muscle fibers. These provide structural support to resist deformation of the puncta upon closing the eyelids.

The canaliculi are small tubes measuring 0.5 mm in diameter. Each is composed of a vertical

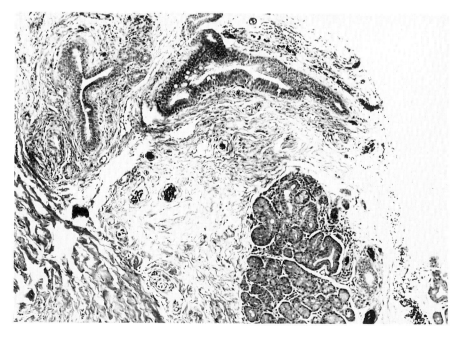

Figure 6-1
NORMAL
LACRIMAL GLAND
Glandular lobule adjacent to ducts lined by pseudostratified epithelium with goblet cells.

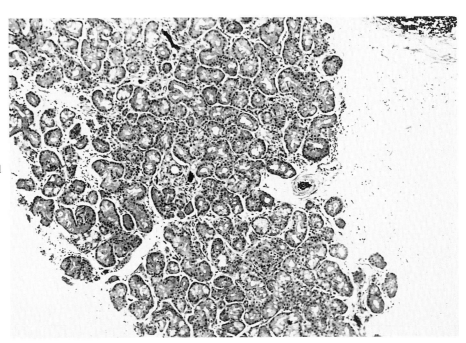

Figure 6-2
NORMAL
LACRIMAL GLAND
Lobule of acinic and mucinous cells.

and a horizontal portion and narrows abruptly to join the counterpart from the other lid, usually just prior to entering the lacrimal sac. The opening of the common canaliculus into the lacrimal sac is the internal lacrimal punctum. Histologically, the canaliculi are tubular structures lined by nonkeratinized, stratified squamous epithelium resting on a stroma containing abundant collagenous and elastic fibers. Like the punctum, the canaliculus is surrounded by the fibers of the orbicularis muscle.

The lacrimal sac is located in the lacrimal fossa in the anterior part of the medial wall of the orbit. The fossa is formed by the lacrimal bone and the frontal processes of the maxilla. Medially and above, the sac is adjacent to the anterior ethmoidal sinuses, and below it lies next to the middle meatus of the nose. The lacrimal sac is lined by a stratified columnar epithelium containing scattered goblet cells; in some areas the epithelium may be ciliated. There is an abrupt transition between the stratified squamous epithelium of the canaliculus to the stratified columnar, goblet cell–containing epithelium of the sac. The underlying connective tissue, just beneath the basement membrane of the epithelium, contains scattered lymphocytes.

The nasolacrimal duct is approximately 12 mm long and 4 mm in diameter. It represents a downward extension of the lacrimal sac. It terminates inferiorly as the lacrimal ostium and opens on the lateral wall of the inferior nasal meatus.

CLASSIFICATION AND FREQUENCY

Benign and malignant lacrimal gland tumors constitute 10 percent of orbital lesions that are biopsied (1). In a series from Wills Eye Hospital that included inflammatory lesions and lymphoid tumors, 78 percent of biopsied lacrimal gland lesions were nonepithelial: inflammatory (64 percent) and lymphoid tumors (14 percent) (2). In a study of 53 lacrimal gland tumors from the Armed Forces Institute of Pathology (AFIP) Registry of Ophthalmic Pathology (ROP) (Table 6-1), not including inflammatory lesions, only 14 (26 percent) were nonepithelial, which is lower than the prevalence at Wills Eye Hospital (39 percent). The prevalence of lymphoid tumors of the lacrimal gland at the AFIP is reduced by the habit of classifying lymphoid tumors that affect the orbit, as well as the lacrimal gland, as orbital tumors. The high prevalence of adenoid cystic carcinomas and pleomorphic carcinomas in the ROP probably reflects the referral of more difficult cases to the AFIP.

Table 6-1

TUMORS OF THE LACRIMAL GLAND*

Type of Tumor	Number of Cases
Epithelial and mixed	
Pleomorphic adenoma (benign mixed tumor)	19
Pleomorphic carcinoma (malignant mixed tumor)	5
Adenoid cystic carcinoma	13
Adenocarcinoma	2
Lymphoid	
Reactive lymphoid hyperplasia	7
Benign lymphoepithelial lesion	1
Lymphoma	5
Plasmacytoma	1

*Frequency distribution of 53 tumors in the AFIP

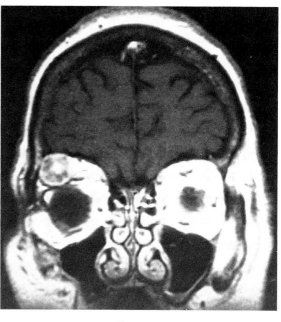

Figure 6-3
PLEOMORPHIC ADENOMA
Magnetic resonance image of a well-circumscribed lacrimal gland tumor.

PLEOMORPHIC ADENOMA (BENIGN MIXED TUMOR)

Pleomorphic adenoma accounts for the majority of epithelial tumors of the lacrimal gland. Most arise from the deep orbital lobe; less commonly, the palpebral lobe is the site of origin (12). Rarely, pleomorphic adenomas arise from accessory or ectopic lacrimal gland tissue (3,10).

The classic clinical history of benign mixed tumor is that of a painless and slowly developing mass in the lacrimal gland region. The tumor occurs in virtually every age group (9), with a mean age at presentation of about 39 years (4).

In addition to proptosis, patients frequently have downward and inward displacement of the globe. In the superotemporal orbital region a firm, smooth mass is usually palpable. Computerized tomography (CT) scans and magnetic resonance imaging (MRI) reveal a round to ovoid tumor (fig. 6-3) that frequently flattens the sclera and may indent bone (7,11).

Grossly, pleomorphic adenomas are pseudoencapsulated tumors (figs. 6-4, 6-5). They typically exhibit small projections beyond their overall contour that are referred to as bosselations;

on their cut surfaces, soft mucinous areas may alternate with fibrous areas. Cystic areas may also be present (fig. 6-5).

Histologic sections reveal the common mixture of epithelial and mesenchymal-like elements that led to the term benign mixed tumor. The epithelial units are classically organized into variably sized ducts containing an inner cuboidal to columnar epithelium and an outer layer of flattened to spindle-shaped cells (fig. 6-6). There is a myoepithelial variant of these tumors characterized by solid sheets of spindle-shaped or ovoid cells with minimal ductal differentiation. The epithelial cells of the outer layer may undergo unusual metaplasias, particularly into myxoid tissue, cartilage (fig. 6-7), and rarely, bone. Focal areas of squamous metaplasia may be observed in the epithelial structures. Tyrosine and collagen crystals occur in a few tumors.

Electron microscopic studies of pleomorphic adenomas have shown that the inner cells lining the tubules have the characteristics of duct cells of the normal lacrimal gland (8). The outer cells are basal germinal cells containing tonofilaments in their cytoplasm; these cells become entrapped in the stroma but still betray their epithelial origin.

217

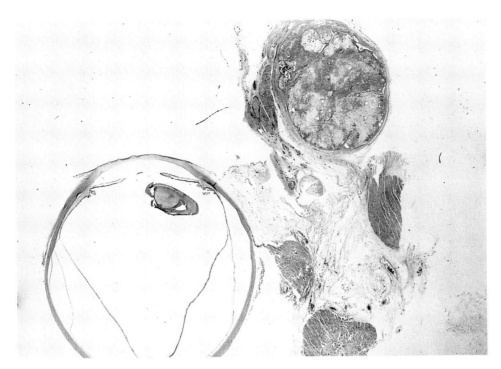

Figure 6-4
PLEOMORPHIC ADENOMA
Well-circumscribed pseudoencapsulated lacrimal gland tumor.

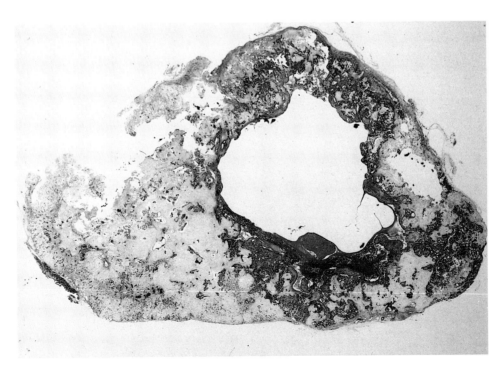

Figure 6-5
PLEOMORPHIC ADENOMA
Tumor composed of a mixture of islands of epithelial cells, myxoid stroma, and cysts.

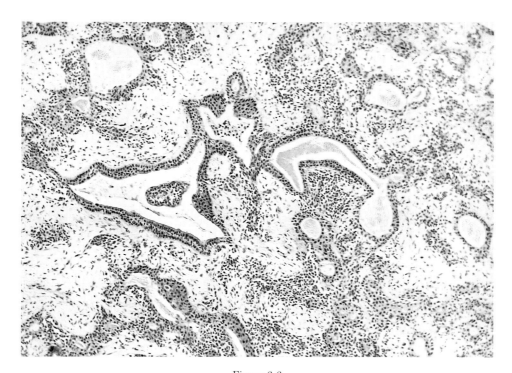

Figure 6-6
PLEOMORPHIC ADENOMA
Tumor composed of ducts lined by a double layer of epithelial cells within a myxoid stroma.

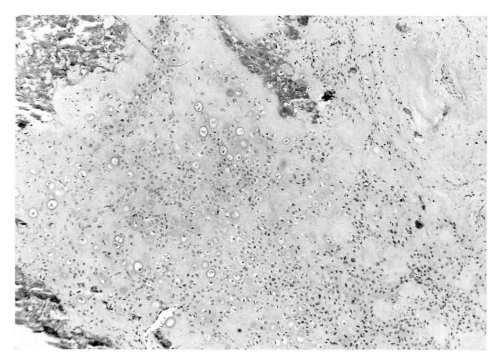

Figure 6-7
PLEOMORPHIC ADENOMA
Area of chondroid differentiation.

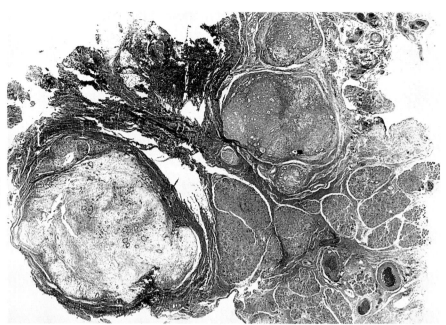

Figure 6-8
PLEOMORPHIC ADENOMA
WITH ADENOCARCINOMA
The large round nodule is a pleomorphic adenoma with multiple smaller nodules of adenocarcinoma that has infiltrated the orbit. (Figures 6-8 and 6-9 are from the same patient.)

Grossniklaus et al. (5) compared the immunohistochemical staining of normal lacrimal glands, pleomorphic adenomas, and pleomorphic carcinomas. Cytokeratin stained occasional myoepithelial cells in the normal glands, ductal epithelium in the normal glands and tumors, and occasional stromal "epithelioid" cells in the tumors. Muscle-specific actin stained myoepithelium in the normal glands and the tumors, and occasional spindle-shaped cells and clusters of stromal cells in the tumors. Glial fibrillary acidic protein (GFAP) stained occasional myoepithelial cells in the normal glands and polyhedral stromal cells in the benign tumors. These findings indicate that benign and malignant pleomorphic adenomas either arise from a progenitor cell capable of both epithelial and myoepithelial differentiation or they arise from more than one type of cell.

The treatment of choice for a presumed pleomorphic adenoma is the complete excision of the lesion with its pseudocapsule via a lateral orbitotomy (6). A biopsy of these lesions through the lid should be avoided because this may lead to local tumor spread. If incompletely excised, pleomorphic adenoma will recur in about one third of cases. Likewise, rupture of the pseudocapsule and piecemeal excision of the tumor has been associated with a high incidence of recurrence.

PLEOMORPHIC CARCINOMA
(MALIGNANT MIXED TUMOR)

A pleomorphic carcinoma (malignant mixed tumor) is a pleomorphic adenoma that has undergone malignant transformation. It is the third most common epithelial tumor of the lacrimal gland (13).

Patients with pleomorphic carcinoma are older than those with benign mixed tumor, probably because a benign tumor must preexist. Patients present in three ways: they have an incompletely excised and recurrent pleomorphic adenoma that recurs every 3 to 5 years; they have a well-tolerated swelling in the lacrimal fossa for many years and develop a rapid enlargement of the mass over a 6- or 12-month period; or their benign mixed tumor is asymptomatic and they appear with rapidly developing symptoms (14,15).

Histopathologically, a pleomorphic carcinoma is an adenocarcinoma (figs. 6-8, 6-9), adenoid cystic carcinoma (fig. 6-10), squamous cell carcinoma, undifferentiated carcinoma, or sebaceous carcinoma in which a preexistent pleomorphic adenoma can be identified.

The prognosis for a patient with malignant mixed tumor is poor, with death usually occurring within a 3-year period. The behavior of a malignant mixed tumor depends on the type of

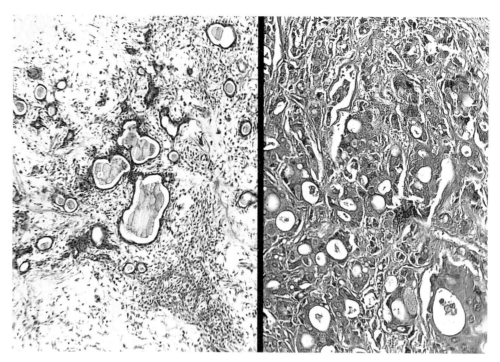

Figure 6-9
PLEOMORPHIC ADENOMA WITH ADENOCARCINOMA
Left: Benign area composed of ducts within a myxoid stroma.
Right: Malignant area with adenocarcinoma pattern.

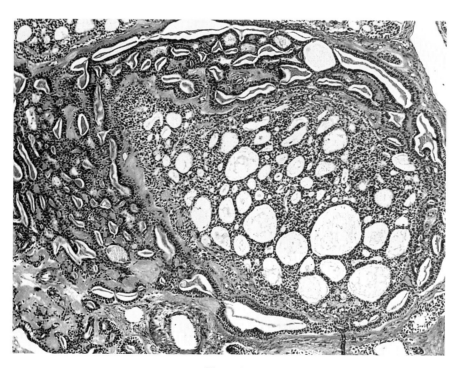

Figure 6-10
PLEOMORPHIC ADENOMA WITH ADENOID CYSTIC CARCINOMA
Within a pleomorphic adenoma, a nodule of carcinoma with a cribriform pattern is present.

cells in its malignant component. Squamous cell carcinoma is probably the least aggressive type. Radical surgery is the best way to treat these lesions (13–15).

ADENOID CYSTIC CARCINOMA

Adenoid cystic carcinomas are highly malignant tumors and they are the second most common epithelial neoplasm of the lacrimal gland (18). Like pleomorphic adenomas, patients average about 40 years of age at presentation, with a range of 12 to 76 years. In contrast to the pleomorphic adenomas, patients are generally symptomatic for short periods of time, typically for less than 6 months. They present with proptosis, numbness, pain, and diplopia because early in its development this lesion invades nerves and extraocular muscles (17).

CT reveals a globular, rounded mass, but with more irregular and serrated borders than pleomorphic adenomas (fig. 6-11). This is due to the infiltrating character of the lesion (fig. 6-12).

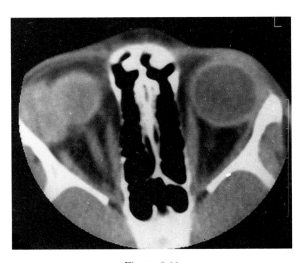

Figure 6-11
ADENOID CYSTIC CARCINOMA
Computed tomograph of a tumor with serrated borders indicative of infiltrative growth in the lacrimal fossa.

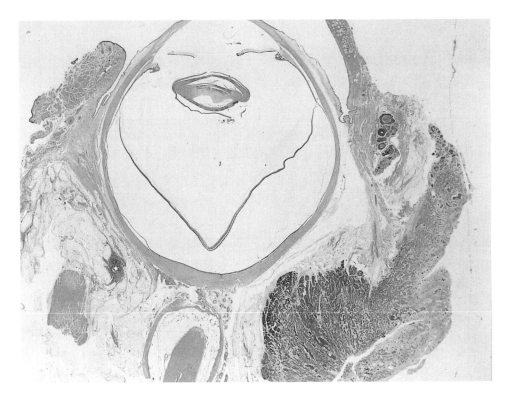

Figure 6-12
ADENOID CYSTIC CARCINOMA
Tumor has infiltrated the orbit.

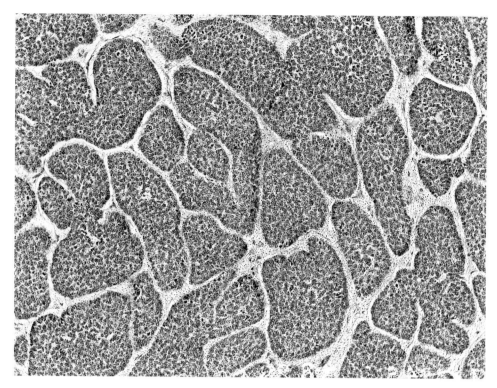

Figure 6-13
ADENOID CYSTIC CARCINOMA
Tumor with a basaloid pattern.

Bone changes occur in about 80 percent of cases; these frequently are destructive or sclerotic rather than the regular well-circumscribed pressure indentation caused by a pleomorphic adenoma (25).

Gross specimens of adenoid cystic carcinoma may appear to be well circumscribed and pseudoencapsulated, but at surgery the dissection of the tumor is more difficult than with a pleomorphic adenoma, indicating invasion beyond the apparent capsule.

Microscopically, most adenoid cystic carcinomas are composed of nests of basaloid cells in which there are foci of cells that have undergone various types of differentiation. When there is no differentiation (fig. 6-13), the carcinoma has an undifferentiated or basaloid pattern. Multiple mucin-filled cysts within the nests of basaloid cells (fig. 6-14) indicate a cribriform pattern. Since these cysts are not true ductules, the term "adenoid" rather than "adeno" is more appropriate. Nests surrounded by sclerotic basement membrane material (fig. 6-15) form a cylindromatous pattern. Within the basaloid nests

there may be areas of central necrosis, comprising the comedo pattern. In one large study (19), there was a poorer prognosis associated with tumors in which less than 30 percent of the basaloid nests had adenoid differentiation (cribriform pattern), however a smaller series did not confirm this association (23). When the nests are small and the sclerotic stroma or cribriform pattern is not evident, distinguishing between a mixed tumor and an adenoid cystic carcinoma may be difficult. In these cases, the margins of the tumor should be carefully examined because adenoid cystic carcinomas are infiltrative, unlike pleomorphic adenomas. Perineural invasion (fig. 6-16) is frequently seen, accounting for the clinical complaint of pain or numbness with adenoid cystic carcinoma. Even early in the course of the disease, neoplastic cells may invade the contiguous bone of the fossa of the lacrimal gland to produce the bony changes observed radiographically.

By electron microscopy, the neoplastic cells of the basaloid and cribriform areas of an adenoid cystic carcinoma frequently have the features of

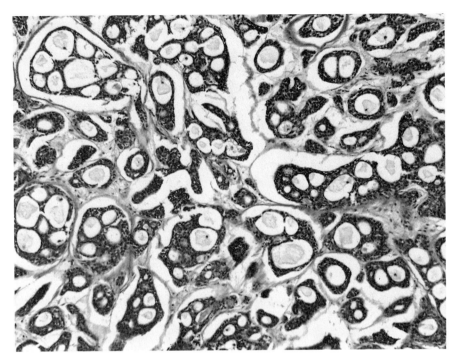

Figure 6-14
ADENOID CYSTIC CARCINOMA
Tumor with a cribriform pattern.

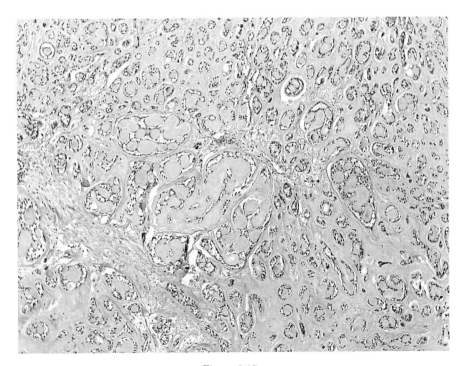

Figure 6-15
ADENOID CYSTIC CARCINOMA
Tumor with a cylindromatous or sclerosing pattern.

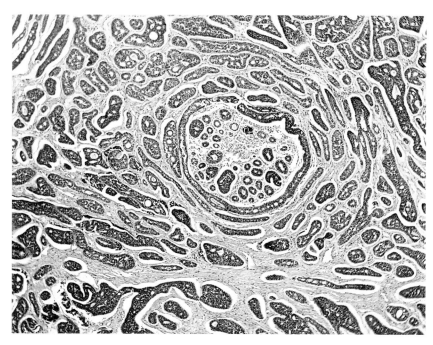

Figure 6-16
ADENOID CYSTIC CARCINOMA
Tumor with nerve invasion.

duct cells of the lacrimal gland, including small secretory granules and tonofilaments. The hyalinized material surrounding the nests and cords of neoplastic cells is composed of redundant basement membrane material and fine collagen fibrils (22).

Most patients with adenoid cystic carcinoma of the lacrimal gland eventually die from tumor-related causes (21). The most common cause of death is tumor extension along nerves (fig. 6-16) through the superior orbital fissure and invasion through the orbital bones (fig. 6-17) into the middle cranial fossa. Hematogenous metastases (fig. 6-18), particularly to the lungs, is the second most common cause of death. Lymphatic spread to regional nodes is uncommon. Deaths due to metastasis may occur many years after initial surgery but is most frequent between the fifth and tenth postoperative years.

The best management of an adenoid cystic carcinoma of the lacrimal gland is still debated. In order to obtain a tissue diagnosis, a biopsy through the lid, without violating the periorbita, is generally performed (26). Exenteration of the orbital contents with removal of any potentially involved bony structures in the lacrimal region was the treatment of choice in the past, but the survival rate was only 20 percent 10 years after orbital surgery. Mainly because of these poor results, removal of the tumor with contiguous bone as a single en bloc excision has been recommended (24). Some ophthalmic oncologists recommend adjunctive postoperative radiotherapy (16).

ADENOCARCINOMA ARISING DE NOVO

Few epithelial tumors of the lacrimal gland (less than 10 percent) are adenocarcinomas arising unassociated with a preexistent benign mixed tumor. These patients have clinical findings similar to those with adenoid cystic carcinoma.

Histopathologically, these tumors may represent a poorly or well-differentiated adenocarcinoma (fig. 6-19). The neoplastic cells are pleomorphic, mitotically active, and arranged in sheets and cords. The tumor may produce mucin or form lumina, depending on its degree of differentiation. Exceptionally, lacrimal gland carcinoma may undergo sebaceous differentiation indistinguishable from carcinoma of the sebaceous glands of the eyelid.

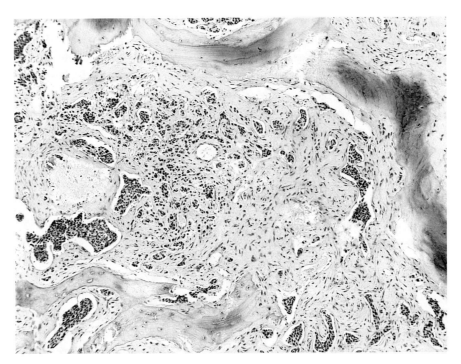

Figure 6-17
ADENOID CYSTIC CARCINOMA
Invasion of orbital bone.

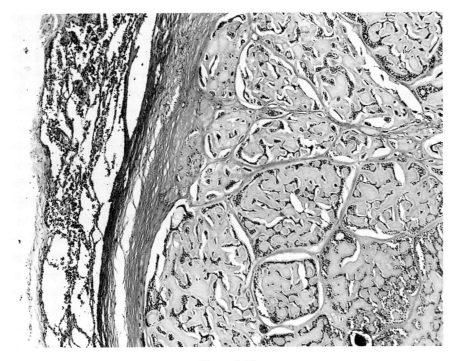

Figure 6-18
ADENOID CYSTIC CARCINOMA
Metastatic nodule in the lung.

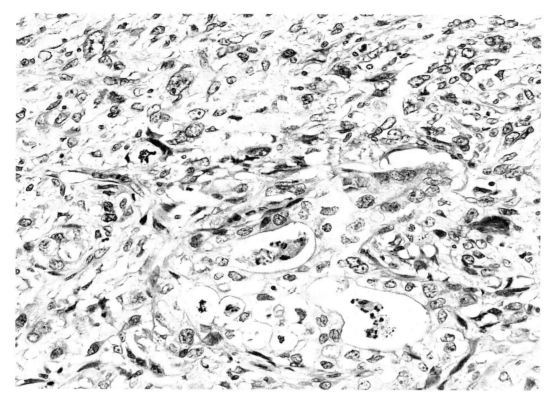

Figure 6-19
ADENOCARCINOMA ARISING DE NOVO
Anaplastic tumor with glandular formation and mitotic activity.

A rare form of carcinoma in the lacrimal gland is *mucoepidermoid carcinoma* (27–29). In this neoplasm there is a mixture of squamous elements frequently arranged in a paving stone fashion and mucin-producing goblet cells. These tumors are generally less threatening than adenoid cystic carcinomas or adenocarcinomas, but they are locally infiltrating.

TUMORS OF THE LACRIMAL SAC

Most lacrimal sac tumors are primary and epithelial in origin. They are either papillomas, adenomas, or carcinomas (32–34,37,38). Oncocytic change may be seen in both benign and malignant epithelial tumors of the lacrimal sac (30,31). Rare primary melanomas of the lacrimal sac have been reported (39) and primary acquired melanosis of the conjunctiva may spread intraepithelially to the lacrimal sac. Primary tumors of mesenchymal origin are rare. Tumors originating in the adjacent maxillary and eth-

moid sinuses or in the nasal mucosa may extend into the lacrimal sac. Metastatic tumors confined to the lacrimal sac are extremely rare, and most metastases also involve adjacent structures such as the eyelid, nose, sinuses, and orbit.

Most patients with a tumor of the lacrimal sac are first examined because of the presence of a mass and signs of obstruction leading to epiphora. With papillomas, the slow growth of the tumor and the obstructive symptoms often masquerade as a chronic dacryocystitis. The presence of hemorrhage associated with pain is highly suggestive of a malignant neoplasm of the lacrimal sac (37).

The age of the patients with a tumor of the lacrimal sac varies according to the histopathologic type of the neoplasm: papillomas are observed in younger patients, whereas those with carcinoma range from 40 to 75 years. The high prevalence of carcinomas in the AFIP ROP probably reflects the referral bias of cases sent there (Table 6-2).

Table 6-2

TUMORS OF THE LACRIMAL SAC*

Type of Tumor	Number of Cases
Epithelial	
Papilloma	9
Oncocytoma	3
Carcinoma	17
Lymphoid	
Reactive lymphoid hyperplasia	2
Lymphoma	4

*Frequency distribution of 35 tumors in the AFIP Registry of Ophthalmic Pathology collected between 1984 and 1989.

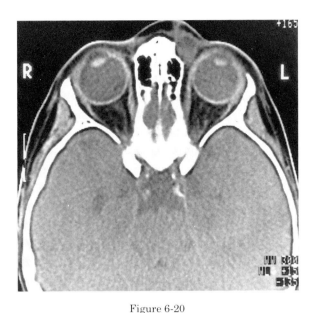

Figure 6-20
PAPILLOMA
Computed tomograph of a well-circumscribed tumor in the lacrimal sac.

Epithelial Tumors
(Papillomas and Carcinomas)

The papillomas of the lacrimal sac may be classified into three groups according to their growth pattern: exophytic, inverted, and mixed.

Exophytic papillomas are fungiform masses with projecting, finger-like proliferations of epithelium that grow into and enlarge the lacrimal sac (figs. 6-20, 6-21). The inverted papillomas have areas of invasive acanthosis of surface epithelium into the underlying stroma (fig. 6-22). Mixed papillomas include tumors showing a combination of exophytic and inverted patterns.

Papillomas of the lacrimal sac may also be classified according to their histopathologic features into three types: squamous cell papillomas are tumors composed of acanthotic, stratified squamous epithelium; transitional cell papillomas are neoplasms composed of stratified columnar epithelium with goblet cells, resembling those normally present in the lacrimal sac mucosa; and mixed cell papillomas are tumors showing a mixture of squamous and transitional types.

Carcinomas of the lacrimal sac (figs. 6-23–6-25) may be divided into papillary and nonpapillary types. Some papillomas are probably precursors of carcinomas because foci of carcinoma may be observed within otherwise benign papillomas (fig. 6-25). Based on the histopathologic features, they may be further classified as squamous, transitional, adenocarcinomatous, and mucoepidermoid (36).

The prognosis of these tumors correlates quite well with their histopathologic features. Inverted papillomas may be locally invasive. Carcinomas of the lacrimal sac are always locally invasive tumors; recurrences are observed in about 40 percent of the cases. If neglected, these carcinomas can invade surrounding structures (nasal cavity, sinuses, orbit, and brain) and metastasize to regional lymph nodes (35). Wide excision is the most effective method of treatment.

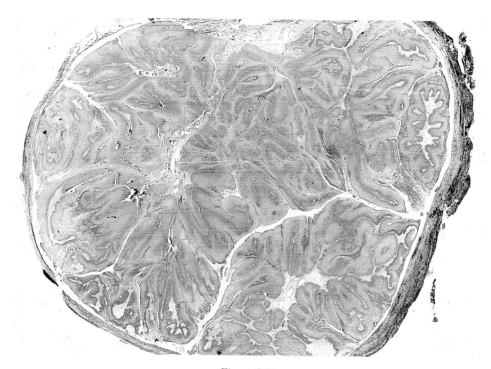

Figure 6-21
PAPILLOMA
Well-circumscribed papillary tumor fills the lacrimal sac.

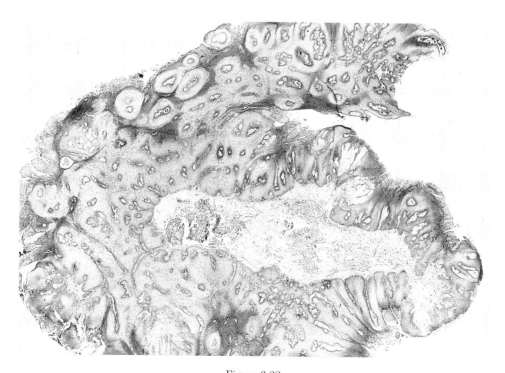

Figure 6-22
PAPILLOMA
Papillary tumor with inverted growth pattern composed of well-differentiated squamous epithelium.

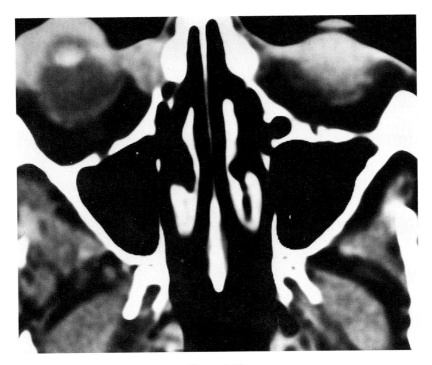

Figure 6-23
CARCINOMA
Computed tomograph of an irregularly shaped tumor in the area of the lacrimal sac.

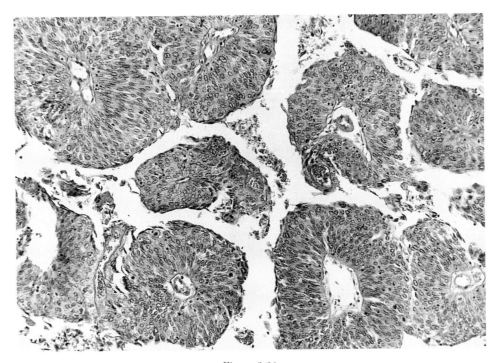

Figure 6-24
CARCINOMA
Papillary tumor with fronds covered by neoplastic transitional epithelium.

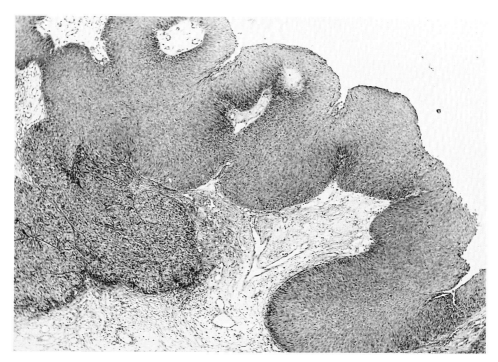

Figure 6-25
PAPILLOMA WITH MALIGNANT TRANSFORMATION
Papillary tumor with an atypical area.

REFERENCES

General References

Font RL, Gamel JW. Epithelial tumors of the lacrimal gland: an analysis of 265 cases. In: Jakobiec FA, ed. Ocular and adnexal tumors. Birmingham: Aesculapius Publishing Company, 1978:787–805.

Iwamoto T, Jakobiec FA. Lacrimal glands. In Jakobiec FA, ed. Ocular anatomy, embryology and teratology. Philadelphia: Harper & Row, 1982:761–82.

Jakobiec FA, Font RL. Orbital tumors. In: Spencer WH, ed. Ophthalmic pathology. An atlas and textbook. 3rd ed. Philadelphia: WB Saunders, 1985:2459–860.

_____, Iwamoto T. The ocular adnexa: lids, conjunctiva and orbit. In Fine BS, Yanoff M, eds. Ocular histology: a text and atlas. 2nd ed. Hagerstown, Md.: Harper & Row, 1979:289–342.

Mafee MF, Haik BG. Lacrimal gland and fossa lesions: role of computed tomography. Radiol Clin North Am 1987; 25:767–80.

Classification and Frequency

1. Kennedy RE. An evaluation of 820 orbital cases. Trans Am Ophthalmol Soc 1984;82:134–57.
2. Shields CL, Shields JA. Review of lacrimal gland lesions. Trans Pa Acad Ophthalmol Otolaryngol 1990;42:925–30.

Pleomorphic Adenoma

3. Bech K, Jensen OA. Mixed tumor of the lower orbital region. Arch Ophthalmol 1965;74:226–8.
4. Font RL, Gamel JW. Epithelial tumors of the lacrimal gland: an analysis of 265 cases. In: Jakobiec FA, ed. Ocular and adnexal tumors. Birmingham: Aesculapius Publishing Company, 1978:787–805.
5. Grossniklaus HE, Abbuhl MF, McLean IW. Immunohistologic properties of benign and malignant mixed tumor of the lacrimal gland. Am J Ophthalmol 1990;110:540–9.
6. Henderson JW, Neault RW. En bloc removal of intrinsic neoplasms of the lacrimal gland. Am J Ophthalmol 1976;82:905–9.
7. Hornblass A, Friedman AH, Yagoda A. Erosion of the orbital plate (frontal bone) by a benign tumor of the lacrimal gland. Ophthalmic Surg 1981;12:737–43.
8. Iwamoto T, Jakobiec FA. A comparative ultrastructural study of the normal lacrimal gland and its epithelial tumors. Hum Pathol 1982;13:236–62.
9. McPherson SD Jr. Mixed tumor of the lacrimal gland in a seven-year-old boy. Am J Ophthalmol 1966;61:561–3.
10. Mueller EC, Borit A. Aberrant lacrimal gland and pleomorphic adenoma within the muscle cone. Ann Ophthalmol 1979;11:661–3.
11. Ni C, Cheng SC, Dryja TP, Cheng TY. Lacrimal gland tumors: a clinicopathological analysis of 160 cases. Int Ophthalmol Clin 1982;22:99–120.

12. Parks SL, Glover AT. Benign mixed tumors arising in the palpebral lobe of the lacrimal gland. Ophthalmology 1990;97:526–30.

Pleomorphic Carcinoma

13. Font RL, Gamel JW. Epithelial tumors of the lacrimal gland: an analysis of 265 cases. In: Jakobiec FA, ed. Ocular and adnexal tumors. Birmingham: Aesculapius Publishing Company, 1978:787–805.
14. Henderson JW, Farrow GM. Primary malignant mixed tumors of the lacrimal gland. Report of 10 cases. Ophthalmology 1980;87:466–75.
15. Perzin KH, Jakobiec FA, LiVolsi VA, Desjardins L. Lacrimal gland malignant mixed tumors (carcinomas arising in benign mixed tumors): a clinico-pathologic study. Cancer 1980;45:2593–606.

Adenoid Cystic Carcinoma

16. Brada M, Henk JM. Radiotherapy for lacrimal gland tumours. Radiother Oncol 1987;9:175–83.
17. Font RL, Gamel JW. Adenoid cystic carcinoma of the lacrimal gland: a clinicopathologic study of 79 cases. In: Nicholson DH, ed. Ocular pathology update. New York: Masson Publishing USA, 1980:277–83.
18. _____. Epithelial tumors of the lacrimal gland: an analysis of 265 cases. In: Jakobiec FA, ed. Ocular and adnexal tumors. Birmingham: Aesculapius Publishing Company, 1978:787–805.
19. Gamel JW, Font RL. Adenoid cystic carcinoma of the lacrimal gland: the clinical significance of a basaloid histologic pattern. Hum Pathol 1982;13:219–25.
21. Henderson JW. Adenoid cystic carcinoma of the lacrimal gland, is there a cure? Trans Am Ophthalmol Soc 1987;85:312–9.
22. Kennedy RE. An evaluation of 820 orbital cases. Trans Am Ophthalmol Soc 1984;82:134–57.
23. Lee DA, Campbell RJ, Waller RR, Ilstrup DM. A clinicopathologic study of primary adenoid cystic carcinoma of the lacrimal gland. Ophthalmology 1985;92:128–34.
24. Marsh JL, Wise DM, Smith M, Schwartz H. Lacrimal gland adenoid cystic carcinoma: intracranial and extracranial en bloc resection. Plast Reconstr Surg 1981;68:577–85.

25. Ni C, Cheng SC, Dryja TP, Cheng TY. Lacrimal gland tumors: a clinicopathological analysis of 160 cases. Int Ophthalmol Clin 1982;22:99–120.
26. Wright JE. Factors affecting the survival of patients with lacrimal gland tumours. Can J Ophthalmol 1982;17:3–9.

Adenocarcinoma and Mucoepidermoid Carcinoma

27. Malhotra GS, Paul SD, Batra DV. Muco-epidermoid carcinoma of the lacrimal gland. Ophthalmologica 1967;153:184–90.
28. Sofinski SJ, Brown BZ, Rao N, Wan WL. Mucoepidermoid carcinoma of the lacrimal gland. Case report and review of the literature. Ophthal Plast Reconstr Surg 1986;2:147–51.
29. Wagoner MD, Chuo N, Gonder JR, Grove AS Jr, Albert DM. Mucoepidermoid carcinoma of the lacrimal gland. Ann Ophthalmol 1982;14:383–6.

Lacrimal Sac Tumors

30. Aurora AL. Oncocytic metaplasia in a lacrimal sac papilloma. Am J Ophthalmol 1973;75:466–8.
31. Barca L. Adenoma ad oncociti del sacco lacrimale. Ann Ottalmol Clin Ocul 1971;97:233–44.
32. Bonder D, Fischer MJ, Levine MR. Squamous cell carcinoma of the lacrimal sac. Ophthalmology 1983;90:1133–5.
33. Flanagan JC, Stokes DP. Lacrimal sac tumors. Ophthalmology 1978;85:1282–7.
34. Hornblass A, Jakobiec FA, Bosniak S, Flanagan J. The diagnosis and management of epithelial tumors of the lacrimal sac. Ophthalmology 1980;87:476–90.
35. Ni C, D'Amico DJ, Fan CQ, Kuo PK. Tumors of the lacrimal sac: a clinicopathological analysis of 82 cases. Int Ophthalmol Clin 1982;22:121–40.
36. _____, Wagoner MD, Wang WJ, Albert DM, Fan CO, Robinson N. Mucoepidermoid carcinomas of the lacrimal sac. Arch Ophthalmol 1983;101:1572–4.
37. Ryan SJ, Font RL. Primary epithelial neoplasms of the lacrimal sac. Am J Ophthalmol 1973;76:73–88.
38. Schenck NL, Ogura JH, Pratt LL. Cancer of the lacrimal sac. Presentation of five cases and review of the literature. Ann Otol Rhinol Laryngol 1973;82:153–61.
39. Yamade S, Kitagawa A. Malignant melanoma of the lacrimal sac. Ophthalmologica 1978;177:30–3.

✧ ✧ ✧

7

TUMORS OF THE ORBIT

ANATOMY AND HISTOLOGY

The orbit is a pear-shaped cavity that contains the eye and its adnexal structures. The optic canal, located posteronasally, corresponds to the stem of the pear (figs. 7-1–7-3). The orbit has a volume of about 30 cm^3 and a length of about 5 cm. Within the orbit are a variety of tissue types: epithelial tissue of the lacrimal gland; white matter of the central nervous system in the optic nerve; peripheral motor, sensory, and autonomic nerves; the ciliary ganglion; striated muscle in the six extraocular muscles; smooth muscle in Müller muscles; arteries and veins; a complicated network of fibroadipose tissue that envelops all the other orbital contents; dense fibrous tissue of the Tenon capsule and periorbita (the periosteum of the orbital bones); and cartilage in the trochlea of the superior oblique tendon. Traditionally, the globe is excluded in discussion of tumors of the orbit, and in this Fascicle we also devote separate chapters to the optic nerve and lacrimal gland.

The orbital contents are bounded by seven bones: frontal, sphenoidal, maxillary, zygomatic, lacrimal, palatine, and ethmoid. The anterior limit of the orbit is formed by the orbital septa in the upper and lower lids, which extend from the periorbita as membranes that blend into the connective tissues of the lids. The orbital walls are interrupted by three major apertures in addition to the anterior opening between the eyelids: the optic canal, the superior orbital fissure, and the inferior orbital fissure. The optic canal (5 to 10 mm in length) contains the optic nerve, sympathetic fibers, and the ophthalmic artery. The superior orbital fissure, between the greater and lesser wings of the sphenoid bone, is separated from the more medial optic canal by a thin strip of bone, the optic strut. It transmits the superior ophthalmic vein to the cavernous sinus; the third, fourth, fifth, and sixth cranial nerves; and some sympathetic fibers. The inferior orbital fissure in the orbital floor permits the inferior ophthalmic vein to empty into the pterygoid plexus

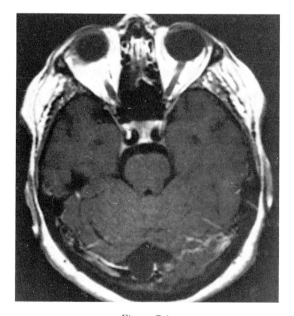

Figure 7-1
NORMAL ORBIT
Gadolinium enhanced T1-weighted magnetic resonance image showing eye and orbital contents.

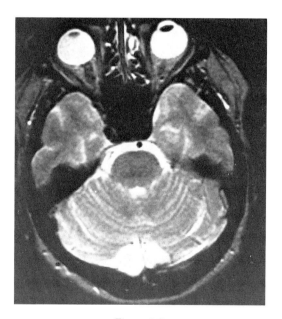

Figure 7-2
NORMAL ORBIT
Gadolinium enhanced T2-weighted magnetic resonance image showing eye and orbital contents.

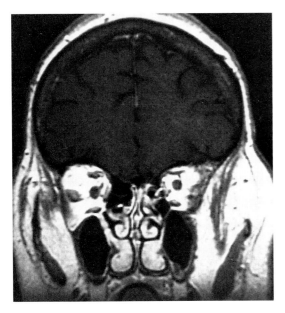

Figure 7-3
NORMAL ORBIT
Gadolinium enhanced T1-weighted magnetic resonance image showing coronal section of orbital contents posterior to the globe.

and ascending branches of the sphenopalatine ganglion to reach their orbital destinations. In addition, there are several vascular foramina, the most important of which are the openings for the anterior and posterior ethmoidal arteries.

The extraocular muscles consist of four rectus muscles and two oblique muscles. The four recti share a common origin from the annulus of Zinn, where the dural sheath of the optic nerve, the periorbita of the bony rim of the optic canal, and the shared tendinous origin of the recti form a foramen for the optic nerve. The four recti are variable in length but average around 40 mm and insert on the globe from 5 to 8 mm behind the limbus (the spiral of Tillaux). The levator palpebrae muscle arises above the superior rectus to end as a broad aponeurotic expansion in the anterior orbit with insertions into the medial and lateral palpebral ligaments as well as into the substance of the upper lid. The superior oblique originates medial to the annulus of Zinn. It travels along the superomedial aspect of the orbit to the trochlea, just behind the orbital rim. Its long tendon passes through the cartilaginous trochlea, which reflects the tendon obliquely and posteriorly to insert on the superior aspect of the globe posterior to the insertion of the superior rectus muscle. The infe-

rior oblique originates at the anterior inferomedial portion of the orbital wall. It crosses the inferior orbit obliquely beneath the inferior rectus muscle and inserts on the globe at the posterior pole in the vicinity of the fovea.

The orbital fat is separated into lobules by fibrous septa that have a highly regular, bilaterally symmetric architecture. The fibrous septa compartmentalize the adipose tissue, connect the extraocular muscles, and support the orbital structures. Within some septa are bundles of smooth muscle cells. For descriptive purposes, it is useful to divide the orbit using the cone formed by the extraocular muscles into a central or intraconal space and a peripheral or extraconal space.

The arterial vascular supply to the orbit is via the ophthalmic artery which is accompanied by sympathetic fibers from the pericarotid sympathetic plexus. In the optic canal, the artery lies inferolateral to the optic nerve. At the orbital optic foramen, the artery curls over the optic nerve to run superomedially. Its first intraorbital branch is the central retinal artery, which perforates the dural sheath of the optic nerve approximately 10 mm from the optic foramen and 8 to 10 mm behind the globe. As it passes superomedially to the nerve, the ophthalmic artery gives off two long posterior ciliary arteries, six to eight short posterior ciliary arteries, the lacrimal artery, the anterior and posterior ethmoidal arteries, and the supraorbital artery. The extraocular muscles are supplied by small branches of the ophthalmic artery which enter their bellies near the annulus of Zinn. The terminal or distal branches of the ophthalmic artery penetrate the orbital septum and emerge beneath the orbital rim as the dorsonasal and frontal arteries. The supraorbital artery passes through the supraorbital foramen above the orbital rim. Major anastomoses occur between branches of the ophthalmic artery and those of the external carotid system, including a branch of the middle meningeal artery which enters the orbit through a lateral foramen or the superior orbital fissure. These anastomoses may save vision when the ophthalmic artery is occluded, if the external carotid system can furnish the central retinal artery with sufficient blood.

The orbital veins readily anastomose with the veins of the face and lids. Like the other veins of the head and neck, they contain no valves. The superior ophthalmic vein is formed by a confluence of the angular, nasofrontal, and supraorbital veins. It runs posterolaterally in the superior orbital space, penetrates the muscle cone in mid-orbit, receives venous drainage from the central retinal vein, and leaves the orbit through the superior orbital fissure to empty into the cavernous sinus. The smaller inferior ophthalmic vein drains the tissues over the floor of the orbit as well as a network of channels in the inferomedial area, including the region of the lacrimal sac. An anastomosis to the superior ophthalmic vein occurs before the inferior vein exits through the inferior orbital fissure into the pterygoid plexus.

The orbital nerves enter the orbit through the superior orbital fissure. Superolaterally, the superior orbital fissure transmits the lacrimal and frontal nerves, which are two major branches of the ophthalmic division of the trigeminal (fifth cranial) nerve, and the trochlear (fourth cranial) nerve. Inferomedially, the fissure transmits the inferior and superior branches of the oculomotor (third cranial) nerve, the abducens (sixth cranial) nerve, and the nasociliary nerve, which is another branch of the ophthalmic division of the trigeminal nerve. The nerves to the various extraocular muscles enter their bellies at the junction of the posterior and middle thirds of the muscle. The ciliary ganglion is located temporal to the optic nerve near the orbital apex. It measures 11 mm in maximal diameter. It receives parasympathetic fibers traveling in the inferior branch of the oculomotor nerve and sends out postsynaptic fibers destined for the ciliary body and iris. Sensory fibers from the nasociliary nerve and sympathetic fibers pass through the ganglion without synapsing to join the ciliary nerves.

Lymphoid tissue is present in the substantia propria of the conjunctiva and the lacrimal gland, but the deep orbital tissue is devoid of lymphoid cells. There are no endothelial-lined lymphatics within the orbit, except those of the lacrimal gland, which drain to the preauricular and cervical nodes.

CLASSIFICATION AND FREQUENCY

The types of tumors that occur in the orbit reflect the diversity of tissues present. The World Health Organization classification provides a framework that divides the tumors of the orbit into groups based on their origin (Tables 7-1–7-5).

Table 7-1

BENIGN SOFT TISSUE TUMORS OF THE ORBIT*

Type of Tumor	Number of Cases
Capillary hemangioma	9
Cavernous hemangioma	11
Lymphangioma	13
Fibromatosis	2
Fibrous histiocytoma	34
Leiomyoma	2
Lipoma	3
Neurofibroma	11
Schwannoma	13

*Frequency distribution of 98 tumors in the AFIP Registry of Ophthalmic Pathology collected between 1984 and 1989.

Table 7-2

MALIGNANT SOFT TISSUE TUMORS OF THE ORBIT*

Type of Tumor	Number of Cases
Hemangiopericytoma	18
Fibrosarcoma	3
Malignant fibrous histiocytoma	5
Leiomyosarcoma	1
Rhabdomyosarcoma	16
Liposarcoma	6
Malignant peripheral nerve sheath tumor	9

*Frequency distribution of 58 tumors in the AFIP Registry of Ophthalmic Pathology collected between 1984 and 1989.

The frequency distribution of tumors of the orbit in the Armed Forces Institute of Pathology (AFIP) Registry of Ophthalmic Pathology (ROP) (Tables 7-1–7-5) is similar to that of other reported series (1,2,4) once differences in classification and referral biases are taken into consideration. Among primary orbital neoplasms, the

Table 7-3

LYMPHOID AND HEMATOLOGIC TUMORS AND PSEUDOTUMORS OF THE ORBIT*

Type of Tumor	Number of Cases
Benign	
Idiopathic inflammation	32
Lymphoid hyperplasia	34
Angiolymphoid hyperplasia with eosinophilia	5
Sinus histiocytosis	3
Malignant	
Lymphoma	76
Plasmacytoma	3
Leukemia (granulocytic sarcoma)	2

*Frequency distribution of 155 tumors in the AFIP Registry of Ophthalmic Pathology collected between 1984 and 1989.

Table 7-4

OTHER PRIMARY TUMORS OF THE ORBIT*

Type of Tumor	Number of Cases
Dermoid cyst	21
Teratoma	1
Endodermal sinus tumor	1
Blue nevus	1
Malignant melanoma	1

*Frequency distribution of 25 tumors in the AFIP Registry of Ophthalmic Pathology collected between 1984 and 1989.

Table 7-5

SECONDARY AND METASTATIC TUMORS OF THE ORBIT*

Type of Tumor	Number of Cases
Secondary	
Carcinoma, eyelid and conjunctiva	13
Meningioma, sphenoid wing	12
Juvenile ossifying fibroma, bone	12
Hemangioma, bone	3
Angiofibroma, nasal cavity	2
Metastatic	
Carcinoma	13
Carcinoid	3
Melanoma	1
Seminoma	1

*Frequency distribution of 60 tumors in the AFIP Registry of Ophthalmic Pathology collected between 1984 and 1989.

frequency of soft tissue tumors and lymphoid and hematopoietic tumors are approximately equal in the series of Kennedy (2), Shields et al. (4), and the AFIP Registry (Tables 7-1–7-5), whereas Henderson (1) reported a higher prevalence of soft tissue tumors. The relative frequency of secondary and metastatic tumors is similar in Kennedy's series and the AFIP Regis-try (Table 7-4), but Shields found a slightly higher prevalence and Henderson a much higher prevalence. Dermoid and epithelial cysts were less frequent in Henderson's series and the AFIP Registry than the other two series. In the AFIP Registry lymphoma, fibrous histiocytoma, and lymphoid hyperplasia were the most common tumors (Tables 7-1–7-5); for Henderson secondary carcinoma, lymphoma, and hemangioma were the most common; for Kennedy these were lymphoma, dermoid cyst, and hemangioma; and Shields found dermoid cyst, lymphoid hyperplasia, and lymphoma to be most frequent. These differences probably reflect the tendency of pathologists to refer difficult and unusual tumors to the AFIP for consultation and referral biases in the hospital-based series. In a series of 99 consecutive cases in which the patients had an orbital exenteration (3), approximately half the tumors were secondary carcinomas of the skin, conjunctiva, and nasal sinuses. Secondary melanomas from conjunctiva, skin, sinuses, and uvea were the next most frequent (16 cases). Only 7 cases were primary orbital soft tissue tumors.

CAPILLARY HEMANGIOMA

Capillary hemangioma has several synonyms. Because this tumor typically develops in the perinatal period, the designation *infantile* or *juvenile hemangioma* has been used. A histologic feature of this hemangioma is enlarged swollen endothelial cells, thus the terms *hemangioblastic hemangioma* and *benign hemangioendothelioma*.

Clinical Features. In 90 percent of cases capillary hemangiomas involve the anterior aspect of the orbit, with frequent lid involvement (5). When the lesion extends into the superficial dermis, an upraised, dimpled, red "strawberry mark" is created. Capillary hemangiomas grow rapidly at the outset and most become apparent within the first 2 weeks after birth. If the hemangioma is large enough to interfere with vision, there is danger of amblyopia developing (9). If the tumor does not interfere with vision, no therapy is advised because the tumor reaches a stationary stage within 1 to 2 years and then involutes spontaneously over the next 5 to 6 years (5). If significant cosmetic or functional impairment is present, the most common therapy is intralesional injection of corticosteroids (8). Low-dose radiation and surgery have been used in severe cases but there is concern that the ocular side effects of these treatments may be more damaging than the sequelae of the involuted capillary hemangioma.

Computerized tomography (CT) and ultrasonography of capillary hemangiomas indicate that these are poorly circumscribed, infiltrating, nonencapsulated tumors (7). The orbit is usually enlarged, implying that the lesions begin to develop in utero and are hamartomas. CT with contrast media reveals greater enhancement of the tumor than the extraocular muscles. Sklar et al. (10) found that the capillary hemangioma that demonstrated the lowest relative enhancement was in the oldest child, suggesting that blood flow decreases with involution. Since capillary hemangiomas cannot always be distinguished clinically from rhabdomyosarcoma, biopsy may be necessary to confirm the diagnosis.

Pathologic Findings. Capillary hemangiomas have an infiltrative pattern of growth that can involve all the orbital structures, including the lacrimal gland, orbital fat, and extraocular muscles. During the phase of rapid growth, the plump endothelial cells proliferate in solid lobules. A reticulin stain may be required to demonstrate the capillary units in which the lumina are inconspicuous. Mitotic figures may be numerous in the endothelial cells. During the involutional phase the endothelial cells flatten with ectasia of the capillary lumina. Fibrosis begins between the lobules, but with time there is complete effacement of the capillary lobules. Electron microscopy has revealed pericytes surrounding the endothelial tubules, indicating the capillary nature of the proliferation (6).

CAVERNOUS HEMANGIOMA

Clinical Features. Orbital cavernous hemangiomas differ significantly from capillary hemangiomas and lymphangiomas. Cavernous hemangioma is a tumor that occurs in adults: Harris and Jakobiec (12) reported that in 66 patients the mean age at onset of symptoms was 42 years with a range of 18 to 67 years. Seventy percent of the patients were women. The typical history is of a slowly developing proptosis over a period of 4 to 5 years. Visual acuity may be reduced slightly, the blind spot may be enlarged, and there may be a scotoma corresponding to where the tumor is pressing on the optic nerve. While most cavernous hemangiomas are located in the retrobulbar region, resulting in axial proptosis, some are located nasally, temporally, or inferiorly with consequent opposite displacement of the globe. CT scans and magnetic resonance imaging (MRI) reveal a sharply circumscribed mass (fig. 7-4) that is usually retrobulbar in location, lying within the muscle cone (11,13,15,16). CT performed 1 to 2 minutes after contrast injection usually does not show enhancement, whereas other well-circumscribed orbital tumors (schwannoma, neurofibroma, hemangiopericytoma) rapidly accumulate the contrast media (15). Ultrasonography demonstrates that the lesion is cystic with high internal reflectivity (fig. 7-5).

Pathologic Findings. Grossly, a cavernous hemangioma has an intense violaceous hue due to the stagnant, poorly oxygenated blood within it. The unfixed specimen is very spongy and during surgery blood can be squeezed from the tumor to facilitate removal. The cut surface of the specimen and low-power microscopy reveal

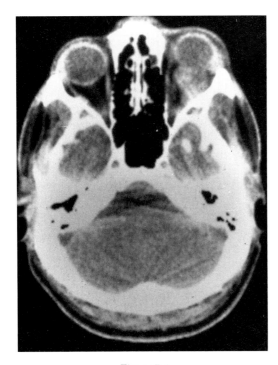

Figure 7-4
CAVERNOUS HEMANGIOMA
CT scan of an intraconal, well-circumscribed, ovoid retrobulbar tumor.

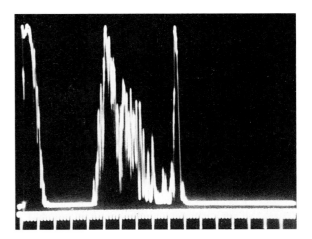

Figure 7-5
CAVERNOUS HEMANGIOMA
Ultrasonogram showing retrobulbar tumor with high internal reflectivity.

a fibrous capsule surrounding a tumor composed of vascular channels measuring 0.5 to 1 mm in diameter (fig. 7-6). The fibrous septa between the vascular channels are of variable thickness (fig. 7-7) and often contain scattered inflammatory cells and hemosiderin-laden macrophages. Large collections of lymphocytes within the septa should raise the possibility of a lymphangioma rather than a cavernous hemangioma. If the patient is less than 20 years of age, the presence of lymphocytic aggregates should be an even stronger signal that the lesion is a lymphangioma. Electron microscopy reveals that the vascular channels of the cavernous hemangioma are lined by a flattened monolayer of endothelial cells surrounded by one to five layers of smooth muscle cells (14).

LYMPHANGIOMA

Lymphangiomas occur in the eyelids, conjunctiva, and orbit; ocular adnexal tumors may be associated with facial lymphangiomas. Lymphangioma is considered a choristoma in the orbit

because normally the orbit does not contain endothelial-lined lymphatic channels, lymph nodes, or even well-defined lymphoid follicles.

Clinical Features. Orbital lymphangiomas typically become symptomatic in the first 15 years of the patient's life. In 29 cases of lymphangioma involving the orbit, Jones (19) found that 10 were present at birth, 11 were diagnosed when the patients were between 1 and 5 years of age, and 5 were diagnosed between the ages of 6 and 15 years. There were only three adults in the series, aged 27, 38, and 44 years when first seen, whereas patients with conjunctival lymphangiomas averaged 25 years of age.

A fluctuating course is common. Hemorrhage into the dilated lymphatic channels of the tumor can result in fulminant proptosis. Infections of the upper respiratory tract can cause hyperplasia of the lymphoid tissue present in the tumor. Orbital lymphangiomas with diffuse involvement that includes the conjunctiva, lids, face, neck, or palate are more common in younger patients. Visual compromise and extraocular muscle dysfunction are more likely to occur with lymphangiomas than capillary or cavernous hemangiomas.

Ultrasonography and CT demonstrate that lymphangiomas are composed of multiple cysts that have diffusely infiltrated the soft tissues (17,18,20). Blood layering may sometimes be detected within cystic structures (fig. 7-8). The orbit may be enlarged on the involved side. Because

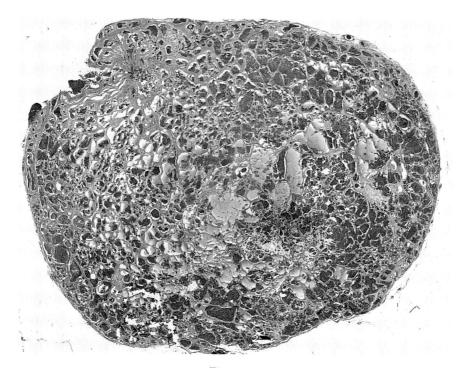

Figure 7-6
CAVERNOUS HEMANGIOMA
Well-circumscribed tumor composed of dilated blood vessels.

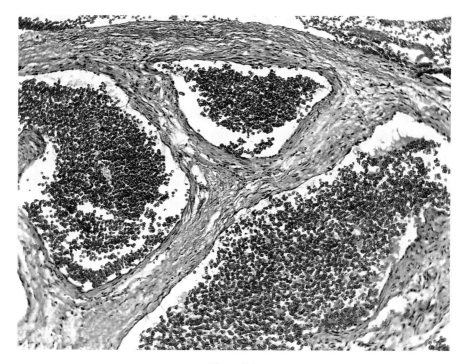

Figure 7-7
CAVERNOUS HEMANGIOMA
Higher power magnification of above tumor showing thick-walled dilated blood vessels.

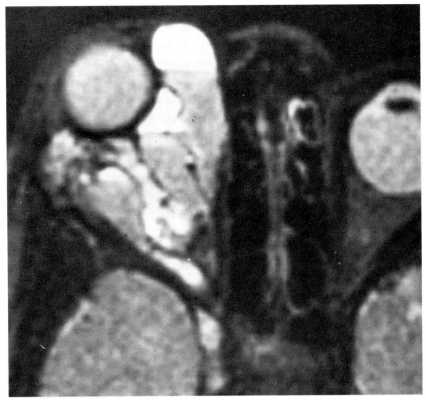

Figure 7-8
LYMPHANGIOMA
Magnetic resonance image showing an ill-defined lobulated mass with blood-fluid levels.

lymphangiomas do not involute like capillary hemangiomas, patients seek corrective surgery. However, since even small lesions often infiltrate extensively and cannot be excised without damage to surrounding structures (17,18), many experienced surgeons recommend doing the minimal excision that will relieve symptoms.

Pathologic Findings. Lymphangioma is an unencapsulated tumor that may diffusely infiltrate the soft tissues of the orbit and ocular adnexa. The lymphatic channels vary markedly in caliber, ranging from capillary to cavernous (figs. 7-9, 7-10). Clear lymph or blood may be present within the lumina of the channels, which are lined by an attenuated endothelium and have a thin wall. The channels have the ultrastructural features of lymphatics, with interrupted basement membrane material, anchoring fibrils, and a general absence of pericytes. The interstitium contains a variable amount of collagen and lymphoid aggregates (fig. 7-10) with occasional

germinal centers. Partially broken-down thrombosed blood from hemorrhage into the lymphangioma can form a chocolate cyst. The wall around the chocolate cyst is typically more fibrotic and may contain hemosiderin-laden macrophages. Older lesions may contain phleboliths.

HEMANGIOPERICYTOMA

Hemangiopericytoma was named by Stout and Murray in 1942 (23). They postulated that the tumor is composed of pericytes, which were first described by Zimmerman in 1923 (23). Although hemangiopericytoma is a relatively rare tumor, it probably has a predilection for the orbit.

Clinical Findings. Hemangiopericytomas affect patients of all ages, with the majority occurring in adults. An orbital hemangiopericytoma that developed congenitally was reported in one case (21). In a series of 30 cases from the AFIP, Croxatto and Font (22) found the median

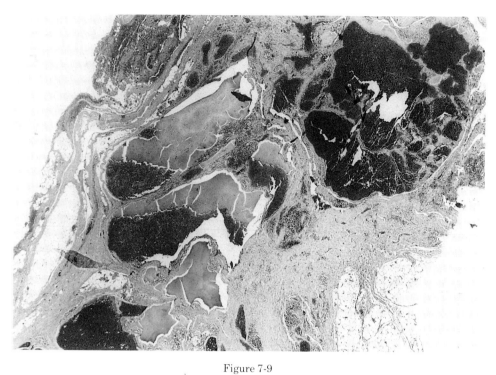

Figure 7-9
LYMPHANGIOMA
Large dilated lymphatic vessels contain serum and layered blood. A large hemorrhage is in the upper right corner.

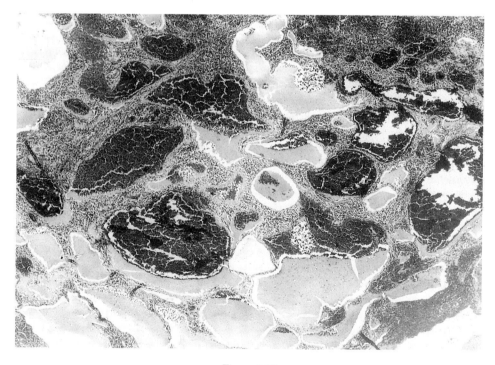

Figure 7-10
LYMPHANGIOMA
Area of same tumor with numerous lymphatics, some of which contain blood. A heavy infiltrate of lymphocytes is present within the connective tissue between the dilated lymphatic channels.

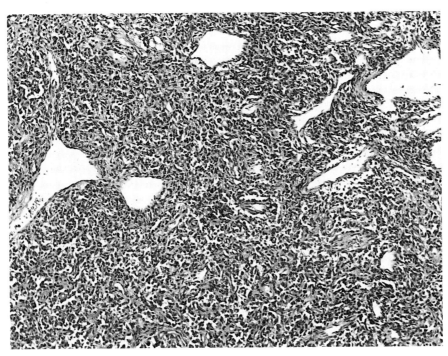

Figure 7-11
HEMANGIOPERICYTOMA
Small polyhedral cells surround vascular spaces.

age to be 42 years; two thirds were men. The most frequent complaints were proptosis, palpable mass, pain, diplopia, and decreased visual acuity.

Patients with hemangiopericytomas differ significantly from patients with cavernous hemangiomas: there is a male predominance, a shorter duration of symptoms, and more severe symptoms. CT reveals a well-circumscribed or encapsulated mass and early dramatic enhancement with injection of contrast media (25). Hemangiopericytoma has a predilection for the superior aspect of the orbit.

Pathologic Findings. Hemangiopericytoma is usually a solitary, well-circumscribed mass with a thin capsule. On cut section, it is grey to red-brown with numerous vascular spaces. Microscopically, the tumor consists of small polyhedral and spindle-shaped cells tightly packed around blood vessels that range from small capillaries to large sinusoidal spaces (fig. 7-11–7-14). The polyhedral cells predominate with small, focal spindle cell areas. The spindle-shaped cells are not arranged in long bundles or fascicles as in a fibrosarcoma or desmoid tumor. Focal fibrous histiocytoma-like areas with a

storiform pattern may be present but this must be a minor component of the tumor since tumors with a significant fibrous histiocytoma component are classified by convention as well-vascularized fibrous histiocytomas (see discussion of fibrous histiocytomas). Tumors with this dual nature seem to be more prevalent in the orbit than at other sites (23). The large sinusoidal vessels are usually more numerous in the periphery of the tumors, where they may have a typical "staghorn" configuration. All of the vessels, including large ones, have the characteristics of capillaries without a muscular wall.

Prognosis. Hemangiopericytomas have been divided into benign and malignant types based on histologic criteria: mitotic activity, cytologic atypia, and necrosis. Although metastasis occurs more frequently in tumors classified as malignant, benign tumors also metastasize (fig. 7-14). Croxatto and Font (22) observed that 1 of 15 benign tumors, 1 of 4 borderline tumors, and 2 of 9 malignant tumors metastasized. Recurrence was seen in 3 of 14 benign tumors, 1 of 4 borderline tumors, and 5 of 9 malignant tumors. Metastasis occurred after recurrence in 3 of 4 fatal cases.

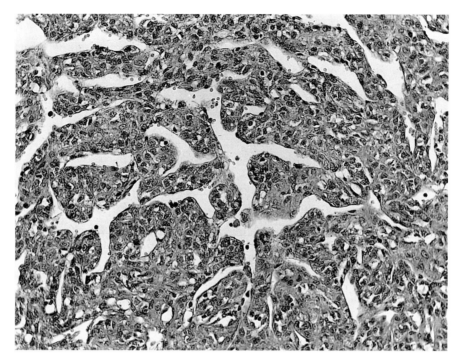

Figure 7-12
HEMANGIOPERICYTOMA
Vascular channels have a staghorn pattern.

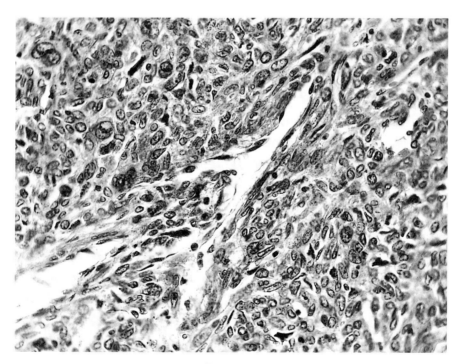

Figure 7-13
HEMANGIOPERICYTOMA
Polyhedral and spindle-shaped cells with mild nuclear atypia.

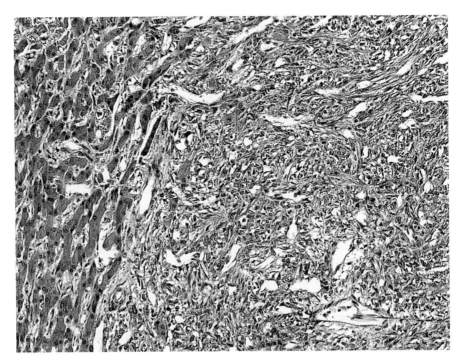

Figure 7-14
HEMANGIOPERICYTOMA
Metastatic nodule in the liver.

These observations are similar to those for hemangiopericytomas in other parts of the body (23). We and others (24) believe that all hemangiopericytomas should be considered malignant and that cytologically they should be divided into low- and high-grade tumors, not benign and malignant ones.

Treatment. Treatment should be complete surgical excision. When complete excision is impossible, adjunctive radiotherapy may be beneficial (26).

FIBROUS HISTIOCYTOMA (FIBROXANTHOMA)

Based on the experience at the AFIP, fibrous histiocytoma is the most common mesenchymal tumor of the orbit in adults (Tables 7-1, 7-2); in other series other tumors are more common (30, 34,36). Fibrous histiocytomas are frequently misdiagnosed as hemangiopericytomas, meningiomas, fibrosarcomas, or peripheral nerve sheath tumors. Not until fibrous histiocytoma was well characterized in the soft tissues elsewhere in the body did its accurate identification

in the orbit become possible. The orbit is probably a site of predilection for this tumor (28,29,33).

Clinical Features. Statistics based on a series of 150 cases from the AFIP provide the most valid and complete information regarding fibrous histiocytoma (29). The median age of the patients at the time of surgery was 43 years, with a range of 4 to 85 years. Males and females were equally affected. The superior orbit was the most frequently involved site (41 percent of cases): nasal involvement tended to occur more frequently than temporal involvement. As with hemangiopericytoma, but unlike cavernous hemangioma, patients were more apt to have evidence of orbital congestion, chemosis of the conjunctiva, motility disturbances, and uncorrectable visual acuity deficits. Patients were symptomatic for about 2.5 years, with a range of 1 month to 20 years.

CT reveals usually well-circumscribed orbital tumors that can be difficult to differentiate from cavernous hemangiomas, hemangiopericytomas, or benign peripheral nerve sheath tumors (fig. 7-15). Locally aggressive tumors are less circumscribed and malignant tumors may invade into the orbital bones (31,32,35).

Pathologic Findings. Grossly, fibrous histiocytomas are rubbery to firm and vary from grayish white to yellow-tan (fig. 7-16). They arise in the orbital fat rather than in the extraocular muscles. Cystic, myxoid, and hemorrhagic areas may also be noted; usually hemorrhage denotes malignancy. Microscopically, the lesion is composed of a mixture of spindle-shaped, fibroblast-like cells and more ovoid, sometimes lipidized histiocytic cells. If lymphocytes and xanthoma cells are prominent and if the orbital condition is bilateral, consideration should be given to a diagnosis of Erdheim-Chester disease rather than fibrous histiocytoma (27).

In most orbital fibrous histiocytomas, elongated fibroblastic cells tend to predominate. The typical architectural feature is the storiform pattern (figs. 7-17–7-19): collections of cells twist about a central focus (spiral-nebular pattern) rather than forming long bundles of spindle-shaped cells typical of pure fibroblastic tumors. Moderate amounts of collagen are deposited in the lesions, and, occasionally, cruciate or hyalinized bands may be seen (33). One third of the 150 lesions in the AFIP series (29) had fields that displayed a hemangiopericytomatous pattern, suggesting a strong histogenetic overlap between

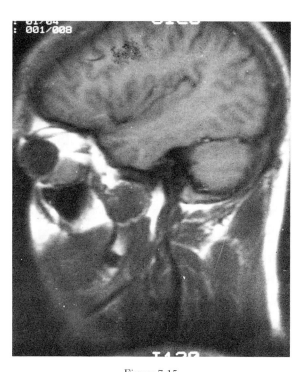

Figure 7-15
FIBROUS HISTIOCYTOMA
Magnetic resonance image of a well-circumscribed tumor in the inferior aspect of the orbit.

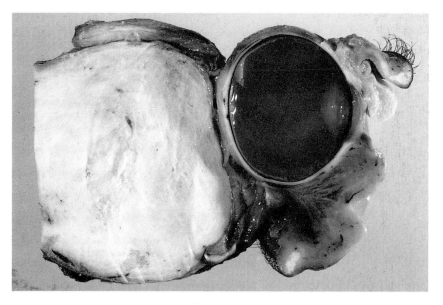

Figure 7-16
FIBROUS HISTIOCYTOMA
Large, retrobulbar, well-circumscribed fibrous tumor.

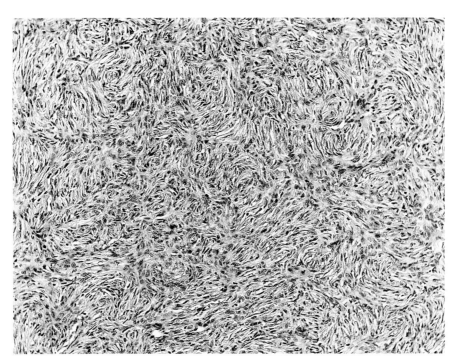

Figure 7-17
FIBROUS HISTIOCYTOMA
Fibrous tumor with a storiform pattern.

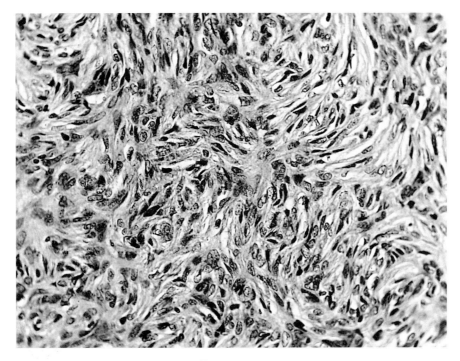

Figure 7-18
FIBROUS HISTIOCYTOMA
Higher power magnification of above tumor with a storiform pattern showing plump spindle-shaped cells.

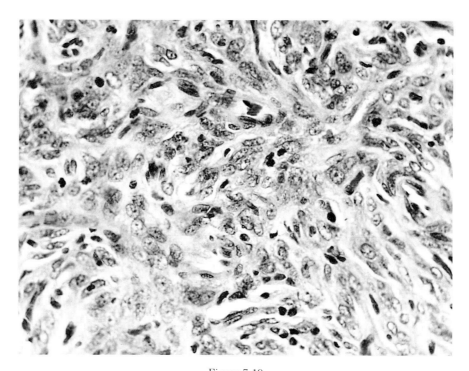

Figure 7-19
FIBROUS HISTIOCYTOMA
Plump spindle-shaped cells have ovoid nuclei with coarse chromatin and small nucleoli.

these two types of tumor. Sometimes a vascular pattern may be exceptionally prominent in both benign and malignant fibrous histiocytomas.

Electron Microscopic Findings. Fibrous histiocytomas of the orbit are composed of a spectrum of cells. At one end of the spectrum are elongated, spindle-shaped cells, usually indistinguishable from fibroblasts. These cells have abundant profiles of rough-surfaced endoplasmic reticulum, absent basement membrane material, and mature collagen fibers in the intercellular spaces. At the other end of the spectrum are cells with a histiocytic character. These cells are ovoid or polyhedral, containing either lipid or electron-dense lysosomal inclusions. Some lesions are composed entirely of fibroblasts arranged in a storiform pattern. In malignant lesions, there may be a population of smaller ovoid cells with features of primitive stem cells. Based on the overlap with hemangiopericytoma and the fact that the predominant cell is fibroblastic, it seems appropriate to consider fibrous histiocytoma as arising from a pluripotential mesenchymal cell (28).

Prognosis. Based on gross and histologic features, the 150 fibrous histiocytomas from the AFIP (29) were divided into three categories: 94 benign lesions, 39 locally aggressive lesions, and 17 malignant lesions. The benign lesions were well circumscribed and small (median diameter 3 cm). The cells were not pleomorphic, and had regular, oval, nonhyperchromatic nuclei; small nucleoli; and few or no mitotic figures. Locally aggressive tumors (fig. 7-20) had increased cellularity and plumper, more hyperchromatic nuclei with more prominent nucleoli; mitotic figures were not atypical and there was generally no more than one per high-power microscopic field. Necrosis was not observed. These tumors had noncircumscribed, infiltrating margins but were about the same size as those in the benign group. In the malignant group, there was far more nuclear pleomorphism (including lesions that were almost entirely composed of pleomorphic giant cells), increased mitotic activity (up to five figures per high-power field), and frequent areas of necrosis. The malignant tumors were somewhat larger (median of 4 cm, with a range of 3 to 15 cm).

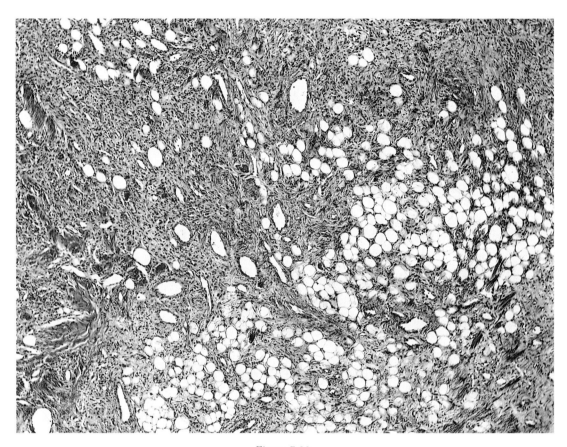

Figure 7-20
FIBROUS HISTIOCYTOMA
Invasion of spindle-shaped neoplastic cells into orbital adipose tissue.

Pathologic grade was correlated with clinical and follow-up data in the 150 cases. The median age of patients with malignant tumors was 53 years versus 42 years for patients with benign tumors; duration of signs and symptoms for patients with malignant tumors was 4 months versus 31 months for benign tumors. Thirty-one percent of the benign fibrous histiocytomas recurred. Patients with locally aggressive lesions had a 57 percent recurrence rate; those with malignant lesions had a 64 percent recurrence rate. None of the 94 patients with benign fibrous histiocytomas died from their disease. Three of the 39 patients with locally aggressive tumors died with invasion into the brain. Six of the 17 patients with malignant fibrous histiocytomas died: 3 had widespread metastases and 3 had local spread into the brain.

Treatment. The best management of fibrous histiocytoma is complete surgical excision. When an incomplete excision is performed for a benign or locally aggressive tumor, and ocular function remains intact, reexcision is not advised since there were no metastases from these lesions in the series from the AFIP. Once a symptomatic recurrence develops, definitive surgery should be performed, including possible exenteration, to prevent spread into the brain and widespread metastases. Histologic examination of the recurrent tumor often reveals more malignant features of increased cellularity, plumper and more pleomorphic nuclei, and increased mitotic figures. For lesions that are unequivocally malignant at the time of first surgery, exenteration should be immediately performed to provide the patient with the best chance for survival. Radiotherapy has not been effective in the management of fibrous histiocytoma: 13 of 18 patients (72 percent) in the AFIP series who received radiotherapy developed recurrences.

FIBROMATOSIS (MYOFIBROMATOSIS, JUVENILE FIBROMATOSIS)

The fibromatoses are a group of locally infiltrative and nonmetastasizing fibrous tumors that tend to recur following local excision (37–39). Fibromatosis in the orbit occurs almost exclusively in children. In a congenital case (38), CT demonstrated a 5-cm enhancing mass that involved the orbit, ethmoid sinuses, sellar region, and middle cranial fossa. This patient was followed for 4 years, during which the tumor regressed spontaneously. Hidayat and Font (37) reported six cases in which the patients ranged in age from 1 to 10 years. Clinically, the children developed a mass in the orbit or eyelid over a period of 2 to 6 months. Grossly, the tumors were firm, rubbery nodules measuring between 1 and 3.5 cm in maximal diameter. Histologically, the tumors were composed of interlacing fascicles of plump spindle-shaped fibroblasts. A moderate amount of fibrous connective tissue separated the tumor cells and each cell was surrounded by heavy reticulin fibers. Mitotic activity was rare or absent. Two of the six patients had a recurrence but all were alive and without disease at last follow-up.

FIBROSARCOMA (JUVENILE FIBROSARCOMA)

Fibrosarcoma of the orbit occurs more commonly in children than adults but several cases in adults have been reported. Weiner and Hidayat (42) described five cases in which the patients ranged in age from newborn to 8 years. The patients presented with proptosis or swelling of the eyelid for up to 5 months' duration. In the congenital case, the infant had massive proptosis at birth. The tumors were grayish white, ranged in diameter from 0.5 to 3.5 cm, and varied from firm to friable. Histologically, they were composed of spindle-shaped fibroblasts with a high nuclear-cytoplasmic ratio. The cells were arranged in a fascicular or herringbone pattern and infiltrated surrounding structures. In four of the five cases there were foci that contained plump cells with atypical pleomorphic nuclei. Although there was minimal fibrous connective tissue between the tumor cells, abundant heavy reticulin fibers surrounded most of them. Mitotic

activity was moderate, ranging from 2 to 10 mitotic figures per 10 high-power fields. Ultrastructural studies (40) confirmed the fibroblastic character of the neoplastic cells. In the congenital case, the infant was treated by exenteration and had no recurrence. One child was treated with radiation after the initial biopsy but there was no response and an exenteration was performed. Two of the patients had a recurrence following local excision. One of these patients had invasion of the orbital floor and this patient had residual tumor at last follow-up. The other four patients were alive and without disease.

Orbital fibrosarcoma is encountered as a second cancer in patients who survive the heritable form of retinoblastoma (41). In these children, orbital radiotherapy is an additional risk factor. Postradiation fibrosarcomas of the orbit are cytologically more anaplastic and behave more aggressively than the juvenile fibrosarcomas described by Weiner and Hidayat.

LEIOMYOMA

Most benign smooth muscle tumors of the orbit are of vascular origin, particularly from the superior ophthalmic vein. Others arise from small foci of smooth muscle cells contained within the larger fibrous connective tissue trabeculae of the orbital fat, the smooth muscle spanning the inferior orbital fissure, or the smooth muscles of Müller associated with the tarsi and lids. Very few leiomyomas have been described in the orbit (45,48); only two tumors were found in the 5-year experience of the AFIP ROP (Table 7-1). Most arise in the third and fourth decades of life. The patients have slowly progressive proptosis; CT reveals a small, well-encapsulated mass. Leiomyomas can recur after incomplete excision.

Histologically, leiomyomas are solid tumors that usually have a conspicuous vascular pattern and a well-developed fibrous capsule. The spindle-shaped tumor cells are arranged in fascicles and have cigar-shaped nuclei. The trichrome and phosphotungstic acid hematoxylin (PTAH) stains demonstrate longitudinally oriented, nonstriated filaments within the cytoplasm. The reticulin and the periodic acid–Schiff (PAS) stains disclose the basement membranes encircling the cells. We have found immunohistochemistry for muscle-specific actin to be especially helpful in differentiating leiomyomas from other spindle cell tumors of nonmuscular origin, but some tumors containing myofibroblasts may also be focally positive.

LEIOMYOSARCOMA

Malignant tumors of smooth muscle are rare in the orbit; most occur in older individuals (46,47). There are two reports of radiation-induced orbital tumors developing in patients who 25 to 30 years earlier had been treated for bilateral retinoblastoma (43,44). Clinically, there is a rapid onset of proptosis and the tumors are found to infiltrate the orbital tissues. Histologically, the diagnosis of malignancy is contingent upon observing an increased nuclear-cytoplasmic ratio, nuclear pleomorphism, foci of necrosis, and mitotic figures in comparison with a leiomyoma. Bizarre cells may be encountered in radiation-induced tumors. The diagnosis of leiomyosarcoma rests upon the demonstration of cytoplasmic filaments with the trichrome stain and electron microscopy, or the identification of muscle-specific antigens (actin or desmin) by immunohistochemistry. Three of four patients with leiomyosarcoma died of metastases at more than 1 year of follow-up (44). The two radiation-induced tumors of the orbit were successfully treated: one by total local excision and the other by subtotal excision with 6000 rads of radiotherapy and adjunctive chemotherapy.

RHABDOMYOSARCOMA

Clinical Features. Rhabdomyosarcoma is the most common primary malignant orbital tumor of childhood (49). It affects younger children preferentially, often with fulminant proptosis. The median age at diagnosis is 7 years. Any quadrant of the orbit may be affected but the superior nasal aspect is the most common. The tumor can arise in the lids, sinuses, or conjunctiva and secondarily involve the orbit. When rhabdomyosarcoma involves submucosal sites, such as the conjunctival stroma, it is designated a botryoid type (fig. 7-21). MRI and CT usually show an invasive tumor (fig. 7-22), but they can reveal a deceptively well-circumscribed mass that enhances following contrast injection (49).

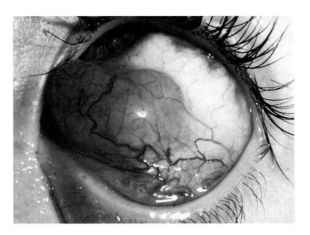

Figure 7-21
RHABDOMYOSARCOMA
Botryoid type with tumor beneath the conjunctiva.

Pathologic Findings. Rhabdomyosarcoma is a yellow or flesh-colored neoplasm that may be red due to hemorrhage into necrotic areas. The tumor is not encapsulated (fig. 7-23) and usually infiltrates the surrounding structures, but occasionally may have a pushing margin. Based on histologic features, rhabdomyosarcomas are divided into embryonal, alveolar, and pleomorphic (differentiated) types.

Embryonal rhabdomyosarcoma (figs. 7-24–7-28) is the most common type in the orbit. The tumor is composed of small polyhedral and spindle-shaped cells arranged in loose fascicles that appear disorganized. Rarely, the nuclei of the spindle-shaped cells are palisaded, creating a problem in differentiation from malignant schwannoma (figs. 7-24, 7-25). The stroma has a myxoid appearance without abundant collagen production (fig. 7-28). The cells have hyperchromatic nuclei with high mitotic activity. Occasionally, one of the bipolar processes of the spindle cells is enlarged, giving the cell a "tadpole" configuration (fig. 7-27). Some cells show rhabdomyoblastic differentiation with the production of eosinophilic cytoplasm. Both spindle-shaped and round rhabdomyoblasts may be present (fig. 7-27). The Masson trichrome stain colors the cytoplasm of the rhabdomyoblasts bright red, the PAS stain demonstrates glycogen within the cytoplasm, and the PTAH stain reveals myofilaments. These stains are helpful in identifying cross striations within the cytoplasm of the spindle cells. Cross striations are rarely found in the

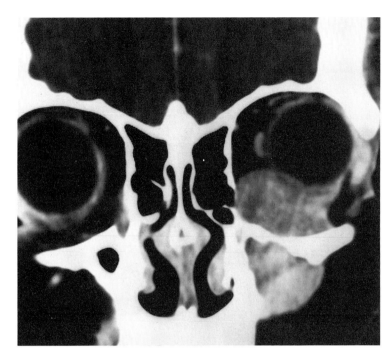

Figure 7-22
RHABDOMYOSARCOMA
Computed tomograph showing a large tumor of the orbital floor invading the maxillary sinus.

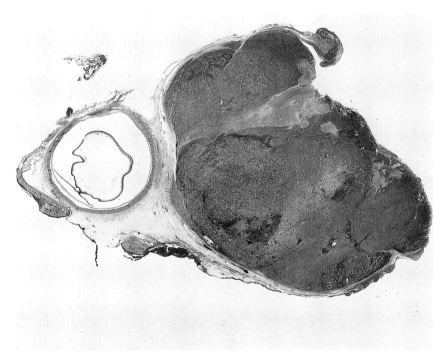

Figure 7-23
RHABDOMYOSARCOMA
A large tumor has infiltrated the orbital tissues.

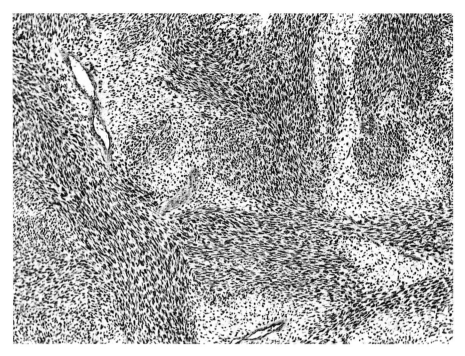

Figure 7-24
RHABDOMYOSARCOMA
Embryonal pattern.

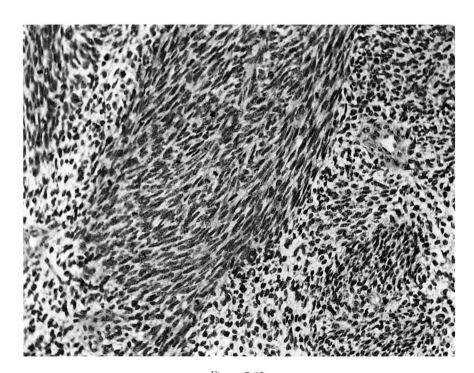

Figure 7-25
RHABDOMYOSARCOMA
Same tumor as in previous figure composed of bundles of spindle-shaped cells with hyperchromatic nuclei and numerous mitotic figures.

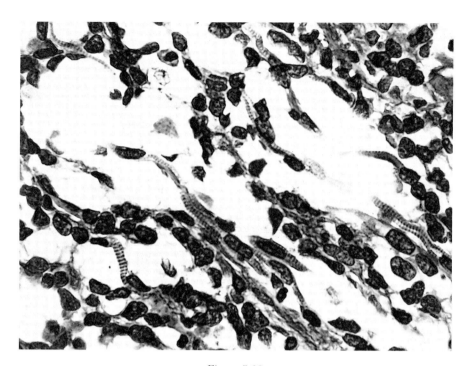

Figure 7-26
RHABDOMYOSARCOMA
Rhabdomyoblasts with cross striations in an embryonal type tumor.

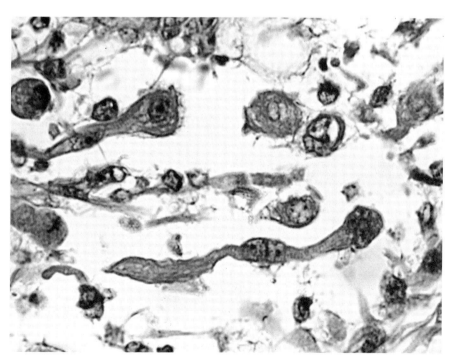

Figure 7-27
RHABDOMYOSARCOMA
Round and tadpole-shaped rhabdomyoblasts.

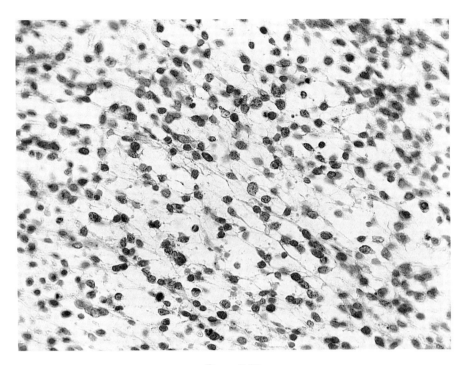

Figure 7-28
RHABDOMYOSARCOMA
Myxoid pattern in an embryonal rhabdomyosarcoma.

round rhabdomyoblasts. Even with the use of these special stains and careful oil immersion microscopy, cross striations can only be identified in about 60 percent of rhabdomyosarcomas. The botryoid variant is always of embryonal histologic type. In this type, the spindle-shaped cells often form a denser layer just beneath the epithelium (Nicholson cambium layer).

Alveolar rhabdomyosarcoma (figs. 7-29–7-32) is the second most common type. This type differs clinically from the embryonal type in that the children are slightly older and the inferior aspect of the orbit is more likely to be involved. Alveolar rhabdomyosarcoma may be attached to an extraocular muscle. Histologically, the tumor is divided into irregular alveolar spaces by dense fibrous septa. The cells are predominately polyhedral and loosely attached in a single layer to the fibrous septa. Numerous cells are shed into the lumen of the alveoli where they are poorly preserved. Multinucleated giant cells with peripherally placed nuclei are seen in some alveolar rhabdomyosarcomas (fig. 7-32). The rhabdomyoblasts are usually round. Cross striations are less common in alveolar tumors than in

embryonal rhabdomyosarcomas. Usually, a small portion of the alveolar tumor has the embryonal pattern. The finding of mixed patterns suggests that the embryonal and alveolar types are closely related.

Pleomorphic (differentiated) rhabdomyosarcoma is the least common type in the orbit. Clinically, this type differs from embryonal and alveolar rhabdomyosarcomas in that the patients are older and more likely to be adults. Histologically, pleomorphic rhabdomyosarcoma can be distinguished from the other types by the presence of numerous large strap cells and large round pleomorphic cells. Despite the abundance of eosinophilic cytoplasm, indicating rhabdomyoblastic differentiation, cross striations may still be difficult to find.

Immunohistochemical Findings. The immunohistochemistry of orbital rhabdomyosarcoma reflects its differentiation towards skeletal muscle (50). We analyzed the reactivity of 10 antibodies in 15 embryonal rhabdomyosarcomas from the ROP (Table 7-6). Cross striations could be identified in only a few tumors. Staining for muscle-specific actin was consistently

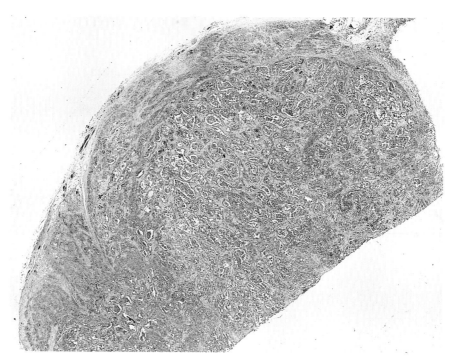

Figure 7-29
RHABDOMYOSARCOMA
Tumor with an alveolar pattern.

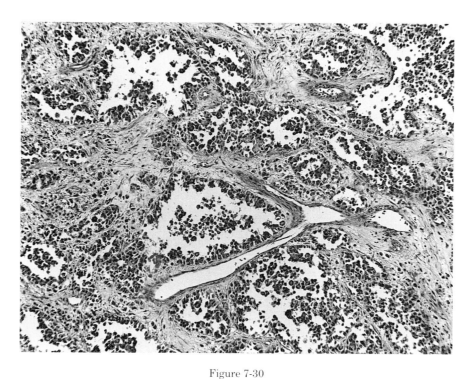

Figure 7-30
RHABDOMYOSARCOMA
Higher power magnification of above tumor showing alveolar spaces containing anaplastic cells.

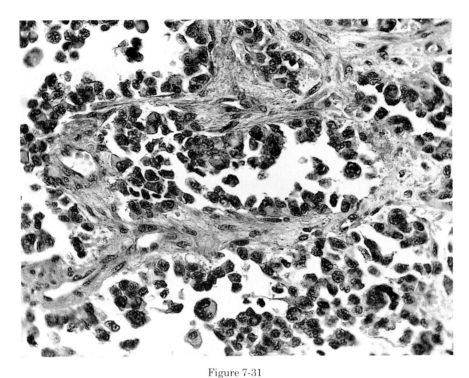

Figure 7-31
RHABDOMYOSARCOMA
Higher power magnification of tumor seen in figure 7-29 illustrating rhabdomyoblasts.

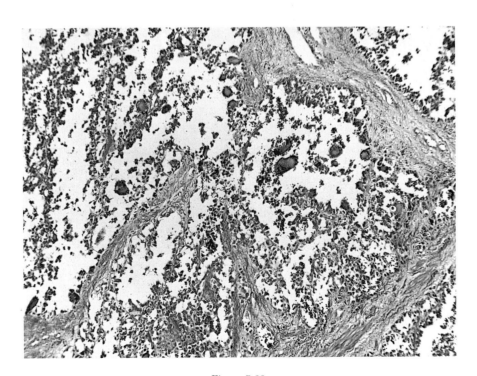

Figure 7-32
RHABDOMYOSARCOMA
Tumor with an alveolar pattern and numerous large anaplastic giant cells.

Table 7-6
IMMUNOHISTOCHEMISTRY OF EMBRYONAL RHABDOMYOSARCOMA OF THE ORBIT: INTENSITY OF STAINING IN 15 CASES FROM THE REGISTRY OF OPHTHALMIC PATHOLOGY

Type of Antibody	Intensity of Immune Reaction		
	Negative	Faint	Positive
Muscle-specific actin	0	1	14
Vimentin	0	2	13
Desmin	2	9	4
Smooth muscle actin	4	6	5
Myoglobin	8	2	5
Cytokeratin mixture	10	1	4
Neuron-specific enolase	13	1	1
Glial fibrillary acidic protein	14	0	1
S-100 protein	15	0	0
Neurofilament protein	15	0	0

positive except for 1 equivocal case. Immunoreactivity for desmin was negative in 2 tumors and equivocal in 9. Myoglobin could not be detected in most tumors. Focal reactivity was observed for cytokeratin in 5 tumors, neuron-specific enolase in 2, and glial fibrillary acidic protein (GFAP) in 1. While muscle-specific actin is the most sensitive antibody for the detection of orbital rhabdomyosarcoma, there is a problem with specificity: some myofibroblastic tumors and pleomorphic carcinomas have weak or focal reactivity. Since much of the orbital mesenchyme is believed to be of neural crest origin, it is interesting that all of the orbital rhabdomyosarcomas were S-100 protein negative.

Electron Microscopic Findings. Even in tumors that do not show light microscopic evidence of rhabdomyoblastic differentiation, electron microscopy may reveal myofilaments in some cells (49). These myosin filaments, measuring 150 Å in diameter, are found in disorganized bundles within the cytoplasm. In the more differentiated tumors the myosin filaments are organized in sarcomeric units. Well-formed sarcomeres have interdigitated thick myosin and thin actin filaments delimited by transverse Z lines.

Treatment and Prognosis. Survival of patients with orbital rhabdomyosarcoma has dra-matically improved over the past 50 years. Orbital exenteration cured about 30 percent of patients; high voltage X-ray therapy, cobalt-60 radiotherapy, or proton beam therapy cured more than 50 percent of patients without the mutilation of an exenteration; and now a combination of modern irradiation plus multidrug chemotherapy cures 90 percent (51,52). The major problems related to modern radiotherapy are its damaging effects on the eye and orbital bones: keratitis, cataracts, retinopathy, and optic neuritis of the globe and growth failure of the orbital bones resulting in a small, shrunken orbit. These complications may subsequently necessitate enucleation.

LIPOMA

Despite its ubiquity, the orbital fat infrequently produces neoplasms (Table 7-1) (54,56, 57). Lipomas of the orbit have been estimated in some series to be responsible for as many as 9 percent of orbital neoplasms, but in all likelihood the excised tissues in some of these cases represent normal orbital fat rather than a true neoplasm. In the orbit, adipose tissue is normally divided into compartments by fibrous septa, and this may be confused with the lobular pattern of a lipoma. There are two reports of spindle cell lipoma in which fascicles of benign-appearing fibroblasts were intermixed with lobules of fully mature adipocytes (53,55). Hibernoma, a tumor of brown or embryonal fat, has never been described in the orbit. Disseminated lipomatosis has been associated with proptosis.

LIPOSARCOMA

Liposarcoma is more common than lipoma in the cases from the ROP (Tables 7-1, 7-2), but even with the AFIP referral bias this is a rare tumor. The clinical course is indolent, with proptosis developing over a period of 1 to 3 years, generally with good preservation of ocular function (58). CTs usually demonstrate well-defined tumors with foci of radiolucency suggestive of a multi-loculated orbital cyst, but in well-differentiated tumors CT may fail to identify a mass (58–60). MRI may show hyperintense signals in T1-weighted images and an abnormally high signal on T2-weighted images, suggesting the presence of abnormal fat within the lesional tissue (58–60).

Histologically, liposarcoma in the orbit is almost always of the well-differentiated or myxoid type. Rarely, the pleomorphic type has been observed in the orbit (60). Well-differentiated lipoma-like liposarcomas of the orbit can be difficult to differentiate histologically from a lipoma. Lipoblasts, which distinguish liposarcoma from lipoma, may be rare in these tumors. Lipoblasts have enlarged, hyperchromatic nuclei and usually multiple lipid vacuoles that indent the nucleus. A major clue regarding the possibility of a liposarcoma is the presence of an abundant plexiform vascularity permeating the tumor. In myxoid liposarcomas, this feature helps distinguish the lesion from a myxoma or other myxoid mesenchymal lesions.

Recommendations for the management of orbital liposarcomas must be based on extrapolation of data from other sites because of the rarity of these tumors. The metastatic potential of liposarcomas in other sites relates to their size; liposarcomas of the thigh and retroperitoneum are often massive compared with those of the orbit. The tumors in the orbit are generally not encapsulated and incomplete excision almost inevitably leads to recurrence. Exenteration probably should not be done for orbital liposarcomas that are of low grade (well-differentiated or myxoid types) and not far advanced because distant metastasis is uncommon with these tumors. The removal of orbital bones at the time of surgery is contraindicated since this might permit easier access of the infiltrating tumor into surrounding compartments. Rare high-grade malignancies (pleomorphic type) that are more likely to metastasize should be exenterated once the pathologic diagnosis is secure.

NEUROFIBROMAS

Three types of neurofibroma are found in the orbit: plexiform neurofibroma, diffuse neurofibroma, and isolated neurofibroma. These three types differ in clinical and histologic findings, and in their association with neurofibromatosis type 1.

Plexiform Neurofibroma

Clinical Features. The plexiform neurofibroma is observed only in patients with neurofibromatosis type 1, and has a distinctive clinical presentation (63,65). It appears within the first decade of life and is an infiltrating lesion that may involve all aspects of the orbital soft tissues, including the extraocular muscles and the lacrimal gland, causing proptosis or orbital-facial disfigurement. Imaging studies (fig. 7-33) confirm the diffuse infiltration by the tumor and differentiate plexiform neurofibromas from other causes of exophthalmos in neurofibromatosis (optic nerve tumors, orbital osseous dysplasia, and buphthalmos) (61,63,64). The enormous overgrowth of the orbital peripheral nerves may cause excessive redundancy of the lid skin, creating the appearance of elephantiasis neuromatosa. Malignant degeneration of a plexiform neurofibroma of the orbit is uncommon, but patients with von Recklinghausen disease are at higher risk of developing malignant peripheral nerve sheath tumors than is the general population.

Pathologic Findings. The plexiform neurofibroma (fig. 7-34) is not an encapsulated tumor but rather, like lymphangioma, grows in a crab grass fashion to involve all the orbital tissues. The tumor is a massive hyperplasia of the peripheral nerve terminal branches and therefore the histopathologic features are highly organoid. Each proliferating unit is surrounded by a perineurium; in the spaces enclosed by the outer perimeters of

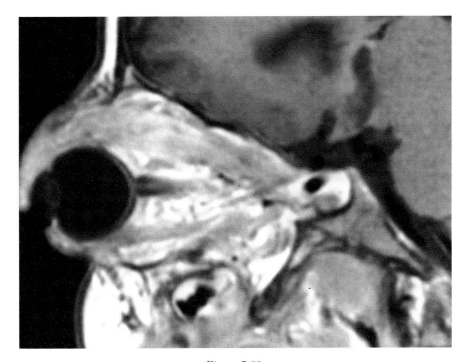

Figure 7-33
NEUROFIBROMATOSIS
Sagittal magnetic resonance image of a large infiltrative tumor of orbit and eyelid.

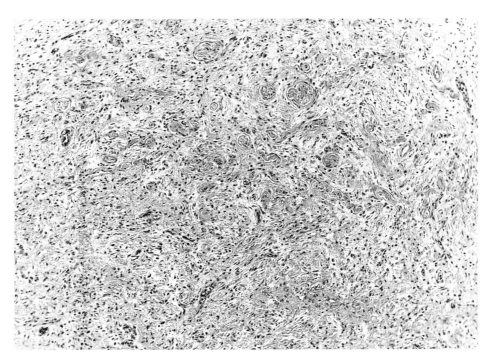

Figure 7-34
NEUROFIBROMATOSIS
Neurofibroma with plexiform pattern.

the perineurium are axons, Schwann cells, and endoneural fibroblasts. Increased vascularity usually accompanies these neuromatous masses, so that at surgery, plexiform neurofibromas bleed profusely. The Bodian stain may reveal axons. Acid mucopolysaccharide rich in hyaluronic acid can be identified in the matrix of the endoneural compartment. There is a distinct tendency to recur after surgical removal.

Diffuse Neurofibroma

The diffuse neurofibroma is the rarest type of neurofibroma in the orbit; it is not always associated with von Recklinghausen disease. It represents an infiltrative, noncircumscribed proliferation of peripheral nerve sheath elements that may replace the orbital fat and permeate the extraocular muscles. Most of these lesions are solid, with an obvious cellularity and only moderate collagenization; others are predominantly myxoid, with a soupy or gelatinous appearance at the time of surgical excision because of abundant mucinous material. Most of the myxoid stroma is rich in hyaluronic acid, in which stellate and elongated peripheral nerve sheath cells are suspended.

Isolated Neurofibroma

Clinical Features. The isolated neurofibroma tends to grow as a circumscribed lesion, although it is not encapsulated. This type of neurofibroma is least likely to be associated with neurofibromatosis type 1. In a large series of patients with isolated neurofibromas in the orbit (62), one fourth had a family history or other signs of systemic neurofibromatosis. Symptoms and signs were generally those of an orbital mass lesion. Pain, visual defect, and peripheral nerve sensory loss were unusual. Within the orbit, most peripheral nerve sheath tumors affect the first division of the trigeminal nerve. Extension of some tumors through the superior orbital fissure limits their surgical resection. Despite incomplete resection of some tumors, and with up to 23 years of follow-up, there were no recurrences requiring further surgery.

Lesions unassociated with neurofibromatosis tend to occur in the third to fifth decades of life. Enlargement of the orbit with fossa formation is not uncommon due to the longstanding nature of these lesions. CT reveals a well-circumscribed lesion (61), and ultrasound examination demonstrates low internal reflectivity with rapid attenuation of the echoes within the lesion. Lesions of the lacrimal fossa may be indistinguishable clinically and radiographically from benign mixed tumors.

Pathologic Findings. On histopathologic examination, the lesions may have a pseudocapsule, but a true perineurium is not discerned. The lesions are composed of wavy bundles of peripheral nerve sheath cells with comma-shaped nuclei; hyaluronic acid and various amounts of collagen are deposited in the stroma. The reticulin stain reveals abundant fiber deposition and the Bodian stain may reveal axon cylinders. In heavily collagenized lesions, differentiation from other soft tissue tumors of the orbit may be difficult. The application of special immunohistochemical methods to identify S-100 protein can be helpful in making the diagnosis.

Electron microscopy has shown that most of the neurofibroma cells have more of the characteristics of perineural cells than Schwann cells. Interrupted segments of basement membrane material, pinocytotic vesicles, and sometimes, cytoplasmic filaments are featured, but long-spacing collagen (Luse bodies or banded basement membrane material) is uncommon. One of the major reasons for distinguishing an isolated neurofibroma from a schwannoma is that only neurofibromas are associated with neurofibromatosis and they are more likely to undergo malignant transformation than schwannomas, although this is quite rare.

SCHWANNOMA (NEURILEMOMA)

Clinical Findings. Like neurofibroma, schwannoma originates from any of the sensory nerves of the orbit, most often the supraorbital nerve. Clinical symptoms are virtually indistinguishable from those of neurofibroma: slowly evolving, well-tolerated symptoms of proptosis; extraocular motility disturbance; and occasional pain (69). If a lesion abuts the optic nerve, there may be optic nerve dysfunction (atrophy, visual field loss, vascular engorgement, and disc edema). Computed tomograms (68) and ultrasonographic findings (65) are those of an encapsulated tumor.

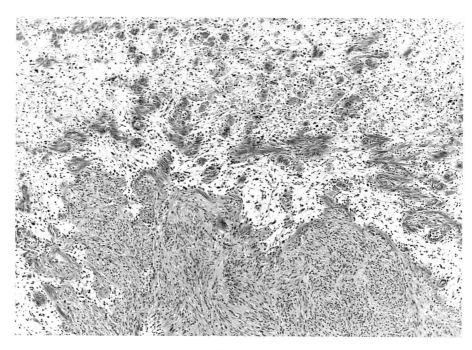

Figure 7-35
SCHWANNOMA
Tumor with cellular solid Antoni A and myxoid Antoni B areas.

Pathologic Findings. Histopathologically, schwannomas are encapsulated by the perineurium of the nerve of origin, which may be eccentrically present in the capsule. The classic feature of a schwannoma is the alternation within the same lesion of solid cellular areas, referred to as the Antoni A pattern, with areas of looser myxoid tissue having stellate or ovoid cells suspended in a mucinous background, the Antoni B pattern (fig. 7-35). In Antoni A areas, nuclear palisading is more common than in neurofibromas, often with fascicles that have highly regimented nuclei arranged in transverse stripes, a pattern referred to as Verocay bodies (fig. 7-36). The reticulin stain discloses abundant fibers, and virtually all the lesions are positive for cytoplasmic S-100 protein. Acid mucopolysaccharides are present only in Antoni B areas where they may be very prominent and create pools. These can be seen grossly as cysts on cross section. Some lesions may display a herringbone pattern, but the nuclei are more oval than those in fibroblastic proliferations; "ancient" schwannomas may exhibit collagenization and atypical nuclei in the absence of mitotic activity. There is a tendency for the capillaries within the lesions to be invested by a thickened, PAS-positive basement membrane; some may be sufficiently fragile to result in intralesional hemorrhage with secondary development of hemosiderin-laden macrophages. Xanthoma cells may also be seen throughout the looser myxoid areas. Electron microscopy has shown these to be transformed, lipidized Schwann cells, as opposed to true macrophages, owing to the presence of basement membranes.

In contrast to neurofibromas, schwannomas display clear-cut ultrastructural evidence of Schwann cell origin (71): an electron-lucent cytoplasm with scant organelles (scattered mitochondria and short segments of rough-surfaced endoplasmic reticulum); cytoplasmic filaments and microtubules; long, delicate cytoplasmic processes; mesaxon and pseudomesaxon formation; and linear, amorphous, and banded basement membrane material (Luse bodies).

Schwannomas, because they are encapsulated, are readily removed from the orbit. If incompletely removed, they, like neurofibromas, are likely to recur, but this can be delayed over decades. Schwannomas are less likely than neurofibromas to undergo malignant degeneration (70,71).

261

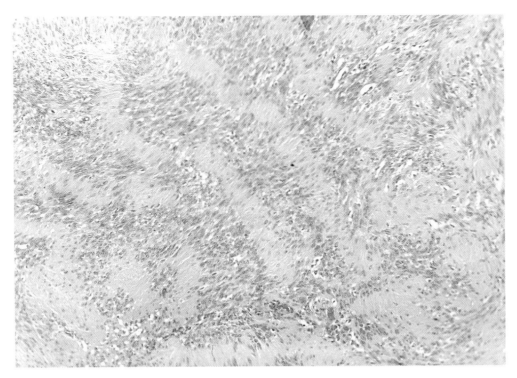

Figure 7-36
SCHWANNOMA
Palisaded nuclei in an Antoni A area form Verocay bodies.

MALIGNANT PERIPHERAL NERVE SHEATH TUMORS

Malignant tumors arising from peripheral nerves have often been designated as either neurofibrosarcomas or malignant schwannomas without evidence that the tumor arose from endoneural or perineural fibroblasts or from Schwann cells. Without such evidence, we recommend designating the tumor as a malignant peripheral nerve sheath tumor. These tumors are rare in the orbit. Jacobiec et al. (70) found only eight well-documented cases in their review of the material in the AFIP ROP prior to 1975. Surprisingly, we found nine cases in our review (Table 7-2), suggesting that some cases may not be well documented. One case was of particular interest because it occurred in a child who previously received radiation therapy for bilateral retinoblastoma. The tumor was biphasic. One portion of the tumor was a benign neurofibroma and the other portion an anaplastic sarcoma, suggesting that the sarcoma arose from the neurofibroma.

Many of the reported orbital malignant peripheral nerve sheath tumors arose from preexistent neurofibromas and about one fourth of the patients had neurofibromatosis (71). Typically, the tumors develop in the superomedial aspect of the orbit in patients between 19 and 75 years of age. Histologically, the neoplasms are composed of a mixture of spindle and epithelioid cells in which there is moderate mitotic activity. Differentiation from an amelanotic melanoma may be difficult by light microscopy. Positive immunohistochemical staining for S-100 protein and negative staining for HMB-45 is helpful in the differential diagnosis. Because malignancies derived from neural fibroblasts and many anaplastic schwannomas are S-100 negative, electron microscopy may be necessary to confirm the diagnosis.

The best treatment is orbital exenteration, combined with craniotomy if there is suspicion of spread through the superior orbital fissure. Postoperative radiation therapy may be added; this probably will not increase the chance of cure but may prolong life.

LYMPHOID TUMORS AND INFLAMMATION

The orbit is a common extranodal site for lymphoid tumors, and such extranodal sites pose special difficulties in staging and diagnosis. Using histologic criteria, reproducible classification of orbital lymphoid tumors is difficult; this limits the ability to predict whether a given lymphoid lesion will be restricted to the orbit or will eventually be part of a systemic disease. An additional problem with orbital lesions is the tendency of some clinicians and pathologists to combine lymphoid tumors with inflammatory pseudotumors. We and others (90) believe that clinically, radiographically, and histologically both benign and malignant lymphoid tumors usually can be distinguished from orbital inflammation.

Inflammatory Pseudotumors

Birch-Hirschfeld (85) introduced the term pseudotumor to describe inflammatory swellings of the orbital contents that produce proptosis and the false clinical impression of a neoplasm. Orbital inflammation can be divided into two broad groups dependent on whether an associated systemic disease or local cause of the inflammation is discovered.

Graves Orbitopathy

In terms of both frequency and severity, Graves disease is the most important cause of orbital pseudotumor (77,86). It causes more than 50 percent of the proptoses seen by ophthalmologists. The work-up of a patient with proptosis should include tests for thyroid dysfunction. Despite its frequency, Graves orbitopathy is rarely seen as a surgical pathology specimen and its etiology remains an enigma. The orbital disease is most often associated with hyperthyroidism, less commonly with Hashimoto lymphocytic thyroiditis, and rarely, with an euthyroid state in which the patient has no detectable thyroid dysfunction (98).

Clinical Features. Men and women are equally affected. Graves disease is usually mild in childhood. Patients have an insidious development of eye irritation (tearing and grittiness), stare or upper lid retraction, and proptosis. The proptosis is virtually always axial without displacement of the eyeball. A late symptom is diplopia from extraocular muscle enlargement

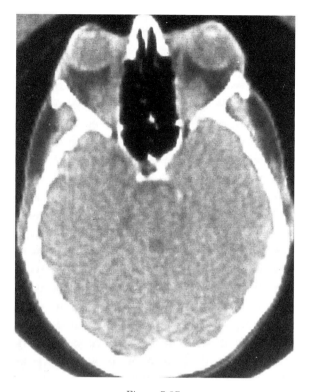

Figure 7-37
GRAVES DISEASE
Computed tomograph showing enlargement of extraocular muscles at orbital apex.

and scarring. When swollen muscles converge at the orbital apex (fig. 7-37), a compressive optic neuropathy with reduction in visual acuity may result. Paradoxically, patients with optic nerve compression from swollen extraocular muscles may not have the highest grades of proptosis because in these patients the posterior third of the muscle bellies are preferentially affected. Less commonly, high-grade proptosis that creates corneal exposure and breakdown can also lead to visual loss.

Patients with Graves ophthalmopathy vary in their manifestations of hyperthyroidism. Most develop proptosis concurrently with tachycardia, weight loss, sweating, and a velvety skin. For some, the ophthalmic signs follow ablation of the thyroid gland. Finally, there is a group of patients with the classic clinical, ultrasonographic, and radiographic findings of orbital Graves disease yet every test of thyroid function is normal. These patients have euthyroid Graves disease but over a 3-year period approximately half will develop thyroid dysfunction (98).

The main technique for the evaluation of Graves orbitopathy is CT (figs. 7-37, 7-38) (78). The inflammation produces swelling of one or more extraocular muscles, which is usually bilateral but may be asymmetric. The inferior rectus muscles are the most frequently affected, followed by the medial rectus and the superior rectus-levator complex; the least involved is the lateral rectus, which is never involved in isolation (fig. 7-38). Generally, the posterior and middle thirds of the muscle bellies are affected; the tendons tend to be spared, so that there is a sharp tapering of the anterior aspect of the enlarged muscle toward the globe. Massive thickening of the medial rectus can cause bowing of the lamina papyracea. Enlargement of the lacrimal glands is frequently seen when there is advanced extraocular muscle swelling. The orbital fat is virtually never inflamed. The sparing of the extraocular muscle tendons and the failure of inflammation to spill over into the orbital fat and track along the intermuscular fibrous membranes help to distinguish Graves disease from other pseudotumors.

Pathologic Findings. The pathologic features of Graves disease are quite consistent with the CT and ultrasonographic findings. The inflammation is virtually always restricted to the muscle bellies of the extraocular muscles. It consists mostly of lymphocytes and plasma cells, with a scattering of mast cells. Germinal centers and eosinophils are usually not present. The earliest inflammation appears to occur in the endomysial connective tissue compartment, with stimulation of the fibroblasts to produce acid mucopolysaccharides. With prolonged inflammation the fibroblasts switch from mucopolysaccharide production to collagen production. The ultimate severity of the disease depends upon the extent to which fibrosis of the extraocular muscles occurs. The tendons inserting onto the globe, the meninges of the optic nerve, and the orbital fat are not generally inflamed. The lacrimal gland shows moderate infiltration of lymphocytes and plasma cells, with interstitial fluid collection but no fibrosis (77,84,86).

Treatment. In the most serious cases, treatment is aimed at preventing visual impairment

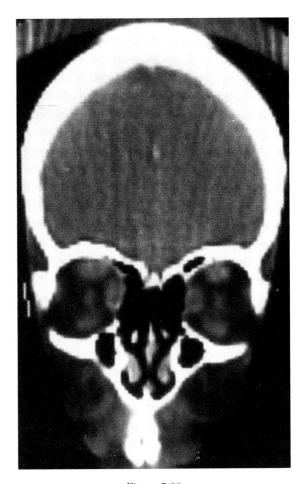

Figure 7-38
GRAVES DISEASE
Coronal computed tomograph showing enlargement of all extraocular muscles except the lateral rectus.

due to optic nerve compression or corneal exposure. Radiotherapy and corticosteroids are the treatments of choice (76,85,86). Orbital decompressive surgery is recommended only for those patients with threatened vision who fail to improve on medical or radiotherapeutic regimes (73). Surgery on the eyelids, as opposed to orbital surgery, is performed only when there is a high degree of proptosis that causes discomfort from tear film evaporation with corneal exposure (86). Therapies aimed at suppression of immunologic hyperreactivity, systemic chemotherapy, serum plasmapheresis, and cyclosporin therapy, have been tried when radiotherapy and orbital decompressive surgery are unsuccessful (86).

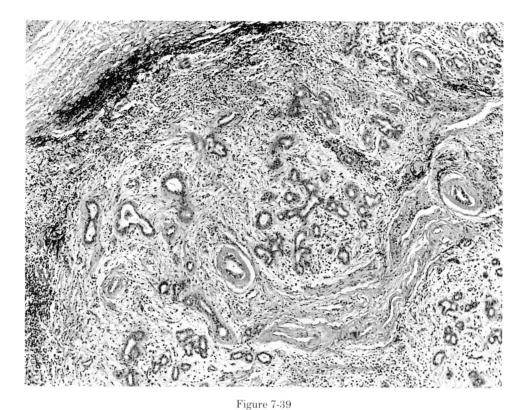

Figure 7-39
ECTOPIC LACRIMAL GLAND
Atrophic glandular tissue with chronic inflammation obtained from the retrobulbar portion of the orbit.

Idiopathic Orbital Inflammation (Pseudotumors)

Idiopathic orbital inflammation has no recognizable local cause in the orbit (infection, ruptured dermoid cyst, ectopic lacrimal gland (fig. 7-39) (74,79), retained foreign body, or hemorrhagic lymphangioma) or any underlying systemic disease such as autoimmune collagen diseases (80), systemic vasculitis, Wegener granulomatosis (87), or Crohn disease (99). In series based on orbital biopsies (see Tables 7-1–7-5) (82,89,96), strictly localized idiopathic orbital inflammation is one of the most common lesions. Since in most instances the diagnosis can be made clinically with ultrasonographic and CT studies, the real incidence of inflammation is far greater. It is probably the second most frequent cause of proptosis after Graves disease.

Clinical Features. Patients with idiopathic orbital inflammation may be of any age, including childhood (91,92). The onset is acute, subacute, or chronic. The disease may recur in one orbit, be

bilateral, or alternate from one orbit to the other. The inflammation can be further classified according to which orbital structure is predominantly involved: myositis (one or more extraocular muscles) (95), dacryoadenitis (lacrimal gland), periscleritis (epibulbar or Tenon-level connective tissue and contiguous orbital fat), trochleitis (inflammation of the trochlear cartilage), and perineuritis (the outer dural sheath of the optic nerve and contiguous periopic orbital fat). The lesions are usually diffuse, involving more than one structure, including the adipose tissue and extraocular muscles, but may be predominantly posterior or anterior (88). Imaging studies are particularly valuable in determining the pattern and extent of orbital involvement (75,81).

The acute form of the disease is the most striking and the easiest to distinguish from other orbital conditions, including Graves disease and lymphoid tumors of the orbit. There is an abrupt onset of periocular pain accompanied by discomfort on movement of the globe, proptosis, chemosis, epibulbar injection, injection over the insertions of the rectus muscles, erythema of the lid skin, and decreased visual acuity or diplopia. Pronounced chemosis, lid swelling, and erythema may occur suggesting an orbital cellulitis, which generally can be ruled out by the absence of sinus disease on radiographic studies.

Subacute cases are characterized by a less fulminant onset, with symptoms and signs developing slowly over weeks to months. In the chronic variety, patients become symptomatic from proptosis, diplopia, or visual loss over months to years with few cutaneous or epibulbar signs of inflammation. If these lesions are situated anteriorly in the orbit and can be palpated through the lids, they have a rock-hard feel that is mimicked only by metastatic scirrhous carcinoma.

In the myositis variant, the entire length of the involved extraocular muscle is enlarged, including the tendon; the latter feature helps distinguish idiopathic inflammation from Graves disease. The inflammation may track along the intermuscular septa from one muscle to another and spill over into the contiguous fat, findings not generally present in Graves disease (95).

In the dacryoadenitis variant, the lacrimal gland is swollen, generally in an oblong fashion, and molded to the shape of adjacent structures, which differs from the rounded appearance of primary epithelial tumors in the lacrimal gland. In the acute and chronic forms, there is generally no erosion of the contiguous orbital bone. Because of frequent involvement of the palpebral and orbital lobes, the gland may have a "V" shape.

The fibrous connective tissue of the orbit and fat are predominantly involved in the diffuse variant. Rarely, inflammation along the medial orbital wall coexists with an ethmoidal inflammatory lesion, with partial dissolution of the medial orbital wall. This may be confused with orbital cellulitis secondary to sinus disease. Chronic sclerosing orbital inflammation rarely extends intracranially. In the subacute or chronic form there is more uniform radiodensity; confluence of the normally streaky infiltrates of orbital fat involvement observed in the acute phase leads to solid radiodensity. Either the anterior or posterior orbital fat may be selectively involved. Sclerosing orbital inflammation can lead to "wall-to-wall" radiodensity, in which the muscles, optic nerve, and globe are totally caught up in a uniform ligneous mass (figs. 7-40, 7-41).

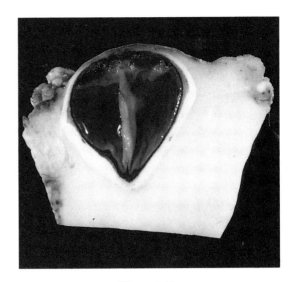

Figure 7-40
IDIOPATHIC INFLAMMATION
Fibrotic mass surrounds the eye.

Pathologic Findings. Edema and a light polymorphic inflammatory infiltrate are highly characteristic in the early stages of inflammation. The infiltrating cells include lymphocytes, plasma cells, eosinophils, and, less often, polymorphonuclear leukocytes. Immunohistochemistry reveals that the lymphocytes are predominately T cells. Eosinophilia may be especially evident in orbital biopsies from children and there may be an elevated absolute count of eosinophils in the peripheral blood.

As the disease progresses, collagen is laid down and the inflammatory cells become more widely separated by fibrous tracts, which radiate outward from the tissue septa and blood vessels into the orbital fat (fig. 7-42). The connective tissues of the muscles thicken (fig. 7-43), and hyperplasia of the periacinal and periductal connective tissues of the lacrimal gland is observed. With progressive fibrosis, extraocular muscle degeneration occurs and the secretory acinar units of the lacrimal gland are obliterated, leading to blind-duct proliferation or hyperplasia. Once the acini of the lacrimal gland are destroyed, they do not regenerate. In inexorably sclerosing inflammation, all the orbital contents, including the optic nerve and sclera, are caught up in the strangulating fibrosis (fig. 7-40, 7-41). There is only a light infiltrate of inflammatory cells and necrosis is not featured, as in a true vasculitis or scleritis.

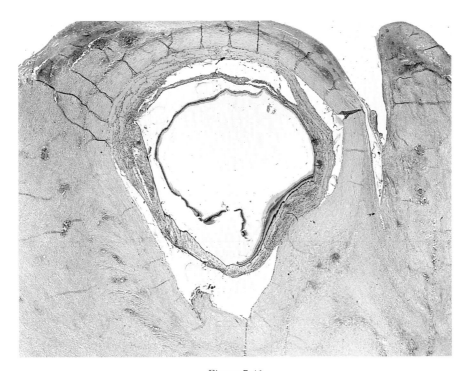

Figure 7-41
IDIOPATHIC INFLAMMATION
Dense fibrotic tissue with focal collections of lymphocytes surrounds the eye.

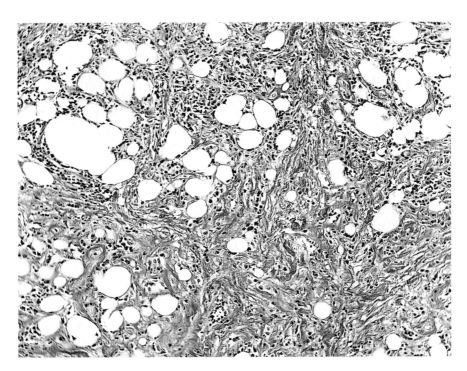

Figure 7-42
IDIOPATHIC INFLAMMATION
Inflammation and fibrosis involve the adipose tissue of the orbit.

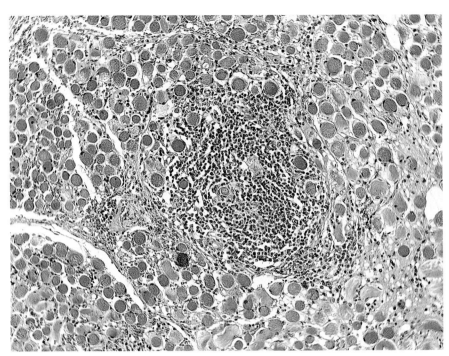

Figure 7-43
IDIOPATHIC
INFLAMMATION
Chronic inflammatory cells
infiltrate an extraocular muscle.

Frequently, perivascular lymphocytic cuffing is a prominent feature of idiopathic orbital inflammation, and occasionally eosinophils may be admixed. Such cuffing represents diapedesis of blood-borne cells into the adventitia of the capillaries and venules and, therefore, does not constitute true vasculitis. In rare instances, a strictly localized idiopathic orbital inflammation appears to be caused by a true vasculitis of the orbital vessels, in which lymphocytes and polymorphonuclear leukocytes cause necrosis of the muscularis of orbital vessels. Henderson (82) pointed out that this subset frequently affects individuals less than 30 years of age. These lesions are less responsive to prednisone and localized orbital radiotherapy and may require systemic administration of chemotherapeutic agents such as cyclophosphamide.

Differential Diagnosis. The involvement of structures other than the extraocular muscles, combined with the presence of eosinophils, helps distinguish idiopathic orbital inflammation from Graves disease. Compared with orbital lymphoid neoplasms, there is hypocellularity and far more cellular polymorphism, fibrosis, and edema. The diffuse, sheetlike hyperplasia of lymphocytes characteristic of lymphoid tumors of the orbit is not seen. Furthermore, lymphoid tumors of the

orbit do not present acute inflammatory signs and are generally unifocal masses rather than the diffuse or multifocal processes of idiopathic orbital inflammation. Locally invasive polymorphic orbital "pseudotumors" should be carefully evaluated microscopically for cytologic atypia of fibrohistiocytic cells to exclude an inflamed malignant fibrous histiocytoma.

Idiopathic orbital inflammation can be indistinguishable clinically and histologically from systemic diseases such as Wegener granulomatosis, rheumatoid arthritis, Crohn regional enteritis, systemic lupus erythematosus, and periarteritis nodosa. Although less than 10 percent of patients with orbital inflammation other than Graves orbitopathy have an underlying disease, it is probably wisest to study patients with inflammation for evidence of a multisystem autoimmune disease. Wegener granulomatosis may only produce orbital signs and symptoms, but patients with this limited form of the disease often have antineutrophilic cytoplasmic antibodies in their serum (87). Bilateral orbital lesions featuring many xanthoma cells should suggest the possibility of Erdheim-Chester disease (72). Lesions with vascular proliferation and eosinophilia may represent Kimura disease (figs. 7-44, 7-45) (83,97).

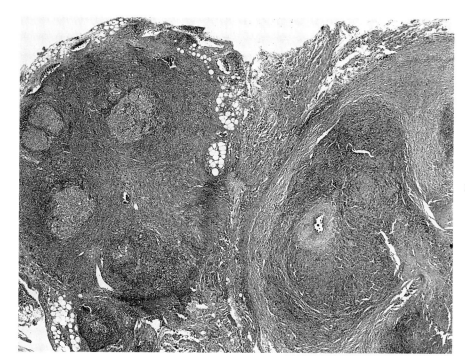

Figure 7-44
KIMURA DISEASE
A mass with lymphoid hyperplasia.

Figure 7-45
KIMURA DISEASE
Higher power magnification of tumor in previous figure showing hyperplastic vessels and eosinophils.

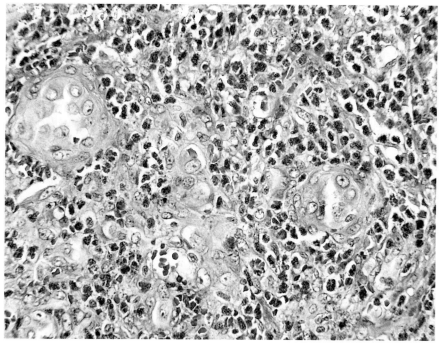

Treatment. High dose corticosteroid therapy for acute fulminant idiopathic orbital inflammation is generally curative. A less dramatic response to corticosteroids is seen in subacute and chronic cases because of the heavy collagenization of the diseased tissues. Radiotherapy is sometimes ad-ministered in cases that are refractory to corticosteroids (93), however, many reports on radiotherapy for orbital inflammation actually deal with lymphoid tumors rather than idiopathic inflammations as defined and described in this section. Immunosuppressive therapy may be helpful in the small subset of patients refractory to corticosteroid therapy and radiotherapy (94). Although idiopathic orbital inflammation generally is not a surgical disease, focal masses of hyalinized connective tissue in end-stage, burned-out cases may be surgically debulked to reduce proptosis or displacement of the eye. In extremely rare cases of refractory sclerosing orbital inflammation, there may be intractable pain and vision may be totally lost from a compressive neuropathy as the fibrous tissue strangulates the optic nerve. Occasionally, when the patient has extraordinary pain and no vision, orbital exenteration may be indicated (figs. 7-40, 7-41).

Lymphoid Tumors

The proportion of patients with systemic lymphoma that have orbital involvement is low (106) but in series of orbital tumors diagnosed by biopsy, orbital lymphoid tumors are among the most prevalent (see Tables 7-1–7-3) (103,113,119).

In considering orbital lymphoid lesions, a few basic anatomic and immunologic features should be kept in mind. Normally, lymphocytes are present in the substantia propria of the conjunctiva and are scattered among the acini of the lacrimal gland but they are not present in the orbit. This may explain why extraorbital manifestations of lymphoproliferative disease are found in approximately 50 percent of patients with orbital lymphoid tumors and in only 10 percent of patients with conjunctival tumors. Other extranodal sites that have associated lymphoid tissue (e.g., bowel and lung) share many biologic features with conjunctival lymphoid tumors (104).

Clinical Features. Precise anatomic distinctions must be made among conjunctival, lid, and orbital lymphoid tumors. Conjunctival tumors are more likely to be a hyperplasia or a well-differentiated lymphoma, whereas preseptal lid tumors are more likely to be a higher grade aggressive lymphoma (108,115). Lymphoid lesions of the conjunctiva present as salmon-colored patches that are generally readily movable over the epibulbar surface because they are limited to the substantia propria. They do not cause extraocular motility problems or proptosis as do orbital lesions. Any lymphoid mass that can be observed subconjunctivally but is essentially located in the orbit has the more serious prognosis

of an orbital lesion. Tumors invading the lid from a deeper orbital location have a prognosis similar to that of orbital lesions. Orbital involvement in these tumors can be confirmed with CT.

Lymphoid tumors of the orbit generally have an insidious onset without overt inflammatory clinical signs, such as erythema, chemosis of the conjunctiva, or orbital or ocular pain (101). Patients are generally older, typically more than 50 years of age at the time of diagnosis; the disease is decidedly rare in children except in areas where Burkitt lymphoma is endemic (100). Patients who are symptomatic for about 6 months usually have moderate proptosis (less than 5 mm), mild motility disorders, and only occasional visual loss. The superior quadrant of the orbit is the most frequent site of involvement, occurring in about 30 percent of cases. The next most frequent site is the lacrimal gland, perhaps due to the scattered population of lymphoid cells normally present between the ducts and acini. These lesions often mold to the globe and orbital septum, and may be palpated through the lids as firm or rubbery masses. If there is a follicular architecture or expansion within preexistent lobules of the lacrimal gland, there may be a pebbly or micronodular consistency. Clinically, there are only a few clues that help distinguish a benign and malignant orbital lymphoid tumor. Recurrences and bilateral lesions not involving the lacrimal gland point toward malignancy (108).

CT discloses a distinctive pattern for orbital lymphoid tumors (fig. 7-46). They mold to the orbital bones, globe, optic nerve, or fascial septa creating straight lines and unusually angulated patterns. Arc-like contours are seen in coronal planes where the lesions abut the orbital bones and sclera, but serrated and irregular margins are seen within the orbital soft tissues because of lack of encapsulation and irregular infiltration of orbital fat. Lymphoid tumors are almost always unifocal masses, differing from many of the multifocal idiopathic inflammations (117,121).

Lymphoid tumors involving the lacrimal gland must be distinguished from epithelial tumors because they are managed differently. They generally create diffuse expansions of the lacrimal gland, which exaggerate its normally oblong and pancake-like character in both axial and coronal CTs. The lesions mold to the globe as well as to the adjacent bone, without destruction of the

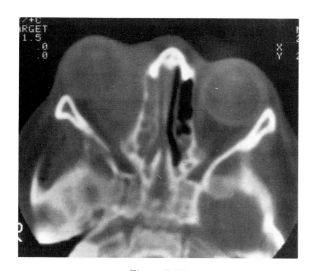

Figure 7-46
LYMPHOID TUMOR
Computed tomograph of a homogeneous tumor that molds to ocular structures causing proptosis.

latter. The anterior portion of the lesion may extend beyond the orbital rim, indicating involvement of the palpebral lobe; the posterior aspect of the lesion abutting the orbital fat often has a straight-line appearance. Epithelial tumors of the lacrimal gland, on the other hand, are oval, globular, or rounded, with arc-like posterior margins. Over 80 percent of epithelial tumors erode adjacent bone, producing a fossa. Erosion of the bone is more common with epithelial tumors because their firm texture contrasts with the putty-like consistency of lymphoid tissue. Rarely do epithelial tumors extend significantly beyond the orbital rim since they tend to arise in the deeper orbital lobe rather than in the palpebral lobe.

Pathologic Findings. At surgery, and grossly in the pathology laboratory, lymphoid tissue has a fish-flesh or creamy to yellow appearance; highly vascularized lesions can appear reddish. A major tip-off that a lesion is a lymphoid tumor is its friability, the result of a paucity of fibrous stroma. From the pathologic point of view, lymphoid tumors of the orbit must be divided into *lymphomas* and *benign lymphoid hyperplasias*. A large size and infiltration of the orbital tissues are not helpful in distinguishing malignant tumors from hyperplasias, since both lesions may exhibit these traits. A major difficulty in the histopathologic interpretation of

lymphoid lesions of the orbit is the inability to use such criteria as the effacement of preexistent architecture or invasion of a capsule, features applicable to the interpretation of lesions arising within lymph nodes (108).

The classification of lymphoid tumors as either benign reactive lymphoid hyperplasia or malignant lymphoma is easy when classic signs of benignity or malignancy exist, but often the degree of cytologic differentiation is not totally clear-cut. Many lymphoid tumors are composed of lymphocytes that are slightly immature or there may be a mixture of mature lymphocytes with a subpopulation of less mature lymphoreticular elements. When it is difficult to make an unequivocal assignment to the benign or malignant category, the lymphoid tumor is referred to as an atypical lymphoid hyperplasia or infiltrate. About 50 percent of orbital lesions have either clear-cut histopathologic features of benign reactive lymphoid hyperplasia or are borderline tumors; the other 50 percent represent various levels of differentiation of malignant lymphoma. In an AFIP study of 66 lesions employing only histologic assessment (110), the most frequent diagnosis was *atypical lymphoid hyperplasia* (30 of the 66 cases), probably reflecting the fact that diagnostically difficult material was sent for consultation.

Almost all of the orbital lymphomas are B-cell non-Hodgkin type (109,115). Despite the fact that about 30 percent of systemic lymphomas are Hodgkin type, Hodgkin disease rarely involves the orbit, and then only late in the course of an already widely disseminated and diagnosed process. Another type of systemic lymphoma that rarely involves the orbit is the T-cell cutaneous lymphoma group, the best example of which is mycosis fungoides (120). These lesions are only rarely identified in the lids and conjunctiva as part of an already well-recognized systemic disease; deep orbital involvement is the rarest manifestation.

The overall skeleton of the National Cancer Institute (NCI) working formulation can be adapted for ophthalmic pathology use (118). The NCI formulation pertains to systemic nodal lymphomas, and therefore separate categories for benign lymphoid tumors must be added. The determination of malignancy is based on the architecture of the lesion and the cytologic differentiation of the cells. Two patterns of growth are recognized: a diffuse pattern in which cells

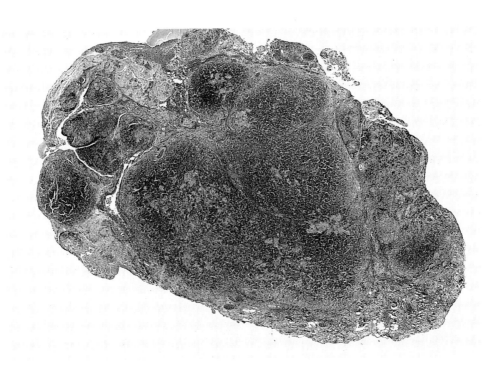

Figure 7-47
LYMPHOID HYPERPLASIA
Multinodular lymphoid tumor.

proliferate in a featureless, sheetlike manner and a follicular or nodular pattern. As a general rule, patients with follicular lymphomas have a better prognosis than patients with diffuse lymphomas. Cytologic atypia is classified by the size of the nucleus, irregularity of the nuclear membrane, chromatin pattern, nucleolar size, hyperchromasia, and mitotic activity. Nuclear shape or configuration has received particular attention: nuclei that are round with only minimal infoldings are characterized as noncleaved, whereas nuclei with infoldings of the nuclear envelope into the center of the nucleus are considered to be cleaved. Based on the degree of atypia, cells are classified as well differentiated (small lymphocytic type), intermediately differentiated (small cleaved cell type), or poorly differentiated (small noncleaved cell, lymphoblastic, large cleaved and noncleaved cells, and immunoblastic types). Lymphomas composed of lymphocytic or small cleaved type cells are not exceptionally mitotically active, whereas large cell and immunoblastic types tend to be the most mitotically active and malignant.

Lymphoid Hyperplasia (Benign Lymphoid Tumor). Several distinctive features are present in these lesions. There is scant fibrous stroma (figs. 7-47–7-49), which distinguishes most lymphoid tumors from inflammation, in which fibrosis is a characteristic feature. Within the solid masses of abnormal lymphoid tissue, the individual cells are small, dark lymphocytes without significant mitotic activity (figs. 7-48, 7-49). There is usually an admixed cell population (polymorphism), consisting of scattered plasma cells and histiocytes (fig. 7-49), or sometimes a subpopulation of eosinophils. Capillary proliferation with plump endothelial cells is a frequent finding. The tumors often have a follicular organization, in which germinal centers contain a mixture of mitotically active, large blastic cells and tingible body macrophages (macrophages that have accumulated cellular and karyorrhectic nuclear debris). The germinal centers are surrounded by a mantle of mature lymphocytes. In lymphoid hyperplasia, the follicles are irregular in size and shape and are highly mitotic (paradoxically, there is usually less mitotic

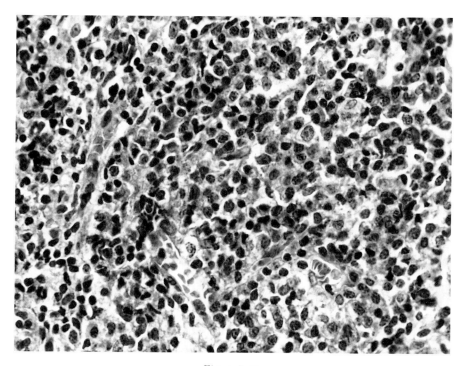

Figure 7-48
LYMPHOID HYPERPLASIA
Higher power magnification of tumor seen in previous figure showing mature lymphocytes and plasma cells.

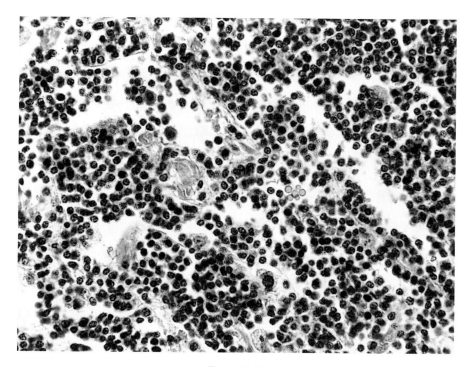

Figure 7-49
LYMPHOID HYPERPLASIA
Tumor composed of mature lymphocytes and plasma cells.

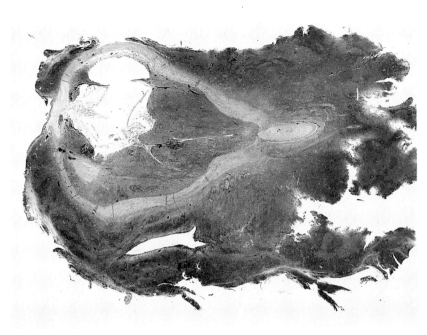

Figure 7-50
MALIGNANT LYMPHOMA
Well-differentiated lymphoma involving orbit, conjunctiva, and uvea.

activity in follicular lymphomas), but mitotic activity is very low in the interfollicular regions and mantle zones (where it is usually identified in follicular lymphomas).

Immunophenotypic studies of lymphoid hyperplasias indicate that these tumors are composed of a mixture of T and B cells. Usually, there is an approximately equal number of T and B cells or a slight B cell predominance. All of these tumors are polyclonal with respect to light chains. Despite immunophenotypic polyclonality, Knowles et al. (114) found that all of 16 lymphoid hyperplasias had clonal immunoglobulin gene rearrangements using molecular genetic analysis. The finding of monoclonality by genetic analysis indicates that lymphoid hyperplasia is a neoplastic rather than reactive process.

Malignant Lymphomas. Most lymphomas in the orbit are diffuse proliferations, with only 10 to 15 percent showing evidence of a follicular or nodular growth pattern.

Follicular Lymphomas. Orbital follicular tumors are almost always of the small cleaved cell or mixed small cleaved and large cell types and have a favorable prognosis (118). These tumors have regularly spaced units often growing in the orbital fat, with delimitations formed by the stretched-out fibrovascular connective tissue septa of the orbit. The cells within the follicles are often of the same type or are slightly less well-differentiated than those in the interfollicular zones. Mitotic activity is not as marked in the germinal centers of lymphomatous follicles or nodules in comparison with the reactive germinal centers of benign lymphoid hyperplasia. Endothelial cell proliferation is not prominent, and tingible body macrophages are rare or absent.

Well-Differentiated and Intermediately Differentiated Diffuse Lymphomas. Most diffuse lesions are well-differentiated (figs. 7-50–7-53) or intermediately differentiated (figs. 7-54–7-56; poorly differentiated lymphomas (figs. 7-57–7-59) are uncommon in the orbit (108,115). In well-fixed specimens, well-differentiated lesions can be separated from intermediately differentiated lesions using thin (4 μm) paraffin sections or 1-μm plastic sections for light microscopy, or by transmission electron microscopy (107). The nuclei in small lymphocytic lymphomas are the same size and shape as the nuclei of small lymphocytes that comprise benign polyclonal lesions. They differ from the nuclei of benign lymphocytes

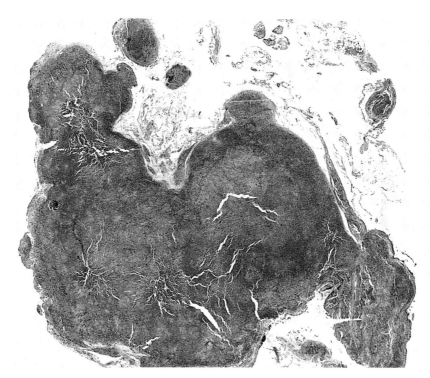

Figure 7-51
MALIGNANT LYMPHOMA
Irregularly shaped mass.

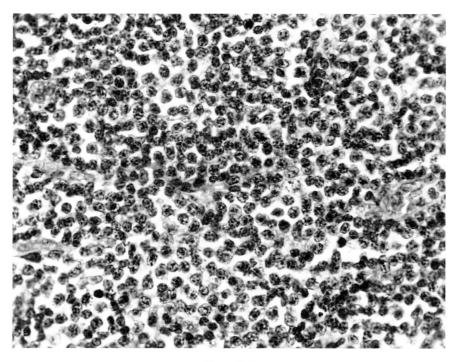

Figure 7-52
MALIGNANT LYMPHOMA
Higher power magnification of above tumor showing a uniform population of well-differentiated lymphocytes.

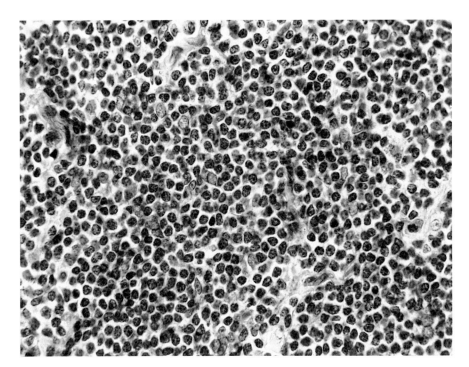

Figure 7-53
MALIGNANT LYMPHOMA
Monotonous proliferation of well-differentiated lymphocytes.

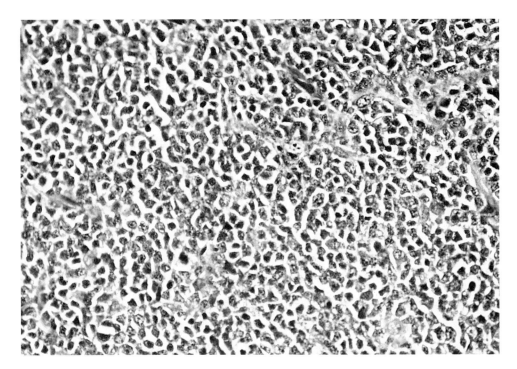

Figure 7-54
MALIGNANT LYMPHOMA
Tumor composed of small cleaved type cells.

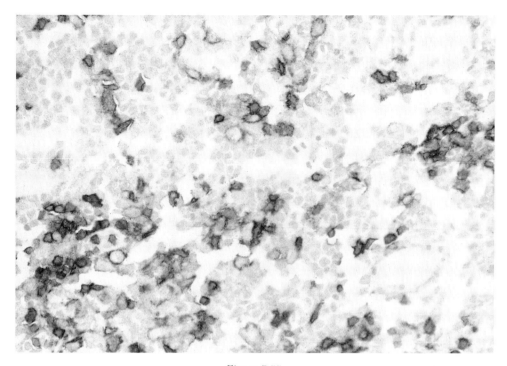

Figure 7-55
MALIGNANT LYMPHOMA
Same tumor as in previous figure with a small population of T cells. (UCHL-1, immunoperoxidase stain)

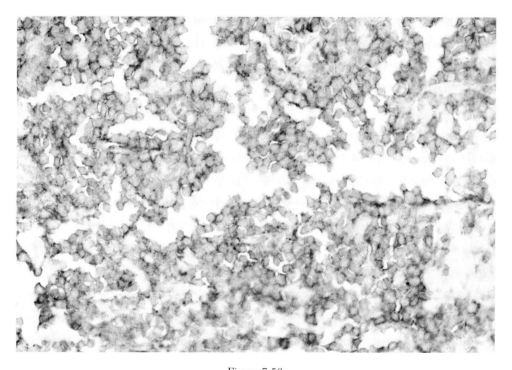

Figure 7-56
MALIGNANT LYMPHOMA
Same tumor as in figure 7-54 with numerous B cells. (L26, immunoperoxidase stain)

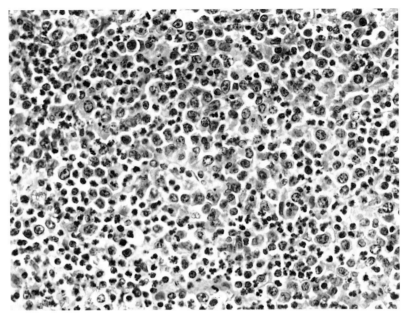

Figure 7-57
MALIGNANT LYMPHOMA
Tumor composed predominantly of large lymphoid cells.

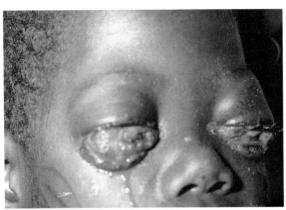

Figure 7-58
BURKITT LYMPHOMA
Bilateral involvement.

Figure 7-59
BURKITT LYMPHOMA
Lymphoblastic tumor with numerous mitotic figures.

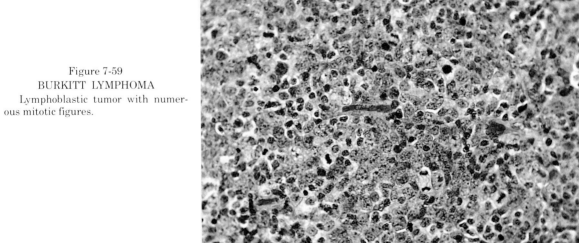

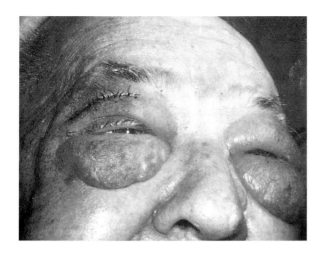

Figure 7-60
WALDENSTRÖM MACROGLOBULINEMIA
Bilateral involvement of orbit and eyelid.

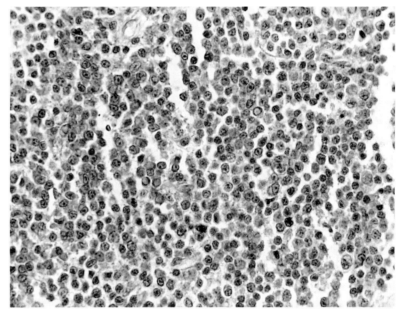

Figure 7-61
LYMPHOPLASMACYTIC
LYMPHOMA
Same case as in previous figure with tumor composed of lymphoid cells with plasmacytic differentiation.

in that their nuclear membranes have slight irregularities, infoldings, or blebs; their nuclear chromatin has slightly less dense clumping; and their nucleoli are more prominent. By transmission electron microscopy, the cytoplasm in small lymphocytic lymphomas shows short strands of rough-surfaced endoplasmic reticulum, scattered mitochondria, and mostly monoribosomes. The intermediately differentiated lesions have larger nuclei (approximately 50 percent larger than a small lymphocyte), more frequent and larger nuclear irregularities with infoldings extending to the center of the nucleus, greater dispersion of the nuclear chromatin, and larger nucleoli. In the cytoplasm are more abundant

mitochondria, more frequent short strands of rough-surfaced endoplasmic reticulum, and a predominance of polyribosomes over monoribosomes. In both groups the mitotic activity is low.

A significant subgroup of well-differentiated small lymphocytic lymphomas have plasmacytic differentiation (figs. 7-60–7-62). These neoplasms are composed of cells with hybrid cellular characteristics, representing a cross between a lymphocyte and a plasma cell. The nucleus frequently has the uniform density of the nucleus of a lymphocyte, but the cytoplasm is more copious and the methyl green pyronine stain may reveal the presence of cytoplasmic RNA, which

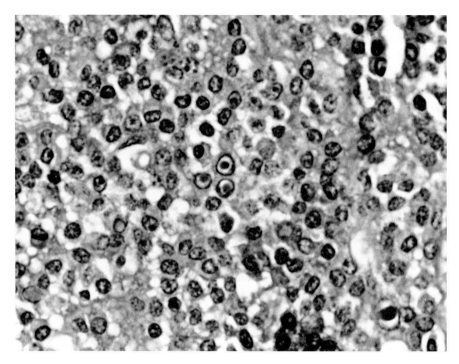

Figure 7-62
LYMPHOPLASMACYTIC LYMPHOMA
Same tumor as in figure 7-60 showing lymphoid cells with plasmacytic differentiation and Dutcher bodies. (PAS and hematoxylin stains)

are characteristics of a plasma cell. Intranuclear eosinophilic inclusions, referred to as Dutcher bodies, represent sequestrations of cytoplasm containing immunoglobulin. When these inclusions contain IgA or IgM, they are PAS positive because of the sugar moieties that these particular immunoglobulin classes possess (fig. 7-62). IgG-containing Dutcher bodies are PAS negative. Lymphoplasmacytic cells may also contain cytoplasmic immunoglobulin crystals. Occasionally, these paracrystalline materials can be extruded into the extracellular space and engulfed by histiocytes. Immunohistochemistry can help the pathologist make the correct diagnosis.

Lymphoplasmacytoid lesions in the orbit may be localized or part of a systemic disease. In a group of 12 lymphoplasmacytoid orbital tumors, only 3 were associated with systemic disease; 2 of 5 orbital lesions displaying Dutcher bodies were associated with systemic disease (110). In one case, the patient had Waldenström macroglobulinemia (figs. 7-60–7-62). In patients with orbital lymphoplasmacytoid lesions, clinical ex-

amination for multisystem disease should include a serum protein immunoelectrophoresis to determine if there is a monoclonal immunoglobulin spike or polyclonal spikes. Some monoclonal gammopathies are benign whereas others are associated with a true malignancy.

Poorly Differentiated Diffuse Lymphomas. The lymphoblastic and small noncleaved cell lymphomas that involve the orbit are more likely to occur in children and young adults than the more differentiated lymphomas, and are almost always part of a systemic disease. Some of these lymphomas are classified as Burkitt type (figs. 7-58, 7-59). This disease preferentially affects children, and it is one of the most common orbital tumors in parts of Africa (100). Unlike the well-differentiated orbital lymphomas, there is usually bone destruction with the maxilla most frequently involved; orbital involvement is often secondary to the bone tumor. Orbital involvement in North American Burkitt lymphoma has also been identified but it is not so consistently associated with a destructive maxillary bone lesion. Histopathologically, Burkitt lymphoma is characterized by a blastic proliferation of immature, immunoglobulin-bearing lymphocytes (fig. 7-59); histiocytes may be regularly interspersed throughout the lesion, conferring a "starry sky" appearance under low-power microscopy.

Orbital large cell lymphomas are usually of the high-grade immunoblastic type (fig. 7-57). In the past, large cell lymphomas displaying hyperchromatic nuclei with prominent nucleoli and conspicuous cytoplasm were referred to as either reticulum cell sarcomas or histiocytic lymphomas (102,105,111). Thirteen orbital large cell lymphomas have been described; half the patients were known to have systemic lymphoma and the other half quickly developed evidence of systemic lymphoma with early deaths (111). All the lesions occurred in adults. Before making the diagnosis of a large cell orbital lymphoma in a child, leukemia (particularly granulocytic sarcoma) should be considered, and a Leder stain for cytoplasmic esterase activity or immunohistochemistry should be done. Most large cell lymphomas, like the better differentiated lymphomas, present with an orbital mass causing proptosis but some are destructive to the medial wall of the orbit. These destructive lesions are more likely to be of T-cell derivation than other orbital lymphomas and have been lumped with lethal midline granulomas in the past (102,105).

Immunologic Findings. Almost all orbital lymphomas are of B-cell type and all B-cell lymphomas are monoclonal for immunoglobulin light chains. Lymphomas expressing kappa light chains are more common than those expressing lambda light chains. In 61 lymphomas studied by cell suspension, the ratio of lambda to kappa light chains in lambda type lymphomas was at least 10 to 1 and the ratio of kappa to lambda in kappa type lymphomas was at least 6.9 to 1 (108). In most of the lymphomas, there was a predominance of B cells, which ranged from 48 to 96 percent (mean 78 percent) (108,116). We find that immunohistochemistry using L26 (pan–B-cell marker) and UCHL-1 (pan–T-cell marker) to distinguish B and T cells in formalin-fixed paraffin-embedded tissue is very helpful in differentiating between benign lymphoid tumors and lymphomas. Most lymphoid hyperplasias contain a preponderance of cells that stain with UCHL-1 and most lymphomas contain cells that stain predomi-

nately with L26 (figs. 7-55, 7-56). Immunostaining of lymphocytes for light chains is unreliable in formalin-fixed paraffin-embedded tissue, unless there is plasmacytic differentiation in the lymphoma.

Despite the important contributions to the biology of ocular adnexal lymphoid tumors provided by newer immunologic techniques, data on polyclonality or monoclonality have not greatly improved the prediction of which patients are likely to have systemic disease. Jakobiec and Knowles (108) found that 29 percent of patients with polyclonal tumors and 35 percent of patients with monoclonal tumors had prior, concurrent, or future nonocular adnexal lymphoma.

Clinical Correlations. The histologic category to which a lymphoid tumor is assigned does not correlate well with whether there is or will be systemic disease (108); 27 percent of patients with lymphoid hyperplasias have prior, concomitant, or subsequent systemic disease. Lesions diagnosed as lymphomas are associated with systemic disease in 33 percent of cases. Subdividing lymphomas into well-, intermediate, and poorly differentiated groups does not help because intermediately differentiated lymphomas in the ocular adnexa have only a slightly higher association with systemic disease than well-differentiated lymphomas, and poorly differentiated lymphomas are uncommon. Jakobiec and Knowles (108) found that only 8 of 117 lymphoid tumors were poorly differentiated using the NCI working formulation. The longer patients with well-differentiated lymphocytic lymphomas are observed, the higher the percentage with systemic disease. The long interval between orbital and systemic involvement in many patients with well-differentiated and intermediate grade lymphomas suggests that these lymphomas may have originated in the orbit.

Of greater prognostic significance than histopathologic classification is staging. In addition to a complete physical exam, the work-up should include a CT scan of neck, chest, and abdomen; bilateral iliac crest biopsies; liver and spleen scans; complete blood count; serum protein immunoelectrophoresis; antinuclear antibodies; antirheumatoid factor; and sedimentation rate. If no nonocular adnexal focus of lymphoma is discovered, the lymphoma is classified as stage I-E. Bilaterality does not appreciably influence

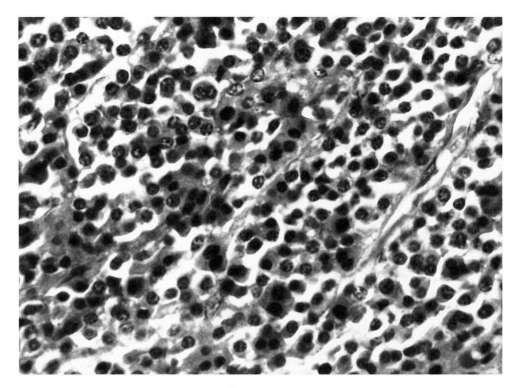

Figure 7-63
PLASMACYTOMA
Tumor composed of atypical plasma cells.

the association with systemic disease and bilateral lymphomas affecting only the ocular adnexa are also classified as stage I-E. In a series of 79 patients with stage I-E lymphoid tumors followed an average of 53 months, 87 percent did not develop systemic disease (115).

Treatment. Management of patients with orbital lymphoid tumors is dependent on the stage. Most patients with stage I-E localized lymphomas should be treated with local radiotherapy to control orbital symptoms and have follow-up examinations for systemic involvement (108,112). For patients with systemic disease or patients with rare diffuse large cell or Burkitt type lymphoma, even if systemic disease is not detected, chemotherapy is usually indicated. The watch and wait program with palliative radiotherapy may be used for disseminated (stage III or IV) well-differentiated small lymphocytic lymphomas in elderly patients or patients in poor general health, because these lymphomas evolve slowly and most of these patients die of causes unrelated to their lymphoma.

PLASMA CELL TUMORS

The orbit may be the site of both benign and malignant plasma cell tumors (122–124). While plasma cell tumors of the orbit vary in their degree of differentiation, it may be impossible to differentiate between a benign and malignant tumor based on histologic findings (fig. 7-63). Because multiple myeloma has a tendency to involve bones, creating punched-out lesions (including the classic multifocal lesions of the skull), it is unusual for the orbit to be the only site of involvement. Thus, systemic work-up and close follow-up is important in the management of patients with plasmacytomas of the orbit. Immunohistochemistry for kappa and lambda light chains should detect a monoclonal plasma cell population in the orbital tumors of multiple myeloma and a polyclonal population in benign plasmacytomas. Even in formalin-fixed, paraffin-embedded tissue, the cytoplasmic immunoglobulins of plasma cells usually provide satisfactory results, unlike the surface immunoglobulins of

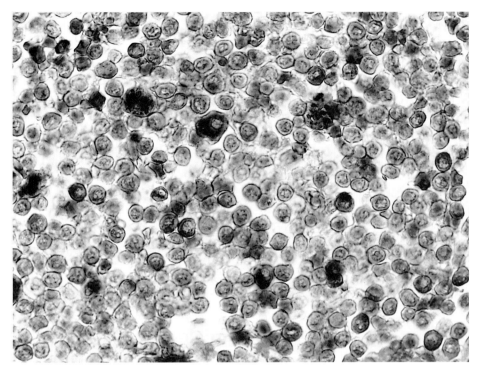

Figure 7-64
GRANULOCYTIC LEUKEMIA
Tumor cells stain positively with the Leder stain.

lymphocytes. Other ophthalmic manifestations of multiple myeloma may be the formation of amyloid around blood vessels and deposition of immunoglobulins in the cornea and beneath the ciliary epithelium.

When orbital involvement occurs as an early manifestation of multiple myeloma, it can be difficult to diagnose both for the clinician and the pathologist. Clinically, multiple myeloma should be considered when there is bone destruction in addition to orbital involvement, which is very unusual in orbital lymphomas. Histologically, very poorly differentiated myelomatous deposits are sometimes difficult to distinguish from undifferentiated carcinoma and histiocytic tumors. The methyl green pyronine stain for cytoplasmic RNA and electron microscopy revealing an abundant, disorganized, rough-surfaced endoplasmic reticulum, may point out the true nature of a poorly differentiated myelomatous deposit. Immunohistochemical reactivity for immunoglobulins, and leukocyte common antigen and lack of reactivity for cytokeratins and lysozyme, should aid in the diagnosis of difficult cases.

LEUKEMIA
(GRANULOCYTIC SARCOMA)

Leukemias are defined as diseases that begin in the bone marrow and secondarily extend into the blood stream, from which multifocal organ and soft tissue involvement, including the orbit, are possible (125–128). It should be recognized, however, that a small number of lymphomas, including Waldenström macroglobulinemia, appear from the outset to have both bone marrow and lymph node involvement, and that a leukemia may eventuate in the late stages of systemic lymphoma. The most common leukemic involvements of the orbit are the result of granulocytic disorders, although acute lymphocytic leukemia in children and chronic lymphocytic leukemia in adults can produce orbital deposits. In a series of 89 patients with acute leukemia, orbital granulocytic sarcomas were observed in 7 (128).

Granulocytic differentiation is signaled by the presence of esterase (fig. 7-64) and other lysosomal enzymes in the cytoplasm and is demonstrated by light microscopy using the Leder stain, by electron microscopy through the demonstration of electron-dense lysosomal granules, and by immunohistochemistry for lysozyme. Histiomonocytic cells are frequently positive for muramidase and alpha-naphthyl acetate esterase (ANAE). Lymphocytic leukemias, on the other hand, are identified immunohistochemically by the presence of leukocyte common antigen and B- or T-cell lineage surface antigens. Unlike lymphomas that affect the orbit, acute lymphocytic leukemias are frequently of T-cell type.

Rarely, leukemias present as a soft tissue or visceral focus of infiltrating leukemic cells in the absence of overt peripheral blood, and sometimes bone marrow, involvement. The orbit, the lacrimal sac region, the lacrimal gland, and the epibulbar tissues may be the first focus of a leukemic disorder in otherwise healthy individuals. This entity, termed *myelocytic* or *granulocytic sarcoma*, was called chloroma in the past because clinically and grossly the lesions have a greenish hue resulting from myeloperoxidase in the granulocytes. Zimmerman and Font (129) studied the largest series, 33 patients, with this entity involving the ocular adnexa. Some of the lesions presented a misleading inflammatory and erythematous character. There was a slight male to female (3 to 2) predominance and a definite predilection for Asians, Africans, and young patients, with a median age at presentation of 7 years.

It is extremely important to diagnose granulocytic sarcoma accurately (125). Total remissions are possible if appropriate chemotherapy is introduced before peripheral blood disease occurs. If clear-cut bone marrow involvement is found, there is no question that immediate systemic chemotherapy should be given; this is often sufficient to cause disappearance of the orbital lesion (128). Sometimes, localized orbital radiotherapy may be given in conjunction with chemotherapy if there is a massive proptosis that is threatening vision.

HISTIOCYTIC DISORDERS

Histiocytic proliferations present major biologic and terminology problems. Macrophages, histiocytes, dendritic cells, and fibrohistiocytes, once lumped together as "histiocytes," are now considered disparate cell types. Two tumors of the orbit that are composed of specialized histiocytes are eosinophilic granuloma and sinus histiocytosis.

Unifocal and Multifocal Eosinophilic Granuloma (Langerhans Cell Histiocytosis)

The entities that were termed histiocytosis X in the past (eosinophilic granuloma, Hand-Schüller-Christian disease, and Letterer-Siwe disease) are all now considered to be tumors of Langerhans cells (130,131). It is now recognized that there are no histopathologic differences between localized and disseminated types. As a rule, the younger the patient with eosinophilic granuloma, the greater the propensity for multifocal involvement. Cases within the first 2 years of life usually display multisystem cutaneous, visceral, lymph node, and rarely, ocular and orbital disease, which in the past was referred to as the Letterer-Siwe form of histiocytosis X. In older children, multifocal bone lesions may produce the rare triad of lytic defects in the skull, proptosis, and diabetes insipidus, which was formerly called Hand-Schüller-Christian disease. Some of the most acute and fulminant cases, particularly in infants, previously diagnosed as Letterer-Siwe disease are now segregated as lymphomas based upon definite evidence of anaplasia and absence of Langerhans cells.

The Langerhans cell is normally present in the epidermis of the skin, which explains the highly characteristic invasive epidermotropism observed in the cutaneous lesions of eosinophilic granuloma. Langerhans cells are large mononucleated histiocytes with bean-shaped nuclei. Electron microscopy reveals that these cells contain distinctive cytoplasmic granules or inclusions referred to as raquet bodies, Birbeck granules, or Langerhans granules. The Langerhans granules are a morphologic marker for the Langerhans type of dendritic histiocytic cell; these cells also stain positively for S-100 protein, and the monoclonal antibody OKT-6 stains the cell surface membrane receptors of Langerhans cells. The multinucleated giant cells that are usually present in the osseous lesions of eosinophilic granulomas are not Langerhans cells because they lack Birbeck granules and are negative for S-100 protein.

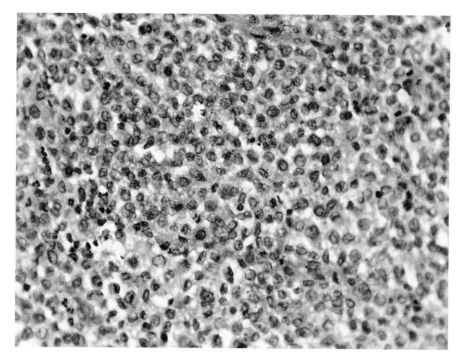

Figure 7-65
EOSINOPHILIC GRANULOMA
Tumor composed predominately of histiocytes.

The orbit is frequently involved secondarily in eosinophilic granuloma, which has a predilection for the bones in superotemporal portion of the orbital rim. An irregular, scalloped, lytic lesion is detected radiographically. When the lesion breaks through the periorbita into the orbit, there are clinical inflammatory signs suggestive of a dacryoadenitis. Involvement of the orbital soft tissue without a lesion of the bony wall is unusual. By light microscopy, the lesion is composed of Langerhans cells intermixed with eosinophils (fig. 7-65). Multinucleated histiocytes, lymphocytes, plasma cells, and neutrophils may also be present. The treatment is usually simple curettage and some lesions spontaneously heal within the bone.

Sinus Histiocytosis with Massive Lymphadenopathy

This condition has a predilection for children of African descent, but adults also may be affected. Bilateral or unilateral proptosis is associated with cervical or retroperitoneal lymphadenopathy. The orbital lesion is produced by massive collections of histiocytes with admixed lymphocytes in the orbital soft tissues (132–135). The viscera and skin are generally spared, in contrast to other histiocytic disorders.

This lesion exhibits a distinctive light microscopic appearance when it occurs in the orbit. Under low power, pale-staining areas composed of sheets of histiocytes, with vesicular nuclei and ample cytoplasm, are seen (fig. 7-66). The pale histiocytes contain scattered, engulfed lymphocytes and plasma cells (lymphophagocytosis or emperipolesis) (fig. 7-67). Focal collections of mature lymphoid tissue, which sometimes are organized into follicles, are scattered throughout the lesion. In lymph nodes, the pale histiocytes pile up along the sinus channels both in the subcapsular and central medullary regions. The pale histiocytes are S-100 protein positive but electron microscopy has failed to demonstrate the cytoplasmic Birbeck granules of Langerhans cells. It appears that this proliferation is a different histiocytic cell line than Langerhans cells and may represent the sinusoidal cells that normally line the sinuses of lymph nodes.

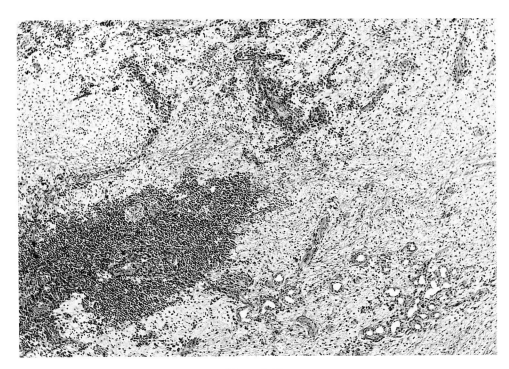

Figure 7-66
SINUS HISTIOCYTOSIS
Tumor composed of sheets of large pale histiocytes and islands of lymphoid tissue.

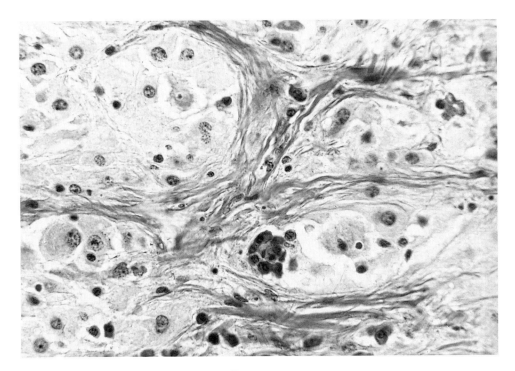

Figure 7-67
SINUS HISTIOCYTOSIS
Higher power magnification of the large pale histiocytes in the previous figure shows phagocytosis of lymphocytes.

The disease is generally self-limited, and neither radiotherapy nor chemotherapy accelerates its resolution. The overall prognosis is good because of the general absence of visceral involvement (135).

DERMOID CYST

Dermoid cysts result from congenital rests of ectoderm that become trapped within the sutures of the orbital bones. They are rounded cystic lesions that usually develop within bone. The majority of dermoid cysts become symptomatic in the first decade of life and represent about one third of the orbital tumors of childhood. Dermoids differ anatomically dependent on their location within the orbit (136). Nasally located dermoids (fig. 7-68) are more likely to be lined by conjunctival-type epithelium (fig. 7-69) and skin appendages are often not present. These dermoids usually contain mucinous fluid. Laterally located dermoids usually have a wall that resembles skin with a lining of epidermis; within the wall there are dermal appendages (fig. 7-70). The lumina of these dermoids are filled with keratin

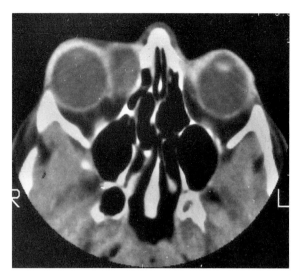

Figure 7-68
DERMOID CYST
Computed tomograph of nasally located cystic lesion.

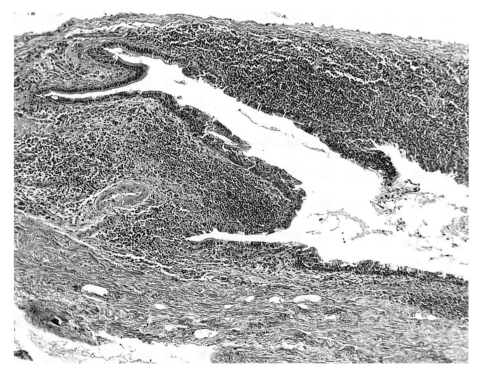

Figure 7-69
DERMOID CYST
Inflamed cyst lined by conjunctival type epithelium.

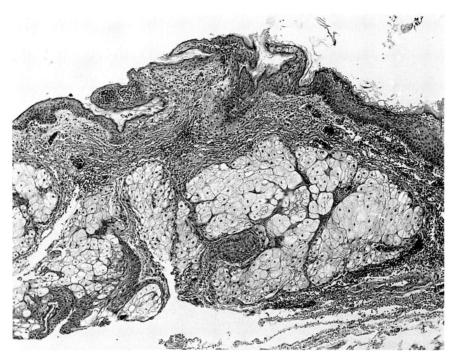

Figure 7-70
DERMOID CYST
Inflamed cyst lined by skin.

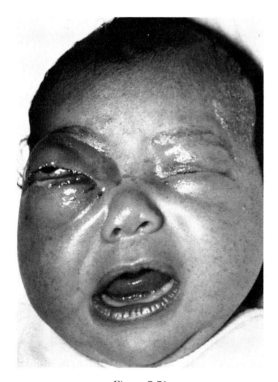

Figure 7-71
TERATOMA
Child with congenital proptosis.

and hairs. Orbital trauma may rupture a clinically inapparent dermoid cyst. The release of the contents of the dermoid can produce an acute inflammatory reaction. The resulting proptosis may simulate an orbital infection or neoplasm. Imaging studies (fig. 7-68) demonstrate the bony involvement and cystic nature of these lesions (137).

TERATOMA

Orbital teratomas arise from misdirected germ cells and are always congenital (138–140). Most orbital teratomas produce massive proptosis (fig. 7-71). Grossly, the tumors are composed of a mixture of solid and cystic areas (fig. 7-72). Orbital teratomas are usually benign and growth is due to the accumulation of secretions within the cystic spaces. Histologically, tissue from all three germ layers can usually be identified. Enteric, respiratory, cartilage, brain, and skin tissues are frequently present (fig. 7-73). Benign teratomas do not infiltrate the orbital tissues and it may be possible in some cases to remove the tumor and retain the eye.

Tumors of the Orbit

CONGENITAL MELANOSIS, CELLULAR BLUE NEVUS, AND PRIMARY MALIGNANT MELANOMA

Primary malignant melanomas of the orbit are rare. Most arise in blue nevi (142,143), often in patients with congenital melanosis involving the orbit (141,144,145). Orbital involvement in melanosis oculi or oculodermal melanocytosis is characterized by diffuse infiltration of the orbital soft tissues by heavily pigmented spindle-shaped and dendritic melanocytes. This infiltration does not produce a detectable mass or proptosis. Two space-occupying lesions may arise in congenital orbital melanosis. The first is composed of cellular islands of tightly packed spindle-shaped cells with ovoid nuclei and abundant lightly pigmented cytoplasm. Mitotic activity is rare and these nodules represent cellular blue nevi (fig. 7-74). The second space-occupying lesion is a malignant melanoma, the malignant counterpart of a cellular blue nevus (fig. 7-75). These tumors are usually composed of spindle-shaped cells, but

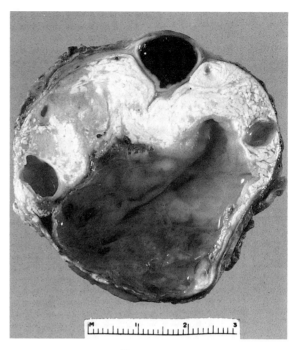
Figure 7-72
TERATOMA
Large tumor with solid and cystic areas.

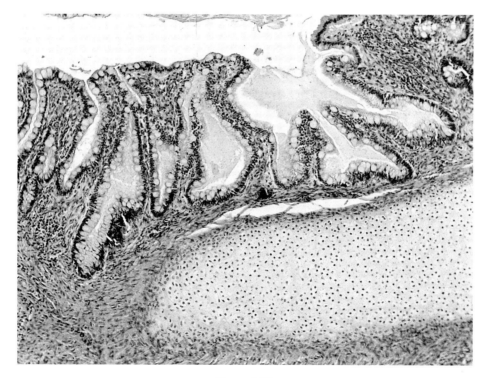
Figure 7-73
TERATOMA
Same tumor as in previous figure has a cyst lined by intestinal-type epithelium with cartilage in the wall.

289

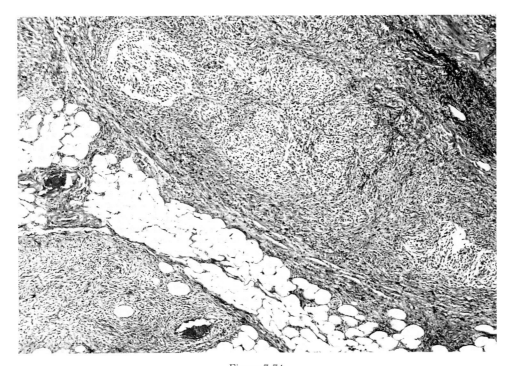

Figure 7-74
CELLULAR BLUE NEVUS
Proliferation of benign-appearing, spindle-shaped melanocytes.

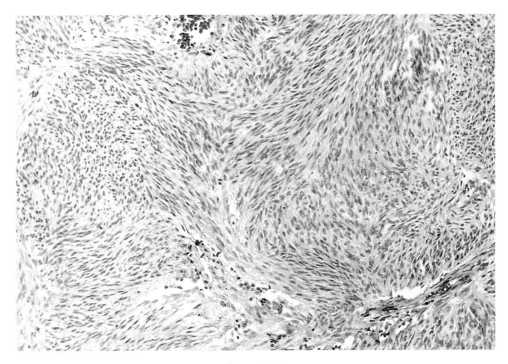

Figure 7-75
MALIGNANT MELANOMA
Same case as in previous figure with an area of malignant spindle-shaped melanocytic cells.

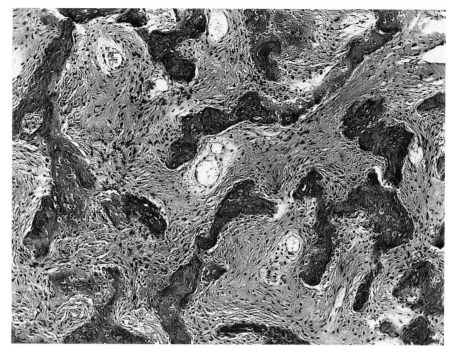

Figure 7-76
FIBROUS DYSPLASIA
Fibrotic tissue containing bone spicules without osteoblastic activity.

some may contain epithelioid cells. They range from amelanotic to heavily pigmented. Mitotic figures are usually present and there may be foci of necrosis. Many of the malignant tumors are of the low-grade spindle cell type; patients often have a long course with multiple recurrences that eventually require an orbital exenteration.

FIBROUS DYSPLASIA

Fibrous dysplasia develops almost exclusively in children, although the full extent of the disease may not occur until early adulthood (146,147). The lesion can arise in any of the orbital bones. The lesions are usually not well demarcated within the bone of origin, and may extend across suture lines to involve multiple bones of the orbital walls. Narrowing of the optic canal is common, but rarely causes optic atrophy. Tearing results from a maxillary lesion impinging upon the nasolacrimal duct. Most of the lesions occurring around the orbit are isolated and not part of multifocal (polyostotic) fibrous dysplasia. There is no malignant degeneration unless there has been radiotherapy. Plain radiographic and CT

studies show a sclerotic margin with a ground-glass appearance and lytic foci. Histologically, there is a prominent fibrous stroma in the lytic areas in which malformed trabeculae are composed of woven (immature) bone; this is best demonstrated with polarized light. The spicules of woven bone often have an irregular shape that resembles Chinese figures (fig. 7-76). The best management is wide local excision with concomitant reconstructive surgery (146).

OSSIFYING FIBROMA
(JUVENILE OSSIFYING FIBROMA, PSAMMOMATOID OSSIFYING FIBROMA)

Ossifying fibroma should not be confused with fibrous dysplasia. Ossifying fibroma is a locally aggressive lesion which typically develops in the first and second decades of life. Any of the orbital bones may be involved, but most frequently the orbital roof is the site of origin (148,149). Radiographically, the lesion is limited to a single bone rather than crossing over suture lines to involve multiple bones, a characteristic of fibrous dysplasia. CT shows a sclerotic margin containing a

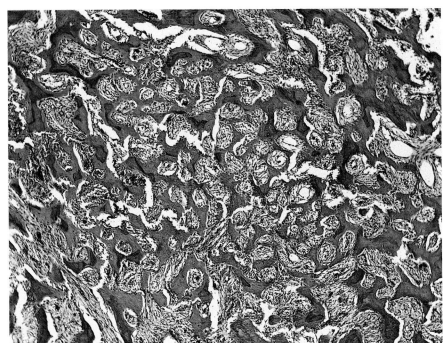

Figure 7-77
OSSIFYING FIBROMA
Bone spicules with osteoblastic activity within fibrous tissue.

less radiodense center with foci of calcification. Ossifying fibromas recur upon incomplete excision and, rarely, expand into one of the intracranial compartments, threatening life or compress the optic nerve, threatening vision. Histologically, within the sclerotic perimeter there is a highly vascularized fibrous stroma in which spicules of lamellar bone are surrounded by osteoblasts (fig. 7-77). Some of the spicules of bone are spherical, mimicking the psammoma bodies of a meningioma. Wide local excision without radiotherapy is the preferred method of treatment for ossifying fibroma.

OSTEOGENIC SARCOMA

Osteogenic sarcoma typically arises in one of the sinuses, generally in younger individuals who usually are survivors of heritable retinoblastoma (150,151). Radiation therapy is an additional risk factor in these patients. It is a massively destructive lesion, which shows calcification on CT. Histopathologic examination reveals a highly anaplastic spindle cell population, which in some areas may resemble a fibrosarcoma; in other areas osteoid and spicules of bone are observed. These lesions require radical local excision, after which adjunctive radiotherapy and chemotherapy may be given.

SECONDARY TUMORS OF THE ORBIT

The most common secondary tumors of the orbit arise in the eye. Both retinoblastoma and uveal melanoma extend out of the eye if there is a delay in treatment. Neoplasms of the skin, eyelid, and conjunctiva may extend posteriorly to involve the orbit (152–155,159). Intracranial meningiomas may extend through the sphenoid wing (see figs. 8-17–8-19), and tumors of the sinuses and nasal cavity frequently invade into the orbit (figs. 7-78, 7-79) (156,157,160). Most fibro-osseous and cartilaginous tumors of the orbit arise from the orbital bones and adjacent sinuses, with the exception of rare chondromas of the trochlear cartilage and malignant mesenchymal chondrosarcomas of the soft tissues of the orbit (158).

METASTATIC TUMORS

Orbital metastatic tumors are different in children and adults. In children, they are most often of embryonal or undifferentiated type. Neuroblastoma (161), Wilms tumor, Ewing sarcoma, and medulloblastoma (167) are important examples. In adults, the most common metastatic tumors to the orbit are carcinomas (162, 163,165,166); the most frequent is carcinoma of

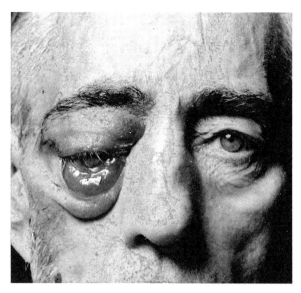

Figure 7-78
SECONDARY CARCINOMA
Paranasal sinus carcinoma involving the orbit.

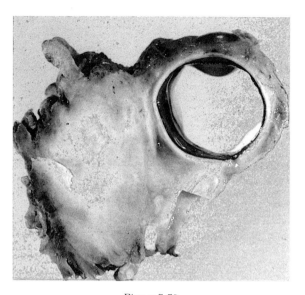

Figure 7-79
SECONDARY CARCINOMA
Same case as previous figure with large tumor invading the nasal aspect of the orbit.

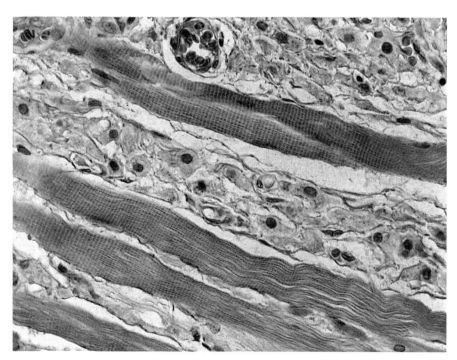

Figure 7-80
METASTATIC CARCINOMA
Histiocytoid breast carcinoma cells have infiltrated an extraocular muscle.

the breast (fig. 7-80) (162,165,166). A frequent finding is enophthalmos, seen in about 25 percent of cases of metastatic carcinoma (163). Enophthalmos is associated with scirrhous carcinomas and is particularly common in patients with metastatic carcinoma from the breast. In men,

the most frequent cause of metastasis is carcinoma of the lung (162). Less common are metastases from the gastrointestinal tract, kidney, and prostate (162,165). Cutaneous malignant melanoma is the most common nonepithelial tumor to metastasize to the orbit (162,164,165).

REFERENCES

General References

Abiose A, Adido J, Agarwal SC. Childhood malignancies of the eye and orbit in northern Nigeria. Cancer 1985;55:2889–93.

Bergen MP. Spatial aspects of the orbital vascular system. In: Jakobiec FA, ed. Ocular anatomy, embryology and teratology. Philadelphia: Harper and Row, 1982:859–68.

Enzinger FM, Weiss SW. Soft tissue tumors. St. Louis: CV Mosby, 1983.

Henderson JW. Orbital Tumors. 2nd ed. New York: B.C. Decker, 1980.

Jakobiec FA, Font RL. Orbital tumors. In: Spencer WH, ed. Ophthalmic pathology. An atlas and textbook. 3rd ed. WB Saunders: Philadelphia, 1985:2459–860.

_____, Iwamoto T. The ocular adnexa: lids, conjunctiva and orbit. In: Fine BS, Yanoff M, eds. Ocular histology: a text and atlas. 2nd ed. Hagerstown, MD: Harper and Row, 1979:289–342.

Kennedy RE. An evaluation of 820 orbital cases. Trans Am Ophthalmol Soc 1984;82:134–57.

Lattes R. Tumors of the soft tissues. Atlas of Tumor Pathology, 2nd Series, Fascicle 1/Revised. Washington, D.C.: Armed Forces Institute of Pathology, 1982.

Levin PS, Dutton JJ. A 20-year series of orbital exenterations. Am J Ophthalmol 1991;112:496–501.

Mafee MF, Putterman A, Valvassori GE, Campos M, Capek V. Orbital space-occupying lesions: role of computed tomography and magnetic resonance imaging. An analysis of 145 cases. Radiol Clin North Am 1987;25:529–59.

Shields JA, Bakewell B, Augsburger JJ, Flanagan JC. Classification and incidence of space-occupying lesions of the orbit. A survey of 645 biopsies. Arch Ophthalmol 1984;102:1606–11.

Classification and Frequency

1. Henderson JW. Orbital Tumors. 2nd ed. New York: B.C. Decker, 1980.
2. Kennedy RE. An evaluation of 820 orbital cases. Trans Am Ophthalmol Soc 1984;82:134–57.
3. Levin PS, Dutton JJ. A 20-year series of orbital exenterations. Am J Ophthalmol 1991;112:496–501.
4. Shields JA, Bakewell B, Augsburger JJ, Flanagan JC. Classification and incidence of space-occupying lesions of the orbit. A survey of 645 biopsies. Arch Ophthalmol 1984;102:1606–11.

Capillary Hemangioma

5. Haik BG, Jakobiec FA, Ellsworth RM, Jones IS. Capillary hemangioma of the lids and orbit: an analysis of the clinical features and therapeutic results in 101 cases. Ophthalmology 1979;86:760–89.
6. Iwamoto T, Jakobiec FA. Ultrastructural comparison of capillary and cavernous hemangioma of the orbit. Arch Ophthalmol 1979;97:1144–53.
7. Jakobiec FA, Font RL. Orbital tumors. In: Spencer WH, ed. Ophthalmic pathology. An atlas and textbook. 3rd ed. WB Saunders: Philadelphia, 1985:2459–860.
8. Kushner BJ. Intralesional corticosteroid injection for infantile adnexal hemangioma. Am J Ophthalmol 1982;93:496–506.
9. Robb RM. Refractive errors associated with hemangiomas of the eyelids and orbit in infancy. Am J Ophthalmol 1977;83:52–8.

10. Sklar EL, Quencer RM, Byrne SF, Sklar VE. Correlative study of the computed tomographic, ultrasonographic, and pathological characteristics of cavernous versus capillary hemangiomas of the orbit. J Clin Neuroophthalmol 1986;6:14–21.

Cavernous Hemangioma

11. Fries PD, Char DH, Norman D. MR imaging of orbital cavernous hemangioma. J Comput Assist Tomogr 1987;11:418–21.
12. Harris GJ, Jakobiec FA. Cavernous hemangioma of the orbit: an analysis of 66 cases. J Neurosurg 1979;51:219-28.
13. Herter T, Bennefeld H, Brandt M. Orbital cavernous hemangiomas. Neurosurg Rev 1988;11:143–7.
14. Iwamoto T, Jakobiec FA. Ultrastructural comparison of capillary and cavernous hemangioma of the orbit. Arch Ophthalmol 1979;97:1144–53.
15. Mafee MF, Putterman A, Valvassori GE, Campos M, Capek V. Orbital space-occupying lesions: role of computed tomography and magnetic resonance imaging. An analysis of 145 cases. Radiol Clin North Am 1987;25:529–59.
16. Sklar EL, Quencer RM, Byrne SF, Sklar VE. Correlative study of the computed tomographic, ultrasonographic, and pathological characteristics of cavernous versus capillary hemangiomas of the orbit. J Clin Neuroophthalmol 1986;6:14–21.

Lymphangioma

17. Graeb DA, Rootman J, Robertson WD, Lapointe JS, Nugent RA, Hay EJ. Orbital lymphangiomas: clinical, radiologic, and pathologic characteristics. Radiology 1990;175:417–21.
18. Harris GJ, Sakol PJ, Bonavolonta G, De Conciliis C. An analysis of thirty cases of orbital lymphangioma. Pathophysiologic considerations and management recommendations. Ophthalmology 1990;97:1583–92.
19. Jones IS. Lymphangioma of the ocular adnexa: an analysis of 62 cases. Trans Am Ophthalmol Soc 1959;57:602–65.
20. Mafee MF, Putterman A, Valvassori GE, Campos M, Capek V. Orbital space-occupying lesions: role of computed tomography and magnetic resonance imaging. An analysis of 145 cases. Radiol Clin North Am 1987;25:529–59.

Hemangiopericytoma

21. Boyle J, Kennedy C, Berry J, Mott MG. Congenital haemangiopericytoma. J R Soc Med 1985;78(Suppl 11):10–2.
22. Croxatto JO, Font RL. Hemangiopericytoma of the orbit: a clinicopathologic study of 30 cases. Hum Pathol 1982;13:210–8.
23. Enzinger FM, Weiss SW. Soft tissue tumors. St. Louis: CV Mosby, 1983.
24. Henderson JW, Farrow GM. Primary orbital hemangiopericytoma: an aggressive and potentially malignant neoplasm. Arch Ophthalmol 1978;96:666–73.
25. Mafee MF, Putterman A, Valvassori GE, Campos M, Capek V. Orbital space-occupying lesions: role of computed tomography and magnetic resonance imaging. An analysis of 145 cases. Radiol Clin North Am 1987;25:529–59.
26. Setzkorn RK, Lee DJ, Iliff NT, Green WR. Hemangiopericytoma of the orbit treated with conservative surgery and radiotherapy. Arch Ophthalmol 1987;105:1103–5.

Fibrous Histiocytoma

27. Alper MG, Zimmerman LE, LaPiana FG. Orbital manifestations of Erdheim-Chester disease. Trans Am Ophthalmol Soc 1983;81:64-85.
28. Enzinger FM, Weiss SW. Soft tissue tumors. St. Louis: CV Mosby, 1983.
29. Font RL, Hidayat AA. Fibrous histiocytoma of the orbit: a clinicopathologic study of 150 cases. Hum Pathol 1982;13:199-209.
30. Henderson JW. Orbital Tumors. 2nd ed. New York: B.C. Decker, 1980.
31. Jacomb-Hood J, Moseley IF. Orbital fibrous histiocytoma: computed tomography in 10 cases and a review of radiological findings. Clin Radiol 1991;43:117-20.
32. Jakobiec FA, Font RL. Orbital tumors. In: Spencer WH, ed. Ophthalmic pathology. An atlas and textbook. 3rd ed. WB Saunders: Philadelphia, 1985:2459-860.
33. _____, Howard GM, Jones IS, Tannenbaum M. Fibrous histiocytoma of the orbit. Am J Ophthalmol 1974;77:333-45.
34. Kennedy RE. An evaluation of 820 orbital cases. Trans Am Ophthalmol Soc 1984;82:134-57.
35. Mafee MF, Putterman A, Valvassori GE, Campos M, Capek V. Orbital space-occupying lesions: role of computed tomography and magnetic resonance imaging. An analysis of 145 cases. Radiol Clin North Am 1987;25:529-59.
36. Shields JA, Bakewell B, Augsburger JJ, Flanagan JC. Classification and incidence of space-occupying lesions of the orbit. A survey of 645 biopsies. Arch Ophthalmol 1984;102:1606-11.

Juvenile Fibromatosis

37. Hidayat AA, Font RL. Juvenile fibromatosis of the periorbital region and eyelid. A clinicopathologic study of six cases. Arch Ophthalmol 1980;98:280-5.
38. Stautz CC. CT of infantile myofibromatosis of the orbit with intracranial involvement: a case report. AJNR Am J Neuroradiol 1991;12:184-5.
39. Waeltermann JM, Huntrakoon M, Beatty EC Jr, Cibis GW. Congenital fibromatosis (myofibromatosis) of the orbit: a rare cause of proptosis at birth. Ann Ophthalmol 1988;20:394-6.

Fibrosarcoma

40. Jakobiec FA, Tannenbaum M. The ultrastructure of orbital fibrosarcoma. Am J Ophthalmol 1974;77:899-917.
41. Liaw CC, Ho YS, Ng KK. Nasopharyngeal carcinoma presenting as a retro-orbital mass: report of three cases. Otolaryngol Head Neck Surg 1990;103:825-8.
42. Weiner JM, Hidayat AA. Juvenile fibrosarcoma of the orbit and eyelid. A study of five cases. Arch Ophthalmol 1983;101:253-9.

Leiomyoma and Leiomyosarcoma

43. Folberg R, Cleasby G, Flanagan JA, Spencer WH, Zimmerman LE. Orbital leiomyosarcoma after radiation therapy for bilateral retinoblastoma. Arch Ophthalmol 1983;101:1562-5.
44. Font RL, Jurco S III, Brechner RJ. Postradiation leiomyosarcoma of the orbit complicating bilateral retinoblastoma. Arch Ophthalmol 1983;101:1557-61.

45. Jakobiec FA, Jones IS, Tannenbaum M. Leiomyoma. An unusual tumor of the orbit. Br J Ophthalmol 1973;57:825-31.
46. Kaltreider SA, Destro M, Lemke BN. Leiomyosarcoma of the orbit. A case report and review of the literature. Ophthal Plast Reconstr Surg 1987;3:35-41.
47. Meekins BB, Dutton JJ, Proia AD. Primary orbital leiomyosarcoma. A case report and review of the literature. Arch Ophthalmol 1988;106:82-6.
48. Sanborn GE, Valenzuela RE, Green WR. Leiomyoma of the orbit. Am J Ophthalmol 1979;87:371-5.

Rhabdomyosarcoma

49. Knowles DM, Jakobiec FA, Potter GD, Jones IS. Ophthalmic striated muscle neoplasms: a clinico-pathologic review. Surv Ophthalmol 1976;21:219-61.
50. Sun XL, Zheng BH, Li B, Li LQ, Soejima K, Kanda M. Orbital rhabdomyosarcoma. Immunohistochemical studies of seven cases. Chin Med J (Engl) 1990;103:485-8.
51. Takahashi N, Minoda K. Prognosis of orbital rhabdomyosarcoma in children in Japan. Jpn J Ophthalmol 1991;35:292-9.
52. Wharam M, Beltangady M, Hays D, et al. Localized orbital rhabdomyosarcoma. An interim report of the Intergroup Rhabdomyosarcoma Study Committee. Ophthalmology 1987;94:251-4.

Lipoma

53. Bartley GB, Yeatts RP, Garrity JA, Farrow GM, Campbell RJ. Spindle cell lipoma of the orbit. Am J Ophthalmol 1985;100:605-9.
54. Henderson JW. Orbital Tumors. 2nd ed. New York: B.C. Decker, 1980.
55. Johnson BL, Linn JG Jr. Spindle cell lipoma of the orbit. Arch Ophthalmol 1979;97:133-4.
56. Kennedy RE. An evaluation of 820 orbital cases. Trans Am Ophthalmol Soc 1984;82:134-57.
57. Shields JA, Bakewell B, Augsburger JJ, Flanagan JC. Classification and incidence of space-occupying lesions of the orbit. A survey of 645 biopsies. Arch Ophthalmol 1984;102:1606-11.

Liposarcoma

58. Jakobiec FA, Rini F, Char D, et al. Primary liposarcoma of the orbit. Problems in the diagnosis and management of five cases. Ophthalmology 1989;96:180-91.
59. Lane CM, Wright JE, Garner A. Primary myxoid liposarcoma of the orbit. Br J Ophthalmol 1988;72:912-7.
60. McNab AA, Moseley I. Primary orbital liposarcoma: clinical and computed tomographic features. Br J Ophthalmol 1990;74:437-9.

Neurofibromas

61. Dervin JE, Beaconsfield M, Wright JE, Moseley IF. CT findings in orbital tumours of nerve sheath origin. Clin Radiol 1989;40:475-9.
62. Rose GE, Wright JE. Isolated peripheral nerve sheath tumours of the orbit. Eye 1991;5(Pt 6):668-73.
63. van der Meulen J. Orbital neurofibromatosis. Clin Plast Surg 1987;14:123-35.
64. Zimmerman RA, Bilaniuk LT, Metzger RA, Grossman RI, Schut L, Bruce DA. Computed tomography of orbital facial neurofibromatosis. Radiology 1983;146:113-6.

Schwannoma

65. Byrne BM, van Heuven WA, Lawton AW. Echographic characteristics of benign orbital schwannomas (neurilemomas). Am J Ophthalmol 1988;106:194–8.
66. Jakobiec FA, Font RL, Zimmerman LE. Malignant peripheral nerve sheath tumors of the orbit: a clinicopathologic study of eight cases. Trans Am Ophthalmol Soc 1985;83:332–66.
67. Lyons CJ, McNab AA, Garner A, Wright JE. Orbital malignant peripheral nerve sheath tumours. Br J Ophthalmol 1989;73:731–8.
68. Mafee MF, Putterman A, Valvassori GE, Campos M, Capek V. Orbital space-occupying lesions: role of computed tomography and magnetic resonance imaging. An analysis of 145 cases. Radiol Clin North Am 1987;25:529–59.
69. Rootman J, Goldberg C, Robertson W. Primary orbital schwannomas. Br J Ophthalmol 1982;66:194–204.

Malignant Peripheral Nerve Sheath Tumors

70. Jakobiec FA, Font RL, Zimmerman LE. Malignant peripheral nerve sheath tumors of the orbit: a clinicopathologic study of eight cases. Trans Am Ophthalmol Soc 1985;83:332–66.
71. Lyons CJ, McNab AA, Garner A, Wright JE. Orbital malignant peripheral nerve sheath tumours. Br J Ophthalmol 1989;73:731–8.

Inflammation (Pseudotumor)

72. Alper MG, Zimmerman LE, LaPiana FG. Orbital manifestations of Erdheim-Chester disease. Trans Am Ophthalmol Soc 1983;81:64-85.
73. Anderson RL, Linberg JV. Transorbital approach to decompression in Graves' disease. Arch Ophthalmol 1981;99:120–4.
74. Appel N, Som PM. Case report: ectopic orbital lacrimal gland tissue. J Comput Assist Tomogr 1982;6:1010–2.
75. Atlas SW, Grossman RI, Savino PJ, et al. Surface coil MR of orbital pseudotumor. AJR Am J Roentgenol 1987;148:803–8.
76. Bartalena L, Marcocci C, Chiovato L, et al. Orbital cobalt irradiation combined with systemic corticosteroids for Graves' ophthalmopathy: comparison with systemic corticosteroids alone. J Clin Endocrinol Metab 1983;56:1139–44.
77. Campbell RJ. Pathology of Graves' disease. In: Gorman C, Waller R, Dyer J, eds. The eye and orbit in thyroid disease. New York: Raven Press, 1984:25–32.
78. Feldon SE, Weiner JM. Clinical significance of extraocular muscle volumes in Graves' ophthalmopathy: a quantitative computed tomography study. Arch Ophthalmol 1982;100:1266–9.
79. Green WR, Zimmerman LE. Ectopic lacrimal gland tissue: report of 8 cases with orbital involvement. Arch Ophthalmol 1967;78:318–27.
80. Grimson BS, Simons KB. Orbital inflammation, myositis and systemic lupus erythematosus. Arch Ophthalmol 1983;101:736–8.
81. Harr DL, Quencer RM, Abrams GW. Computed tomography and ultrasound in the evaluation of orbital infection and pseudotumor. Radiology 1982;142:395–401.
82. Henderson JW. Orbital Tumors. 2nd ed. New York: B.C. Decker, 1980.
83. Hidayat AA, Cameron JD, Font RL, Zimmerman LE. Angiolymphoid hyperplasia with eosinophilia (Kimura's disease) of the orbit and ocular adnexa. Am J Ophthalmol 1983;96:176–89.

84. Hufnagel TJ, Hickey WF, Cobbs WH, Weaver K, Greenspan F, Sheline G. Immunohistochemical and ultrastructural studies on the exenterated orbital tissues of a patient with Graves' disease. Ophthalmology 1984;91:1411–9.
85. Hurbli T, Char DS, Harris J, Weaver K, Greenspan F, Sheline G. Radiation therapy for thyroid eye disease. Am J Ophthalmol 1985;99:633–7.
86. Jakobiec FA, Font RL. Orbital tumors. In: Spencer WH, ed. Ophthalmic pathology. An atlas and textbook. 3rd ed. WB Saunders: Philadelphia, 1985:2459–860.
87. Kalina PH, Garrity JA, Herman DC, DeRemee RA, Specks U. Role of testing for anticytoplasmic autoantibodies in the differential diagnosis of scleritis and orbital pseudotumor. Mayo Clin Proc 1990;65:1110–7.
88. Kennerdell JS, Dresner SC. The nonspecific orbital inflammatory syndromes. Surv Ophthalmol 1984; 29:93–103.
89. Lattes R. Tumors of the soft tissues. Atlas of Tumor Pathology, 2nd Series, Fascicle 1/Revised. Washington, D.C.: Armed Forces Institute of Pathology, 1982.
90. Mauriello JA Jr, Flanagan JC. Pseudotumor and lymphoid tumor: distinct clinicopathologic entities. Surv Ophthalmol 1989;34:142–8.
91. Mottow LS, Jakobiec FA. Idiopathic inflammatory orbital pseudotumor in childhood. I. Clinical characteristics. Arch Ophthalmol 1978;96:1410–7.
92. Mottow-Lippa L, Jakobiec FA, Smith M. Idiopathic inflammatory orbital pseudotumor in childhood. II. Results of diagnostic tests and biopsies. Ophthalmology 1981;88:565–74.
93. Orcutt JC, Garner A, Henk JM, Wright JE. Treatment of idiopathic inflammatory orbital pseudotumours by radiotherapy. Br J Ophthalmol 1983;67:570–4.
94. Paris GL, Waltuch GF, Egbert PR. Treatment of refractory orbital pseudotumors with pulsed chemotherapy. Ophthal Plast Reconstr Surg 1990;6:96–101.
95. Ross WH. Myositic pseudotumor of the orbit. Can J Ophthalmol 1983;18:199–201.
96. Shields JA, Bakewell B, Augsburger JJ, Flanagan JC. Classification and incidence of space-occupying lesions of the orbit. A survey of 645 biopsies. Arch Ophthalmol 1984;102:1606–11.
97. Smith DL, Kincaid MC, Nicolitz E. Angiolymphoid hyperplasia with eosinophilia (Kimura's disease) of the orbit. Arch Ophthalmol 1988;106:793–5.
98. Tamai H, Nakagawa T, Ohsako N, et al. Changes in thyroid function in patients with euthyroid Graves' disease. J Clin Endocrinol Metab 1980;50:108–12.
99. Weinstein JM, Koch K, Lane S. Orbital pseudotumor in Crohn's colitis. Ann Ophthalmol 1984;16:275–8.

Lymphoid Tumors

100. Abiose A, Adido J, Agarwal SC. Childhood malignancies of the eye and orbit in northern Nigeria. Cancer 1985;55:2889–93.
101. Alper MG, Bray M. Evolution of a primary lymphoma of the orbit. Br J Ophthalmol 1984;68:225–60.
102. Cheij G, Cooper JL, Wesley RE. Orbital histiocytic lymphoma arising from the ethmoid sinus. Ophthalmic Surg 1987;18:95–6.
103. Henderson JW. Orbital Tumors. 2nd ed. New York: B.C. Decker, 1980.
104. Isaacson P, Wright DH. Extranodal lymphoma arising from mucosa-associated lymphoid tissue. Cancer 1984;53:2515–24.

105. Ishii Y, Yamanaka N, Ogawa K, et al. Nasal T-cell lymphoma as a type of so-called "lethal midline granuloma". Cancer 1982;50:2336–44.

106. Jakobiec FA, Font RL. Orbital tumors. In: Spencer WH, ed. Ophthalmic pathology. An atlas and textbook. 3rd ed. WB Saunders: Philadelphia, 1985:2459–860.

107. _____, Iwamoto T, Knowles DM II. Ocular adnexal lymphoid tumors. Correlative ultrastructural and immunohistochemical studies. Arch Ophthalmol 1982; 100:84–8.

108. _____, Knowles DM. An overview of ocular adnexal lymphoid tumors. Trans Am Ophthalmol Soc 1990;87:420–42.

109. _____, Lefkowitch J, Knowles DM II. B- and T-lymphocytes in ocular disease. Ophthalmology 1984; 91:635–54.

110. _____, McLean I, Font RL. Clinicopathologic characteristics of orbital lymphoid hyperplasia. Ophthalmology 1979;86:948–66.

111. _____, Williams P, Wolff AM. Reticulum cell sarcoma (histiocytic lymphoma) of the orbit: a clinicopathologic review of 13 cases. Surv Ophthalmol 1978;22: 255–70.

112. Keleti D, Flickinger JC, Hobson SR, Mittal BB. Radiotherapy of lymphoproliferative diseases of the orbit. Surveillance of 65 cases. Am J Clin Oncol 1992;15:422–7.

113. Kennedy RE. An evaluation of 820 orbital cases. Trans Am Ophthalmol Soc 1984;82:134–57.

114. Knowles DM, Athan E, Ubriaco A, et al. Extranodal noncutaneous lymphoid hyperplasias represent a continuous spectrum of B-cell neoplasia: demonstrated by molecular genetic analysis. Blood 1989;73:1635–45.

115. _____, Jakobiec FA, McNally L, Burke JS. Lymphoid hyperplasia and malignant lymphoma occurring in the ocular adnexa (orbit, conjunctiva, and eyelids): a prospective multiparametric analysis of 108 cases during 1977 to 1987. Hum Pathol 1990;21:959–73.

116. Knowles DM II, Jakobiec FA. Quantitative determination of T cells in ocular lymphoid infiltrates: an indirect method for distinguishing between pseudolymphomas and malignant lymphomas. Arch Ophthalmol 1981;99:309–16.

117. Mafee MF, Putterman A, Valvassori GE, Campos M, Capek V. Orbital space-occupying lesions: role of computed tomography and magnetic resonance imaging. An analysis of 145 cases. Radiol Clin North Am 1987;25:529–59.

118. Rosenberg S. National Cancer Institute-sponsored study of classifications of non-Hodgkin's lymphomas. Summary and description of a working formulation for clinical usage. Cancer 1982;49:2112–35.

119. Shields JA, Bakewell B, Augsburger JJ, Flanagan JC. Classification and incidence of space-occupying lesions of the orbit. A survey of 645 biopsies. Arch Ophthalmol 1984;102:1606–11.

120. Stenson S, Ramsay DL. Ocular findings in mycosis fungoides. Arch Ophthalmol 1981;99:272–7.

121. Yeo JH, Jakobiec FA, Abbott GF, Trokel SL. Combined clinical and computed tomographic diagnosis of orbital lymphoid tumors. Am J Ophthalmol 1982;94:235–45.

Plasmacytoma

122. Jonasson F. Orbital plasma cell tumours. Ophthalmologica 1978;177:152–7.

123. Khalil MK, Huang S, Viloria J, Duguid WP. Extramedullary plasmacytoma of the orbit: Case report with results of immunocytochemical studies. Can J Ophthalmol 1981;16:39–42.

124. Knowles DM II, Halper JA, Trokel S, Jakobiec A. Immunofluorescent and immunoperoxidase characteristics of IgD myeloma involving the orbit. Am J Ophthalmol 1978;85:485–94.

Leukemia

125. Davis JL, Parke DW II, Font RL. Granulocytic sarcoma of the orbit. A clinicopathologic study. Ophthalmology 1985;92:1758–62.

126. Kincaid MC, Green WR. Ocular and orbital involvement in leukemia. Surv Ophthalmol 1982;27:211–32.

127. Rubinfeld RS, Gootenberg JE, Chavis RM, Zimmerman LE. Early onset acute orbital involvement in childhood acute lymphoblastic leukemia. Ophthalmology 1988;95:116–20.

128. Shome DK, Gupta NK, Prajapati NC, Raju GM, Choudhury P, Dubey AP. Orbital granulocytic sarcomas (myeloid sarcomas) in acute nonlymphocytic leukemia. Cancer 1992;70:2298–301.

129. Zimmerman LE, Font RL. Ophthalmologic manifestations of granulocytic sarcoma (myeloid sarcoma or chloroma). Am J Ophthalmol 1975;80:975–90.

Eosinophilic Granuloma

130. Chu A, Eisinger M, Lee JS, Takezaki S, Kung PC, Edelson RL. Immunoelectron microscopic identification of Langerhans cells using a new antigenic marker. J Invest Dermatol 1982;78:177–80.

131. Feldman RB, Moore DM, Hood CI, Hiles DA, Romano PE. Solitary eosinophilic granuloma of the lateral orbital wall. Am J Ophthalmol 1985;100:318–23.

Sinus Histiocytosis

132. Burton EM, Hickman M, Boulden TF, Joyner RE, Tierney MB. Orbital sinus histiocytosis: MR appearance. J Comput Assist Tomogr 1989;13:696–9.

133. Foucar E, Rosai J, Dorfman RF. The ophthalmologic manifestations of sinus histiocytosis with massive lymphadenopathy. Am J Ophthalmol 1979;87:354–67.

134. Karcioglu ZA, Allam B, Insler MS. Ocular involvement in sinus histiocytosis with massive lymphadenopathy. Br J Ophthalmol 1988;72:793–5.

135. Zimmerman LE, Hidayat AA, Grantham RL, et al. Atypical cases of sinus histiocytosis (Rosai-Dorfman disease) with ophthalmological manifestations. Trans Am Ophthalmol Soc 1988;86:113–35.

Dermoid Cyst

136. Jakobiec FA, Bonanno PA, Sigelman J. Conjunctival adnexal cysts and dermoids. Arch Ophthalmol 1978;96:1040–9.

137. Nugent RA, Lapointe JS, Rootman J, Robertson WD, Graeb DA. Orbital dermoids: features on CT. Radiology 1987;165:475–8.

Teratoma

138. Levin ML, Leone CR Jr, Kincaid MC. Congenital orbital teratomas. Am J Ophthalmol 1986;102:476–81.

139. Neiger R, Sacks LM. Massive orbital and intracranial teratoma in the newborn: a case report. J Med Assoc Ga 1989;78:811–3.

140. Weiss AH, Greenwald MJ, Margo CE, Myers W. Primary and secondary orbital teratomas. J Pediatr Ophthalmol Strabismus 1989;26:44–9.

Melanoma

141. Dutton JJ, Anderson RL, Schelper RL, Purcell JJ, Tse DT. Orbital malignant melanoma and oculodermal melanocytosis: report of two cases and review of the literature. Ophthalmology 1984;91:497–507.
142. Jakobiec FA, Ellsworth R, Tannenbaum M. Primary orbital melanoma. Am J Ophthalmol 1974;78:24–39.
143. Löffler KU, Witschel H. Primary malignant melanoma of the orbit arising in a cellular blue naevus. Br J Ophthalmol 1989;73:388–93.
144. Rice CD, Brown HH. Primary orbital melanoma associated with orbital melanocytosis. Arch Ophthalmol 1990;108:1130–4.
145. Wilkes TD, Uthman EO, Thornton CN, Cole RE. Malignant melanoma of the orbit in a black patient with ocular melanocytosis. Arch Ophthalmol 1984;102:904–6.

Fibrous Dysplasia

146. Moore AT, Buncic JR, Munro IR. Fibrous dysplasia of the orbit in childhood: clinical features and management. Ophthalmology 1985;92:12–20.
147. Sevel D, James HE, Burns R, Jones KL. McCune-Albright syndrome (fibrous dysplasia) associated with an orbital tumor. Ann Ophthalmol 1984;16:283–97.

Ossifying Fibroma

148. Johnson LC, Yousef M, Vinh TN, Heffner DK, Hyams VJ, Hartman KS. Juvenile active ossifying fibroma. Its nature, dynamics and origin. Acta Otolaryngol (Stockh) 1991;488(Suppl):1–40.
149. Margo CE, Ragsdale BD, Perman KI, Zimmerman LE, Sweet DE. Psammomatoid (juvenile) ossifying fibroma of the orbit. Ophthalmology 1985;92:150–9.

Osteogenic Sarcoma

150. Abramson DH, Ellsworth RM, Zimmerman LE. Non-ocular cancer in retinoblastoma survivors. Trans Am Acad Ophthalmol Otolaryngol 1976;81(3 Pt 1):451–7.
151. Roarty JD, McLean IW, Zimmerman LE. Incidence of second neoplasms in patients with bilateral retinoblastoma. Ophthalmology 1988;95:1583–7.

Secondary Tumors

152. Amoaku WM, Bagegni A, Logan WC, Archer DB. Orbital infiltration by eyelid skin carcinoma. Int Ophthalmol 1990;14:285–94.

153. Clouston PD, Sharpe DM, Corbett AJ, Kos S, Kennedy PJ. Perineural spread of cutaneous head and neck cancer. Its orbital and central neurologic complications. Arch Neurol 1990;47:73–7.
154. Cohen BH, Green WR, Iliff NT, et al. Spindle cell carcinoma of the conjunctiva. Arch Ophthalmol 1980; 98:1809–13.
155. Glover AT, Grove AS Jr. Orbital invasion by malignant eyelid tumors. Ophthal Plast Reconstr Surg 1989;5:1–12.
156. Graamans K, Slootweg PJ. Orbital exenteration in surgery of malignant neoplasms of the paranasal sinuses. The value of preoperative computed tomography. Arch Otolaryngol Head Neck Surg 1989;115:977–80.
157. Gullane PJ, Conley J. Carcinoma of the maxillary sinus. A correlation of the clinical course with orbital involvement, pterygoid erosion or pterygopalatine invasion and cervical metastases. J Otolaryngol 1983; 12:141–5.
158. Jakobiec FA, Font RL. Orbital tumors. In: Spencer WH, ed. Ophthalmic pathology. An atlas and textbook. 3rd ed. WB Saunders: Philadelphia, 1985:2459–860.
159. Khalil MK, Duguid WP. Neurotropic malignant melanoma of right temple with orbital metastasis: a clinicopathological case report. Br J Ophthalmol 1987;71:41–6.
160. Liaw CC, Ho YS, Ng KK. Nasopharyngeal carcinoma presenting as a retro—orbital mass report of three cases. Otolaryngol Head Neck Surg 1990;103:825–8.

Metastatic Tumors

161. Alfano JE. Ophthalmological aspects of neuroblastomatosis: a study of 53 verified cases. Trans Am Acad Ophthalmol Otolaryngol 1968;72:830–48.
162. Font RL, Ferry AP. Carcinoma metastatic to the eye and orbit: III. A clinicopathologic study of 28 cases metastatic to the orbit. Cancer 1976;38:1326–35.
163. Goldberg RA, Rootman J. Clinical characteristics of metastatic orbital tumors. Ophthalmology 1990;97:620–4.
164. Orcutt JC, Char DH. Melanoma metastatic to the orbit. Ophthalmology 1988;95:1033–7.
165. Shields CL, Shields JA, Peggs M. Tumors metastatic to the orbit. Ophthal Plast Reconstr Surg 1988;4:73–80.
166. Stefanyszyn MA, DeVita EG, Flanagan JC. Breast carcinoma metastatic to the orbit. Ophthal Plast Reconstr Surg 1987;3:43–7.
167. Vanneste JA. Subacute bilateral malignant exophthalmos due to orbital medulloblastoma metastases. Arch Neurol 1983;40:441–3.

8
TUMORS OF THE OPTIC NERVE AND OPTIC NERVE HEAD

ANATOMY AND HISTOLOGY

The optic nerve emerges from the eye just above and somewhat nasal to the posterior pole and connects the retina and the brain. Its total length averages 50 mm: the intraorbital portion measures 33 mm, the intracanalicular portion measures 10 mm, and the intracranial portion is 7 mm. The diameter of the intraorbital segment of the optic nerve with its meningeal sheaths is 3 to 4 mm.

The optic nerve head is formed by the convergence of axons from the retinal ganglion cells at the optic disc (fig. 8-1). The intraocular portion of the optic nerve extends from the surface of the optic disc to the posterior border of the lamina cribrosa. The intraorbital portion emerges from the back of the eye and courses in an upward and inward direction, entering the optic foramen at the apex of the orbit. This segment is longer than the distance from the back of the eye to the apex of the orbit. This excess of nerve permits normal eye movements and even a considerable proptosis without damage to the nerve fibers.

As with the brain, three sheaths enclose the optic nerve (fig. 8-2). The outermost is the dura mater, a dense collagenous and elastic tunic continuous anteriorly with the sclera. At the orbital apex, there is a close relationship of the optic nerve and its sheaths to the insertion of the rectus muscles. The dura of the intracanalicular segment is continuous with that covering the brain. Branches of the ophthalmic artery supplying the optic nerve parenchyma pass through the dura en route to the middle sheath, the arachnoid.

The arachnoid is composed of delicate connective tissue trabeculae that join the dura and the underlying pia mater. The trabeculae of the arachnoid contain fibroblasts, histiocytes, and numerous blood vessels. Nests of meningothelial cells cover the trabeculae, which are identical to the arachnoid villi found elsewhere in the meninges of the brain.

The pia mater is the most vascular of the meningeal sheaths and is the only one that is firmly attached to the nerve. Fibrovascular connective tissue septa extending from the surface of the nerve subdivide the nerve parenchyma into compartments that contain bundles of axons.

The main blood supply to the intraorbital and intraocular portions of the optic nerve is from the

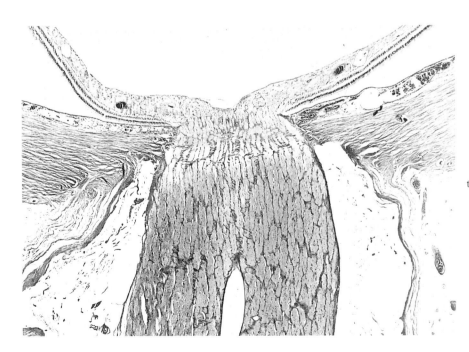

Figure 8-1
NORMAL OPTIC NERVE
Intraocular and orbital portions of the optic nerve.

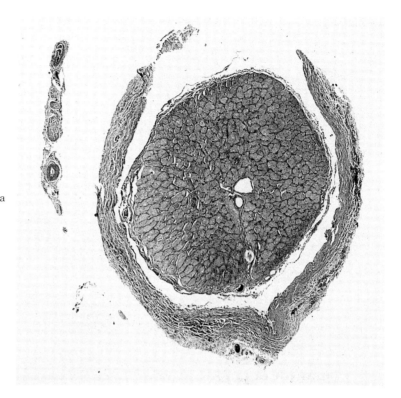

Figure 8-2
NORMAL OPTIC NERVE
Cross section of optic nerve parenchyma and meninges.

ophthalmic artery via the vessels of the pia mater. Recurrent branches from the posterior ciliary arteries and juxtapapillary choroid add to the anterior pial supply. The pia of the intracranial portion of the optic nerve derives its blood supply from the internal carotid, anterior cerebral, anterior communicating, and ophthalmic arteries.

In the region of the lamina cribrosa and optic nerve head, an extensive network of arterioles and capillaries originate from the short posterior ciliary arteries, the pia mater, and the choroid with minimal contribution from the central retinal artery.

CLASSIFICATION AND FREQUENCY

The relative frequency of the different types of tumors received at the Armed Forces Institute of Pathology (AFIP) are classified using the schema of the World Health Organization (Table 8-1). Astrocytomas are the most common type of tumor in this series, which differs from the data reported by Henderson (1), who found that meningiomas were slightly more common. The rare melanocytoma of the optic nerve head is a lesion that is unique to ophthalmic pathology and may be atavistic because many reptiles normally have similar pigmentation of their optic nerve heads.

Table 8-1

TUMORS OF THE OPTIC NERVE AND DISC*

Type of Tumor	Number of Cases
Nerve	
Astrocytoma	17
Meningioma	8
Hemangiopericytoma (angioblastic meningioma)	2
Melanoma	1
Lymphoma	1
Carcinoma, metastatic	1
Disc	
Melanocytoma	3
Astrocytoma	1

*Frequency distribution of 34 tumors in the AFIP Registry of Ophthalmic Pathology collected between 1984 and 1989.

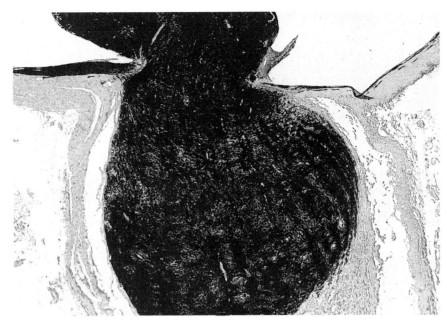

Figure 8-3
MELANOCYTOMA
Heavily pigmented tumor involving the optic nerve head, optic
nerve, and peripapillary choroid.

MELANOCYTOMA
(MAGNOCELLULAR NEVUS)

This benign melanocytic tumor is the most common primary tumor of the optic nerve head (2,4,6,7). It is a distinctive nevus composed of large polyhedral cells that are packed with melanosomes. Melanocytomas differ from melanomas in almost every aspect (4,6,7).

Clinically, melanocytomas most often occur in nonwhite and heavily pigmented individuals (7); malignant melanomas are uncommon in heavily pigmented races. Melanocytomas of the nerve head are usually small and always deeply pigmented (pl. XV), while other nevi and malignant melanomas of the uveal tract vary enormously in size and pigmentation. Rarely do melanocytomas become much larger than the nerve head itself, and they seldom protrude into the vitreous more than 1 or 2 mm. They often extend posteriorly a few millimeters behind the lamina cribrosa. Most frequently, they are situated eccentrically in the lower temporal quadrant (7). When they extend from the nerve head into the adjacent retina, the tumor has a feathery border.

Microscopically, unlike other melanocytic tumors, the cytoplasm of every cell in a melanocytoma is completely stuffed with melanosomes (fig. 8-3). Morphologically, two types of melanoctyes are present: the first type has giant melanosomes and the second contains the small round melanosomes that are characteristic of uveal melanocytes. Neither type contains the large ovoid melanosomes that are found in retinal pigment epithelial cells. Melanocytomas are also remarkably uniform in their cytologic characteristics, without the pleomorphism of spindle and epithelioid type cells that is observed in uveal melanomas. Melanocytomas are composed of tightly packed, moderately plump polyhedral cells (fig. 8-3, 8-4) that may be compressed and distorted by the nerve fibers, lamina cribrosa, and other anatomic structures of the nerve head. Their nuclei, which are generally small and round, contain fine dispersed chromatin and small inconspicuous nucleoli. Although melanocytoma cells may superficially resemble melanophages, they can usually be differentiated from macrophages by their uniform melanin granules. Melanophages contain degenerated phagocytosed pigment, which characteristically varies markedly in size and shape. By electron microscopy, melanophages contain melanosome complexes bound within lysosomal membranes.

Tumors of similar cellular composition whose clinical features and natural history closely resemble optic nerve head melanocytomas have been observed throughout the uveal tract (fig. 8-5) (3,5). Some optic nerve head melanocytomas also involve the juxtapapillary choroid, causing difficulties in determining where such tumors originate.

PLATE XV
MELANOCYTOMA

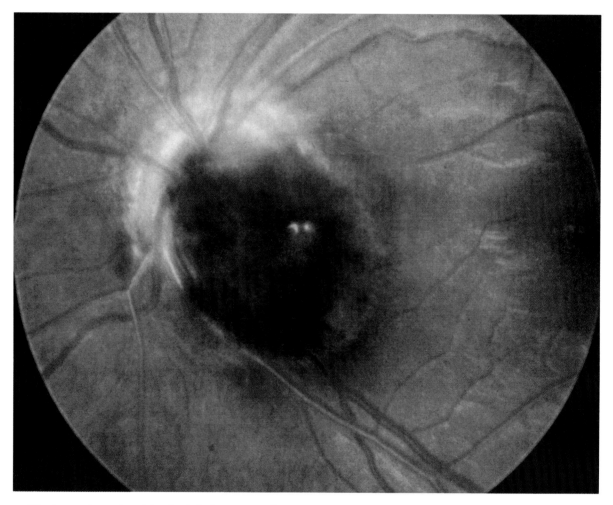

The tumor is centered in the inferior temporal quadrant of the optic nerve head and has a feathery border where it infiltrates the retina.

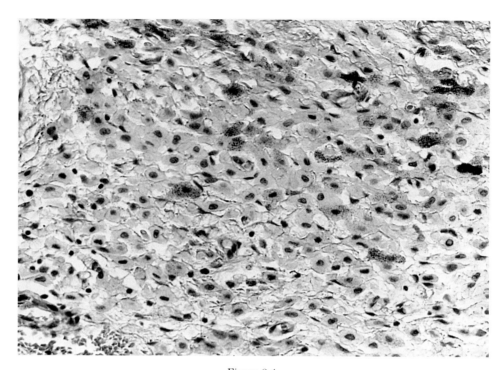

Figure 8-4
MELANOCYTOMA
Bleached preparation showing plump polyhedral melanocytes with small ovoid nuclei.

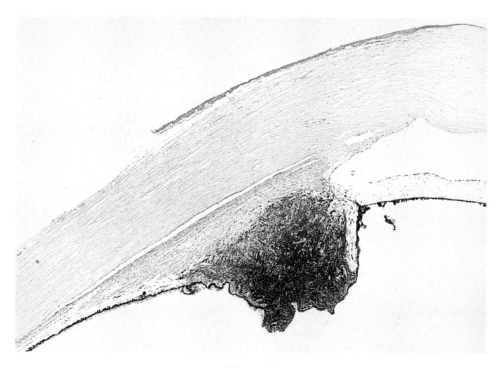

Figure 8-5
MELANOCYTOMA
Pigmented tumor located in the ciliary body.

Melanocytomas have never been reported to metastasize or even to extend out of the ocular tissues into the orbit. Zimmerman and Garron (7) documented the benign nature of these tumors in 34 cases. In 20 patients the involved eye was enucleated and in 14 patients the melanocytoma was followed without treatment. In none of the cases was there metastasis. The 14 tumors that were not treated showed little or no growth during follow-up periods ranging from 1 to 34 years.

In most instances, melanocytoma cells seem to be able to mingle with the axons, glia, and vessels of the disc without producing functional loss or histologic evidence of cellular injury. Nevertheless, slow growth of some melanocytomas occurs and a few have infiltrated the adjacent retina and choroid or extended posteriorly into the nerve, to surround the central retinal vessels and invade the pia. Enlargement of the melanocytoma may result in compression of axons, which are pressed against the unyielding scleral margins of the optic nerve head, but this usually does not cause measurable visual loss. Rarely, there is loss of vision due to necrosis within the tumor, central retinal vein occlusion, or maculopathy. In a few cases, malignant melanomas have been interpreted as originating in melanocytomas of the optic nerve head, however almost all malignant melanomas of the optic nerve head represent extensions of juxtapapillary choroidal tumors.

MALIGNANT MELANOMA

Rare primary melanomas and several cases of metastatic melanoma to the optic nerve have been reported (8). Secondary invasion of the optic nerve by uveal malignant melanoma is far more common. Spread of uveal melanoma within the nerve to the brain is almost never the cause of death as it is with retinoblastoma. Primary melanomas arise from the rare melanocytes in the meninges of the optic nerve and may develop in patients with congenital melanosis oculi or nevus of Ota.

JUVENILE PILOCYTIC ASTROCYTOMA

Most "gliomas" of the optic nerve and chiasm are benign pilocytic astrocytomas. They can be present at birth (9,10,17,19). Ninety percent become evident during the first two decades with a median age of 5 years. There is a 60 percent female predominance. Optic nerve astrocytomas are uncommon and have been estimated to represent 1 to 2.5 percent of orbital tumors by Kennedy (15) and Henderson (12) and 4 percent in the AFIP Registry of Ophthalmic Pathology. Approximately 48 percent involve only the orbit, 24 percent both the orbital and intracranial portions of the nerve, and 28 percent only the intracranial portion (19).

It has been estimated that up to 50 percent of patients with juvenile pilocytic astrocytomas of the optic nerve have neurofibromatosis type 1 (17,18). The frequency of the association in many reported series is probably underestimated because cafe-au-lait spots and other manifestations of neurofibromatosis may not be recognized until after puberty, while optic nerve gliomas most often produce symptoms in the first decade. There are many families with neurofibromatosis in which there is more than one member with an optic nerve glioma. These gliomas are usually unilateral, but bilateral intraorbital optic nerve gliomas in association with neurofibromatosis type 1 have been observed. Multicentric gliomas within the anterior optic pathways are extremely rare except in patients with neurofibromatosis.

Clinical Features. Pilocytic astrocytomas of the optic nerve are slow-growing tumors and signs and symptoms usually develop insidiously (9,10,17). In approximately half the patients the tumor appears to stop growing without treatment. In this group the tumor is either stable when first seen, or it enlarges slowly (occasionally in an episodic fashion) and then stops growing, remaining unchanged for many years. In the remaining patients the growth continues, resulting in progressive proptosis requiring surgical intervention. Even in neglected situations a huge optic nerve pilocytic astrocytoma is never seen, suggesting that even in progressive tumors the growth is self-limiting. Pilocytic astrocytomas of the optic nerve do not undergo malignant change or metastasize. Cytologically benign intracranial gliomas may result in death because of elevated intracranial pressure or interference with hypothalamic and pituitary function. Since pilocytic astrocytomas arise from elements normally found in the optic nerve and do not grow relentlessly, they have been considered by some to be hamartomatous lesions.

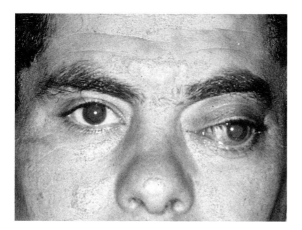

Figure 8-6
PILOCYTIC ASTROCYTOMA
Orbital tumor causing proptosis.

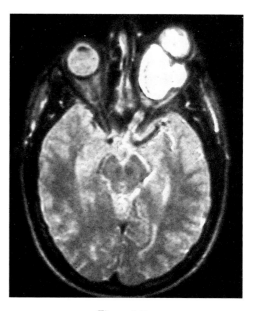

Figure 8-7
PILOCYTIC ASTROCYTOMA
Magnetic resonance image of a large retrobulbar optic nerve tumor causing massive proptosis.

Loss of vision is usually an early symptom in patients with juvenile pilocytic astrocytoma involving any portion of the optic nerve. This differentiates gliomas from meningiomas in which loss of vision is usually a late symptom. Early loss of vision probably results from early destruction of axons, because astrocytomas are tumors of the parenchyma of the nerve, whereas meningiomas rarely involve the parenchyma. Other clinical signs and symptoms depend on location. Astrocytomas that arise in the orbit usually produce proptosis (figs. 8-6, 8-7). Tumors that are anteriorly located are more likely to cause papilledema and may interfere with retinal circulation by causing an artery or vein occlusion. Astrocytomas arising in the intracranial portion of the optic nerve may cause hypothalamic and pituitary dysfunction, headache, abnormalities of gait, and polyuria. The diagnosis of pilocytic astrocytoma of the orbital optic nerve is aided by imaging studies, either computerized tomography (CT) or magnetic resonance imaging (MRI), which demonstrate fusiform enlargement of the optic nerve without signs of invasion of orbital soft tissue (13).

Pathologic Findings. Grossly, gliomas of the orbital portion of the optic nerve are typically fusiform, although those arising near the optic canal may extend through each end of the canal and have a dumbbell shape. The dura overlying the tumor may be stretched and thin, but it is almost always intact. At the tapered margins of the

tumor it is often difficult, and sometimes impossible, to see the junction between the tumor and uninvolved nerve. The usual appearance during surgery is of a firm, tan, fusiform swelling of the optic nerve. Vascular congestion within the tumor may cause it to appear dusky red.

Cross sections of excised optic nerve gliomas are more informative than are longitudinal sections. It is helpful to obtain cross sections at each end of the specimen and at several levels through the middle. Sections through the middle portion often show the whitish nerve to be enlarged and surrounded by a cuff of arachnoidal tissue of varying thickness, which in turn is covered by stretched intact dura mater. Near the tapered ends of the mass the nerve itself may be of normal thickness, but the overall diameter may still be increased because of the perineural component. Occasionally, the entire cross section will have a gelatinous appearance.

Microscopically, pilocytic astrocytomas of the optic nerve are composed of elongated, spindle-shaped, hair-like astrocytes (figs. 8-8–8-11). These spindle-shaped astrocytes are relatively cohesive and form intersecting bundles that distend the pial septa of the optic nerve. They have a benign histologic appearance, with a notable absence of mitotic

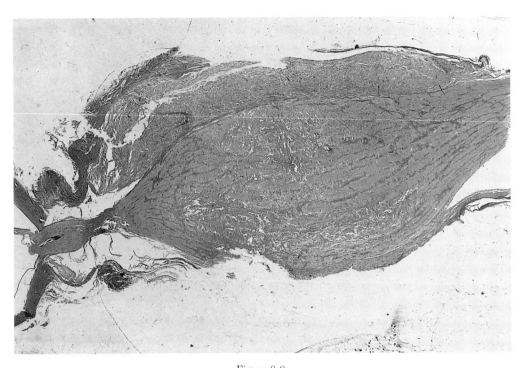

Figure 8-8
PILOCYTIC ASTROCYTOMA
Tumor of optic nerve parenchyma with infiltration of meninges.

figures. The nuclei are rarely hyperchromatic and are usually uniform and oval. The elongated cytoplasm contains glial filaments demonstrable by phosphotungstic acid hematoxylin (PTAH) staining, immunohistochemistry for glial fibrillary acidic protein (GFAP), and electron microscopy. The reticulin stain is also helpful in differentiating gliomas from peripheral nerve tumors because there is no intercellular basement membrane material between astrocytes, whereas basement membrane is abundant between Schwann cells, resulting in a positive reticulin stain. Rosenthal fibers are frequently seen in pilocytic astrocytomas of the optic nerve (fig. 8-10), although they may be absent or vary in number in different areas of the same tumor. This degenerative change is an eosinophilic cylindrical or spherical swelling within astrocytic cell processes.

Ultrastructurally, Rosenthal fibers are composed of electron-dense granular material and glial filaments (14). Foci of calcification occur in gliomas much less commonly than psammoma bodies in meningiomas. Frequently interspersed among the astrocytes are paler staining areas that appear cystic on hematoxylin and eosin (H&E) stained sections. With special stains, the cystic spaces are shown to contain mucopolysaccharides, which are partially sensitive to hyaluronidase digestion. Most of the vessels in the tumor are of capillary size and are located either in the pial septa or between bundles of astrocytes. On occasion, dilated congested sinusoidal vascular channels are seen.

Many optic nerve gliomas contain areas in which the proliferation of neoplastic glia is impossible to differentiate from reactive gliosis, particularly where the tumor merges with normal nerve. In such areas, the astrocytic nuclei may appear to be more numerous and less orderly arranged than in the normal nerve. In gliomas, each affected nerve bundle may be considerably enlarged by the increase in glial cells, which differentiates them from reactive gliosis in which the neuronal bundles are atrophic.

Longstanding untreated tumors in adults and incompletely excised tumors in children may contain large cystic areas filled with blood, serous exudate, or mucin. Areas of hemorrhagic necrosis may also occur as a consequence of vascular

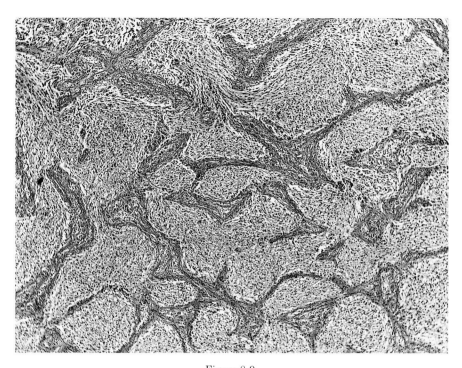

Figure 8-9
PILOCYTIC ASTROCYTOMA
Intraparenchymal tumor with hypercellularity and enlargement of axonal bundles.

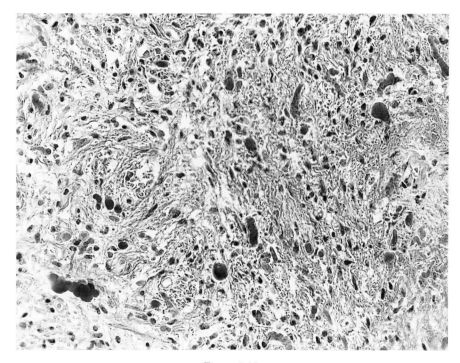

Figure 8-10
PILOCYTIC ASTROCYTOMA
Tumor contains numerous Rosenthal fibers.

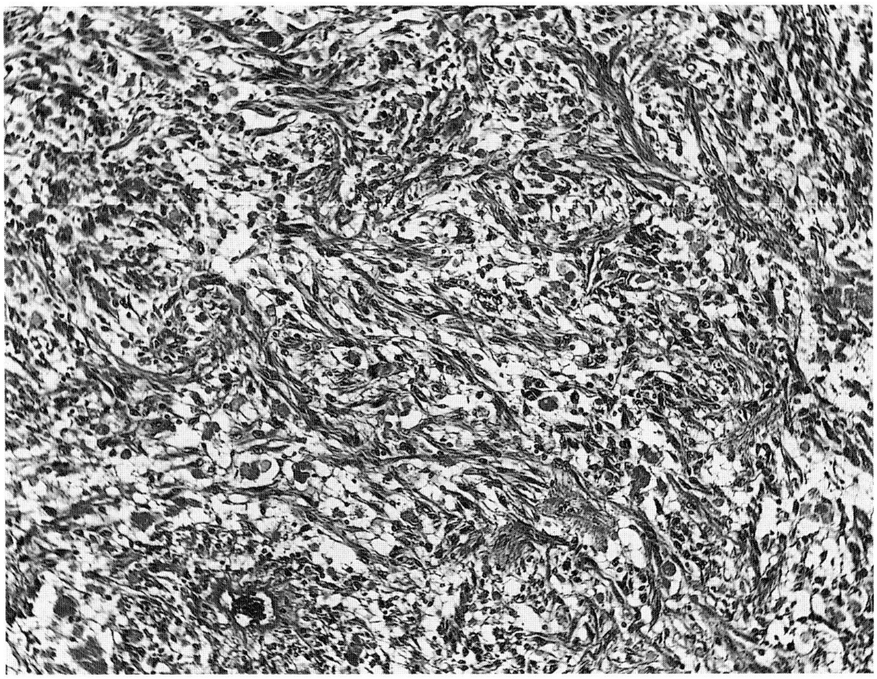

Figure 8-11
PILOCYTIC
ASTROCYTOMA
Astrocytes infiltrating the meninges are accompanied by fibroblasts and meningothelial cells.

occlusion. In these older gliomas, the degenerative features may be quite marked and neoplastic astrocytes difficult to recognize. These "ancient" gliomas may be largely fibrotic and contain lipoidal histiocytes and thick-walled fibrotic blood vessels suggestive of an angiomatous lesion. Such tumors are reminiscent of ancient schwannomas of peripheral nerves.

Some pilocytic astrocytomas extensively invade the leptomeninges, stimulating an exuberant proliferation of fibrous tissue and meningothelial cells, and leading to an increased diameter of the nerve and distension of the overlying dura (figs. 8-8, 8-11). The leptomeningeal thickening may spread anterior and posterior to the site of the intraneural glioma and contribute to the characteristic fusiform configuration. Verhoeff (18) reported that this thickening is caused by a proliferation of meningothelial cells and fibroblasts intermingled with astrocytes and called it arachnoidal hyperplasia. Ultrastructural studies by Stern et al. (18) confirmed the admixture of meningothelial cells, fibroblasts, and neoplastic astrocytes, but these investigators found a preponderance of astrocytes. They proposed the term arachnoidal gliomatosis to emphasize that tumor astrocytes, rather than fibroblasts or meningothelial cells, constitute the majority of

the circumferential proliferation. They found that circumferential arachnoidal gliomatosis is usually associated with neurofibromatosis type 1 and that purely intraneural growth with intact pial boundaries is more characteristic of optic nerve gliomas that are not associated with neurofibromatosis. However, a more recent study was unable to confirm this observation (16).

Increased size of an optic nerve glioma occurs not only from proliferating neoplastic glia but also from mucin production, cystic changes, reactive gliosis, meningeal hyperplasia, and congestion within dilated vascular channels. In several cases of rapidly evolving optic nerve gliomas, the cause of the increased size was the accumulation of mucin or bleeding into necrotic or cystic areas of the tumor.

In most cases, the clinical signs and symptoms and imaging studies are sufficiently explicit to permit the appropriate diagnosis without necessitating biopsy. Nevertheless, meningiomas arising within the orbital optic nerve can produce signs and symptoms closely resembling those of optic nerve gliomas. Since orbital meningiomas can extend intracranially and cause death, they should be recognized and excised while still within the orbit. When clinical doubt exists, some have advocated biopsy of the optic nerve

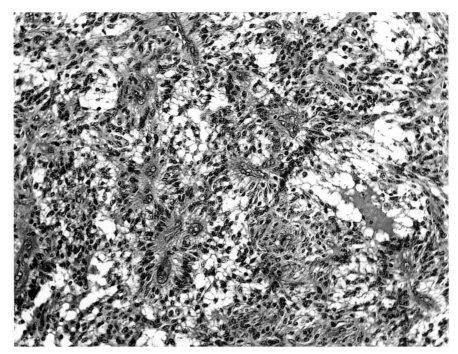

Figure 8-12
ASTROCYTOMA
Higher grade tumor with palisading cells around blood vessels and myxoid areas.

sheaths; however, difficulty with histopathologic interpretation of the biopsy specimen on occasion has resulted in diagnostic confusion between arachnoidal gliomatosis associated with glioma and meningioma (11). Immunostaining for GFAP may be useful in distinguishing fibrillary glial cells from fibroblasts or fibrous meningiomas. Most orbital meningiomas extend through the dura at one point or another, whereas in arachnoidal hyperplasia associated with glioma the cellular proliferation remains intradural. Therefore, the presence of transdural tumor extension is strong evidence in favor of meningioma. The alert surgeon who observes transdural tumor extension may obtain a frozen section diagnosis and then proceed with resection.

MALIGNANT ASTROCYTOMA OF OPTIC NERVE AND CHIASM

Rare, highly lethal astrocytomas usually arise from the intracranial portion of the optic nerve in adults (20–24). These neoplasms are composed of malignant astrocytes that proliferate rapidly and invade surrounding tissues. Extension through the optic canal into the orbital portion of the optic nerve, with invasion through the dura into the orbital soft tissues, is a feature of malignant gliomas that is not seen with benign tumors. The

clinical course usually begins with unilateral visual loss or a condition resembling acute unilateral optic neuritis and progresses to bilateral blindness within a few months and death in less than 1 year. Involvement of the posterior visual pathways may cause visual field loss in addition to other signs of progressive intracranial malignancy. The disc may appear normal throughout the illness or may develop papilledema. The age of affected individuals in published series ranges from 22 to 79 years (mean, 52).

Histologic examination of these tumors shows atypical pleomorphic astrocytes (fig. 8-12). Numerous mitoses and areas of necrosis may be present. Secondary vascular and endothelial proliferation are additional characteristics (20).

MENINGIOMA

Almost all meningiomas in the orbit either originate from the meninges of the optic nerve (figs. 8-13–8-16) or invade the orbit secondarily from an intracranial site of origin near the sphenoid wing (figs. 8-17–8-19) (28,31). Ectopic (extradural) meningiomas arising in the orbit constitute an exceedingly rare third type. Ectopic tumors are believed to arise from congenitally displaced rests of meningothelial cells (30).

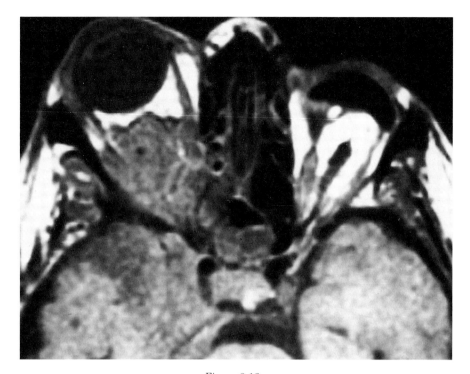

Figure 8-13
MENINGIOMA
Magnetic resonance image of large tumor at orbital apex causing proptosis.

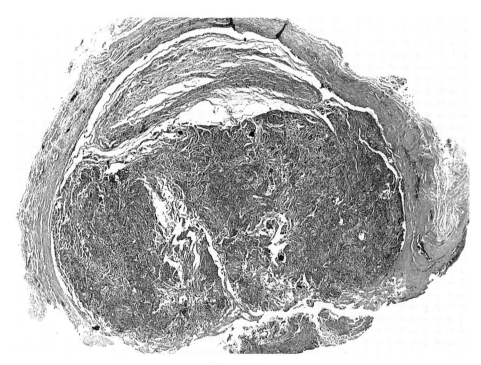

Figure 8-14
MENINGIOMA
Tumor growing within the dura has caused marked compression of the optic nerve.

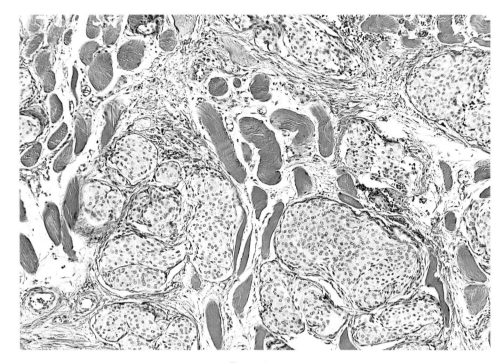

Figure 8-15
MENINGIOMA
Islands of meningothelial cells infiltrating extraocular muscle.

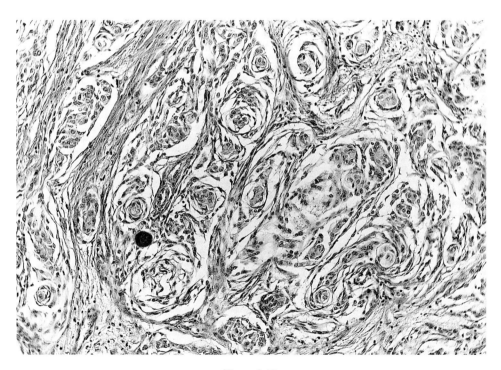

Figure 8-16
MENINGIOMA
Meningothelial cells arranged in small nests with a whorled pattern.

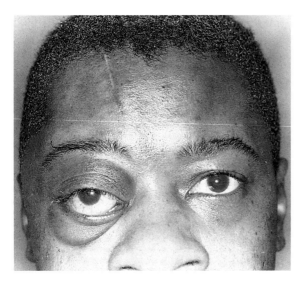

Figure 8-17
MENINGIOMA

Tumor that has arisen adjacent to the sphenoid wing has invaded the superior lateral aspect of the orbit causing downward displacement and proptosis. (Figures 8-17–8-19 are from the same patient.)

Clinical Features. The age of patients with primary optic nerve meningioma is substantially younger than for patients with meningioma arising from the coverings of the brain and spinal cord. This may be because slowly enlarging intracranial meningiomas do not produce symptoms until adulthood, whereas a meningioma occurring in the smaller orbital bony cavity may produce exophthalmos and visual symptoms that are apparent while the tumor is still small. Optic nerve meningiomas at a young age may also be a manifestation of the central form of neurofibromatosis type 2. Multiple intracranial and optic nerve meningiomas in a child is suggestive of neurofibromatosis type 2 even in the absence of other stigmata. Meningiomas associated with acoustic neuromas are diagnostic of neurofibromatosis type 2. Whatever the explanation, orbital meningiomas do arise in children and must be considered in the differential diagnosis of any lesion producing unilateral progressive

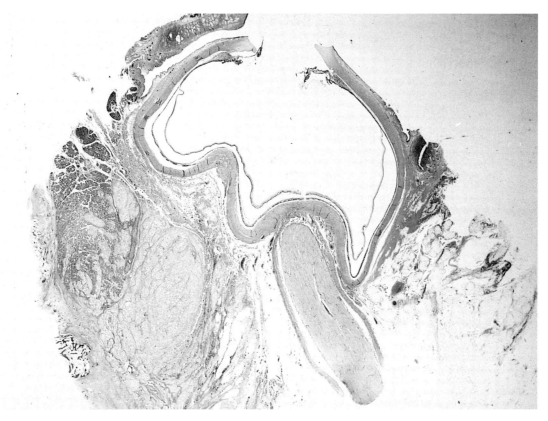

Figure 8-18
MENINGIOMA

A tumor unrelated to the meninges of the optic nerve is located in the superior lateral aspect of the orbit.

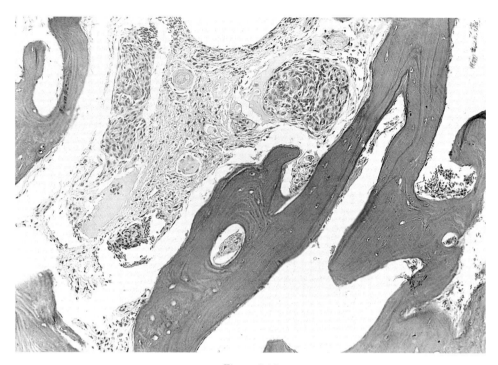

Figure 8-19
MENINGIOMA
Invasion of the sphenoid bone.

exophthalmos and visual loss, even in the first few years of life (32).

The characteristic clinical course is that of slowly progressive axial proptosis with flattening of the posterior pole of the eye, causing increased hyperopia and striae that are visible ophthalmoscopically. Anteriorly located meningiomas usually cause proptosis before limitation of eye motion; however, meningiomas situated in the posterior orbit quickly invade the nerves and muscles, causing an early onset of strabismus.

Meningiomas arising in the region of the optic canal may cause signs simulating retrobulbar neuritis (29). The patient may have a central or a centrocecal scotoma that slowly enlarges over a period of months to years. Proptosis can be minimal or absent. CT can show slight enlargement of the optic canal, minute calcium deposits within the intracanalicular nerve or its sheaths, or hyperostosis adjacent to the orbital or intracranial meatus of the optic canal.

Disc edema is a frequent finding, especially when the meningioma arises in the arachnoid at the anterior end of optic nerve. In longstanding cases, the disc swelling subsides as the nerve undergoes atrophy. Rarely, tumor cells may invade the sclera, the peripapillary vascular channels, the choroid, and the optic nerve head. On the surface of the disc, optociliary (retinochoroidal) shunt vessels may be seen (26). This is explained by the slow expansion of a "sleeve" meningioma that compromises retinal venous outflow by the central retinal vein and induces collateral flow via retinochoroidal channels. Optociliary shunt vessels are commonly seen with anteriorly located meningiomas, but they are rare with retrobulbar gliomas.

CT and MRI with gadolinium enhancement have become essential in the diagnosis and management of optic nerve tumors (25,27). The most common tomographic appearance of meningioma is a diffuse swelling of the optic nerve with a bulbous enlargement at the orbital apex, with or without bone erosion (fig. 8-13). "Railroad tracking" in the subarachnoid space and focal or extensive calcification due to psammoma bodies are features more typical of meningioma than glioma. Hyperostosis at the orbital apex is more in keeping with meningioma than with glioma. Irregular excrescences along the nerve signify invasion of the dura, an indication that the lesion is a meningioma.

Imaging studies provide information necessary to plan the best surgical approach to excise meningiomas of the optic nerve (25,27). Intracranial tumors and tumors involving the optic canal are best approached intracranially, whereas tumors confined to the orbit should be approached by a lateral orbitotomy. Patients with primary optic nerve meningiomas have a poor prognosis for retention of vision on the affected side, but with appropriate treatment there is a good prognosis for life. Meningiomas that are diagnosed early and completely excised are cured. Complete excision is most likely when the meningioma is confined within the orbit. A difficult decision faces the surgeon when the tumor has not yet resulted in severe visual loss; however, slow progression of visual loss with eventual intracranial extension is almost certain if the tumor is left untreated. Growth of meningiomas has been slowed by radiation therapy, but this form of treatment is not curative.

Pathologic Findings. Unlike orbital optic nerve gliomas, meningiomas usually extend through the dura. The tumor usually does not invade the parenchyma of the optic nerve but grows mainly within the meninges in a sleeve-like manner and through the dura into the orbit. The optic nerve is often compressed and may undergo atrophy, especially if the meningioma involves the portion of the optic nerve within the bony canal connecting the orbit to the brain (fig. 8-14). Meningiomas may infiltrate all of the orbital tissues (fig. 8-15) but invasion through the sclera into the eye is uncommon.

Optic nerve meningiomas originate from a variety of cellular elements residing in the perineural space. They have histologic features similar to those of intracranial meningiomas. The most common types arise from meningothelial cells. Meningothelial type meningiomas are composed of polyhedral cells that form small nodules in which the cells wrap around more centrally lo-cated ones, forming densely packed whorls. Psammomatous meningiomas have numerous calcific (psammoma) bodies in the center of the meningothelial whorls. The meningothelial cells have uniform, small, oval nuclei that lack prominent nucleoli (figs. 8-15, 8-16). A highly characteristic feature is the presence of intranuclear vacuoles of herniated cytoplasm. Mitotic activity is rare and mitotic figures are usually not seen.

The arachnoidal trabeculae and vessels of the meninges are of mesodermal origin and may give rise to fibroblastic, angioblastic, or transitional (containing meningothelial and fibroblastic features) meningiomas, but these types of meningiomas are extremely rare in the optic nerve. Fibrous histiocytomas and hemangiopericytomas arise much more commonly from the soft tissues of the orbit and may be mistaken for meningiomas.

SECONDARY AND METASTATIC OPTIC NERVE TUMORS

Secondary optic nerve tumors are more common than primary tumors (33). This statistic is slightly deceptive because almost all of the secondary tumors represent optic nerve invasion by either uveal melanoma or retinoblastoma. In the case of uveal melanoma, the optic nerve invasion is usually confined to the optic nerve head and is of little clinical significance. In the case of retinoblastoma, invasion of the optic nerve represents the pathway by which retinoblastoma spreads to the brain, killing the patient. The optic nerve is frequently involved in leukemia. In a series based on autopsy findings, Kincaid and Green (34) reported optic nerve involvement in 18 percent and 16 percent of patients with acute and chronic leukemia, respectively. Most lymphomas of the optic nerve probably represent primary tumors or extensions from ocular or intracranial primaries. Hematogenous metastasis of solid tumors to the optic nerve are rare. Most are carcinomas usually from breast or lung (33).

REFERENCES

General References

Azar-Kia B, Naheedy MH, Elias DA, Mafee MF, Fine M. Optic nerve tumors: role of magnetic resonance imaging and computed tomography. Radiol Clin North Am 1987;25:561–82.

Eggers H, Jakobiec FA, Jones IS. Tumors of the optic nerve. Doc Ophthalmol 1976;41:43–128.

Fine BS, Yanoff M. Ocular histology: a text and atlas. 2nd ed. Hagerstown, Md.: Harper and Row, 1979:271–88.

Glaser JS, Shipkin PM. Visual sensory system. In Jakobiec FA, ed. Ocular anatomy, embryology and teratology. Philadelphia: Harper and Row, 1982:869–84.

Henderson JW. Orbital tumors. 2nd ed. New York: B. C. Decker, 1980.

Jakobiec FA. Ocular and adnexal tumors. Birmingham, Ala.: Aesculapius Publishing Company, 1978.

_____, Depot MJ, Kennerdell JS, et al. Combined clinical and computed tomographic diagnosis of orbital glioma and meningioma. Ophthalmology 1985;91:137–55.

_____, Font RL. Orbit. In: Spencer WH, ed. Ophthalmic pathology. An atlas and textbook. 3rd ed. Philadelphia: WB Saunders, 1985:2459–860.

Kennedy RE. An evaluation of 820 orbital cases. Trans Am Ophthalmol Soc 1984;82:134–57.

Marquardt MD, Zimmerman LE. Histopathology of meningiomas and gliomas of the optic nerve. Hum Pathol 1982;13:226–35.

Spencer WH. Optic nerve. In: Spencer WH, ed. Ophthalmic pathology. An atlas and textbook. 3rd ed. Philadelphia: WB Saunders, 1985:2409–45.

Classification and Frequency

1. Henderson JW. Orbital tumors. 2nd ed. New York: B. C. Decker, 1980.

Melanocytoma

2. Howard GM, Forrest AW. Incidence and location of melanocytomas. Arch Ophthalmol 1967;77:61–6.
3. Shammas HJ, Minckler DS, Hulquist R, Sherins RS. Melanocytoma of the ciliary body. Ann Ophthalmol 1981;13:1381–3.
4. Shields JA. Melanocytoma of the optic nerve head: a review. Int Ophthalmol 1978;1:31-7.
5. _____, Augsburger JJ, Bernardino V Jr, Eller AW, Kulczycki E. Melanocytoma of the ciliary body and iris. Am J Ophthalmol 1980;89:632–5.
6. Zimmerman LE. Melanocytes, melanocytic nevi, and melanocytomas (The Jonas S. Friedenwald Memorial Lecture). Invest Ophthalmol 1965;4:11–41.
7. _____, Garron LK. Melanocytoma of the optic disc. Int Ophthalmol Clin 1962;2:431–40.

Malignant Melanoma

8. Spencer WH. Optic nerve. In: Spencer WH, ed. Ophthalmic pathology. An atlas and textbook. 3rd ed. Philadelphia: WB Saunders, 1985:2409–45.

Juvenile Pilocytic Astrocytoma

9. Bilgic S, Erbengi A, Tinaztepe B, Onol B. Optic glioma of childhood: clinical, histopathological, and histochemical observations. Br J Ophthalmol 1989;73:832–7.

10. Borit A, Richardson EP Jr. The biological and clinical behavior of pilocytic astrocytomas of the optic pathways. Brain 1982;105:161–87.
11. Cooling M, Wright JE. Arachnoid hyperplasia in optic nerve glioma: confusion with orbital meningioma. Br J Ophthalmol 1979;63:596–9.
12. Henderson JW. Orbital tumors. 2nd ed. New York: B. C. Decker, 1980.
13. Jakobiec FA, Depot MJ, Kennerdell JS, et al. Combined clinical and computed tomographic diagnosis of orbital glioma and meningioma. Ophthalmology 1985;91:137–55.
14. _____, Font RL. Orbit. In: Spencer WH, ed. Ophthalmic pathology. An atlas and textbook. 3rd ed. Philadelphia: WB Saunders, 1985:2459–860.
15. Kennedy RE. An evaluation of 820 orbital cases. Trans Am Ophthalmol Soc 1984;82:134–57.
16. Rush JA, Younge BR, Campbell RJ, MacCarty CS. Optic glioma: long term follow-up of 85 histopathologically verified cases. Ophthalmology 1982;89:1213–9.
17. Seiff SR, Brodsky MC, MacDonald G, Berg BO, Howes EL Jr, Hoyt WF. Orbital optic glioma in neurofibromatosis. Magnetic resonance diagnosis of perineural arachnoidal gliomatosis. Arch Ophthalmol 1987;105:1689–92.
18. Stern J, Jakobiec FA, Housepian EM. The architecture of optic nerve gliomas with and without neurofibromatosis. Arch Ophthalmol 1980;98:505–11.
19. Yanoff M, Davis RL, Zimmerman LE. Juvenile pilocytic astrocytoma ("glioma") of the optic nerve: clinicopathologic study of sixty-three cases. In: Jakobiec FA, ed. Ocular and adnexal tumors. Birmingham, Ala.: Aesculapius Publishing Company, 1978:685–707.

Malignant Astrocytomas

20. Hamilton AM, Garner A, Tripathi RC, Sanders MD. Malignant optic nerve glioma: report of a case with electron microscope study. Br J Ophthalmol 1973; 57:253–64.
21. Harper CG, Stewart-Wynne EG. Malignant optic gliomas in adults. Arch Neurol 1978;35:731–5.
22. Manor RS, Israeli J, Sandbank U. Malignant optic glioma in a 70-year-old patient. Arch Ophthalmol 1976; 94:1142–4.
23. Spoor TC, Kennerdell JS, Martinez AJ, Zorub D. Malignant gliomas of the optic nerve pathways. Am J Ophthalmol 1980;89:284–92.
24. Wulc AE, Bergin DJ, Barnes D, Scaravilli F, Wright JE, McDonald WI. Orbital optic nerve glioma in adult life. Arch Ophthalmol 1989;107:1013–6.

Meningioma

25. Azar-Kia B, Naheedy MH, Elias DA, Mafee MF, Fine M. Optic nerve tumors: role of magnetic resonance imaging and computed tomography. Radiol Clin North Am 1987;25:561–82.
26. Hollenhorst RW Jr, Hollenhorst RW Sr, MacCarty CS. Visual prognosis of optic nerve sheath meningiomas producing shunt vessels on the optic disk: the Hoyt-Spencer syndrome. Trans Am Ophthalmol Soc 1979;75:141–63.
27. Jakobiec FA, Depot MJ, Kennerdell JS, et al. Combined clinical and computed tomographic diagnosis of orbital glioma and meningioma. Ophthalmology 1985;91:137–55.
28. Karp LA, Zimmerman LE, Borit A, Spencer W. Primary intraorbital meningiomas. Arch Ophthalmol 1974;91:24–8.

29. Sanders MD, Falconer MA. Optic nerve compression by an intracanalicular meningioma. Br J Opthalmol 1964;48:13–8.

30. Wolter JR, Benz SC. Ectopic meningioma of the superior orbital rim. Arch Ophthalmol 1976;94:1920–2.

31. Wright JE, Call NB, Liaricos S. Primary optic nerve meningiomas. Br J Ophthalmol 1980;64:553–8.

32. Zimmerman LE. Arachnoid hyperplasia in optic nerve glioma [Letter]. Br J Ophthalmol 1980;64:638–40.

Secondary and Metastatic Tumors

33. Christmas NJ, Mead MD, Richardson EP, Albert DM. Secondary tumors of the optic nerve. Surv Ophthalmol 1991;36:196–206.

34. Kincaid MC, Green WR. Ocular and orbital involvement in leukemia. Surv Ophthalmol 1983;27:211–32.

Index*

Actinic keratosis
  conjunctiva, **51**, 55, **56–58**
  eyelid, **9**, 14, **16**
Acquired neuroepithelial tumors of the ciliary body,
  retina, 145
Adenocarcinoma
  apocrine, eyelid, **10**, 28
  conjunctiva, **51**
  eccrine, eyelid, 24, **25–27**
  lacrimal gland, **217**
    arising de novo, 225, **227**
    arising in pleomorphic adenoma, 220, **220, 221**
  sebaceous gland, eyelid, 28
Adenoid cystic carcinoma, lacrimal gland, **217**, 222, **222–226**
Adenoma
  coronal (Fuchs), ciliary epithelium, 145
  oncocytic, conjunctiva, 69, **70, 71**
  oxyphilic, conjunctiva, 69, **70, 71**
  pigmented ciliary epithelium, 148, **149**
  retinal pigmented epithelium, 148
  nonpigmented ciliary epithelium, 145
Adnexal carcinoma, eyelid, 38
Adnexal tumors, conjunctiva, 69
  oncocytoma, 69, **70, 71**
Alveolar rhabdomyosarcoma, orbit, 254, **255, 256**
Anatomy and histology
  conjunctiva, 49, **50**
  eyelid, 7, **7, 8**
  lacrimal gland and sac, 215, **215, 216**
  optic nerve and optic nerve head, 299, **299, 300**
  orbit, 233, **233, 234**
  retina, 97, **98–100**
  uveal tract, 155, **155–158**
    choroid, 157, **158**
    ciliary body, **155**, 157
    iris, 155, **155**
Angiofibroma, nasal cavity, orbit, **236**
Angiolymphoid hyperplasia with eosinophilia, orbit, **236**
Angiomatosis retinae, 136, **137**
Apocrine adenoma, conjunctiva, **51**
Apocrine, tumors, eyelid, **10**
  adenocarcinoma, 28
  hidrocystoma, **10**, 22
  pleomorphic adenoma, 24
APUDoma, cutaneous, eyelid, 41, **42–44**
Astrocytic hamartoma (tuberous sclerosis), retina, **101**
Astrocytoma
  juvenile pilocytic, optic nerve, **300**, 304,
    305–308
  optic nerve and chiasm, 309, **309**
  retina, **101**, 135
Atypical lymphoid hyperplasia
  conjunctiva, **51**
  eyelid, **11**
  orbit, 271
Atypical melanocytic hyperplasia, conjunctiva, 78, **79–81**

Basal cell carcinoma
  conjunctiva, **51**
  eyelid, **9**, 18, **19–21**
Basal cell papilloma, eyelid, **9**, 11
Benign acquired melanosis, conjunctiva, 78, **79–81**
Benign hemangioendothelioma
  eyelid, 38
  orbit, 237
Benign lymphoid hyperplasia, orbit, 271, **272, 273**
Benign lymphoid tumor, orbit, 272, **272, 273**
Benign mixed tumor, lacrimal gland, 217, **217–219**
Blue nevus, orbit, **236**
Bowen disease, eyelid, **9**, 16
Brooke tumor, eyelid, 35

Calcifying epithelioma of Malherbe, eyelid, 36, **37**
Capillary hemangioma
  eyelid, 38
  orbit, **235**, 237
  retina, **101**, 136, **137**
Carcinoid tumor, metastatic
  orbit, **236**
  uveal tract, **207**, 209
Carcinoma, histologic type
  adenoid cystic, lacrimal gland, 222, **222–226**
  basal cell, eyelid, **9, 10**, 18, **19–21**
  mucoepidermoid
    conjunctiva, 65, **67–69**
    lacrimal gland, 227
  squamous cell
    conjunctiva, 60, **63–67**
    eyelid, 17, **17, 18**
    lacrimal sac, 228, **230**
  sebaceous
    caruncle, 28, 69
    eyelid, 28, **29–35**
Carcinoma in situ
  conjunctiva, **51**, 59, **60–63**
  eyelid, 16
Carcinoma, metastatic,
  eyelid, **27**, 42
  orbit, **236**, 292, **293**
  uveal tract, 207, **207–210**
Carcinoma
  lacrimal sac, **228**
  nonpigmented ciliary epithelium, retina, 145, **147**
  retinal pigment epithelium, 148, **149–151**
Cavernous hemangioma
  eyelid, 39
  orbit, **235**, 237, **238**
  retina, **101**, 136
Cellular blue nevus, orbit, 289, **290**
Chondroid syringoma, eyelid, 24, **24**
Choroidal osteoma, uveal tract, **196**, 198
Classification and frequency of tumors
  anatomic site, 1, **2**

*Numbers in boldface indicate table and figure pages.

conjunctiva, 50, **51, 52**
eyelid, 9, **9–11**
lacrimal gland and sac, 216, **217**
optic nerve and optic nerve head, 300, **300**
orbit, 235, **235, 236**
retina, 100, **101**
uveal tract, 159, **159**
Clear cell hidradenoma, eyelid, 22, **23**
Clear cell myoepithelioma, eyelid, 22, **23**
Choristomas, conjunctiva, **52**
complex, **52**, 90, **93**
dermolipoma, **52**, 91, **93**
limbal dermoid, 91, **92, 93**
Chromosomal deletion retinoblastoma, 103, **104**
Coats disease, retina, **101**, 130, **131, 133**
Complete spontaneous regression, retinoblastoma, 111, **113, 114**
Congenital melanosis
conjunctiva, **51**, 76, **76, 77**
orbit, 289, **290**
uveal tract, 162, **162–164**
Conjunctiva
anatomy and histology, 49, **50**
classification and frequency of tumors, **2**, 50, **51, 52**
Coronal adenoma, retina, 145
Cutaneous APUDoma, eyelid, 41, **42–44**
Cystic epithelioma, multiple benign, eyelid, 35

Dendritic-lentiginous melanosis, conjunctiva, 78, **79–81**
Dermoid cyst
conjunctiva, **52**
orbit, **236**, 287, **287, 288**
Dermolipoma, conjunctiva, **52**, 91, **93**
Diffuse infiltrating retinoblastomas, 111
Diktyoma, ciliary epithelium, 143, **144–146**
Dyskeratosis, hereditary benign intraepithelial, conjunctiva, 53
Dysplasia, conjunctiva, **51**, 55, **59**

Eccrine tumors, eyelid, **10**, 22
acrospiroma, **10**, 22, **23**
adenocarcinoma, **10**, 24, **25–27**
hydrocystoma, 22
poroma, eyelid, 22
pleomorphic adenoma, **10**, 24, **24**
syringoma, **10**, 22
Embryonal rhabdomyosarcoma, orbit, 250, **252–254**
Endodermal sinus tumor, orbit, **236**
Endophytic retinoblastomas, 108, **107–110**
Eosinophilic granuloma, unifocal and multifocal, orbit, 284, **285**
Ephelis, conjunctiva, 76, **76**
Epidermal tumors, eyelid, **9**
actinic keratosis, 14, **16**
basal cell carcinoma, 18, **19–21**
Bowen disease, 16
inverted follicular keratosis, 13, **13, 14**
keratoacanthoma, 14, **15**
pseudocarcinomatous (pseudoepitheliomatous) hyperplasia, 13
seborrheic keratosis, 11, **12**
squamous cell carcinoma, 17, **17, 18**

squamous cell papilloma, 11
Epithelial congenital melanosis, conjunctiva, **51**, 76, **76**
Epithelial tumors
conjunctiva
benign, 52, **53, 54**
intraepithelial, 55, **56–63**
malignant, 60, **63–69**
lacrimal gland, 217, **217–227**
lacrimal sac, 228, **228–231**
Epithelioma adenoides cysticum, eyelid, 35
Exophytic retinoblastoma, 108, **111, 112**
Eyelid
anatomy and histology, 7, **7, 8**
classification and frequency of tumors, **2**, 9, **9, 10, 11**

Fibroepithelial papilloma, eyelid, 11
Fibroma, juvenile ossifying, orbit, 291, **292**
Fibroma, psammomatoid ossifying, orbit, 291, **292**
Fibromatosis, orbit, **235**, 249
Fibrosarcoma, orbit, **235**, 249
Fibrous dysplasia, orbit, 291, **291**
Fibrous histiocytoma
conjunctiva, **52**
eyelid, **11**
Fibrous histiocytoma (fibroxanthoma), orbit, **235**, 244
clinical features, 244, **245**
electron microscopic findings, 247
pathologic findings, 245, **245–247**
prognosis, 247, **248**
treatment, 248
Follicular lymphomas, orbit, 274
Fuchs adenoma, retina, 145

Glial tumors and tumorlike conditions, retina
astrocytoma, 135
massive gliosis, 136
Glioneuroma, ciliary epithelium, 143, **143**
Granular cell tumor, eyelid, **11**
Granulocytic sarcoma, orbit, 283, **283**
Graves orbitopathy, 263
clinical features, 263, **263, 264**
pathologic findings, 264
treatment, 264

Hair follicle, tumors, eyelid, 35
pilomatrixoma, 36, **37**
trichilemmoma, 36, **37**
trichoepithelioma, 35, **36**
trichofolliculoma, 35
Hemangioblastic hemangioma, orbit, 237
Hemangioblastoma, retina, 136, **137**
Hemangioendothelioma of childhood, benign, eyelid, 38
Hemangioma, hemangioblastic, orbit, 237
Hemangioma
conjunctiva, **52**
eyelid, **11**, 38
capillary, 38
cavernous, 39
juvenile, 38
nevus flammeus, 38, **195**
orbit, **236**
capillary, 237
cavernous, 237, **238, 239**

infantile, 237
juvenile, 237
uveal tract, **159**, 195, **195–197**
Hemangiopericytoma, orbit, **235**, 240
clinical findings, 240
pathologic findings, 242, **242–244**
prognosis, 242, **244**
treatment, 244
Hereditary benign intraepithelial dyskeratosis,
conjunctiva, **51**, 53
Histiocytic disorders, orbit, 282
sinus histiocytosis with massive lymphadenopathy,
285, **286**
unifocal and multifocal eosinophilic granuloma, 284, **285**
Histiocytoma, fibrous (fibroxanthoma), orbit, **235**, 244,
245–248
Histiocytosis, Langerhans cell, orbit, 282, **285**
Hutchinson freckle, conjunctiva, 78, **79–81**
Hyperplasia, lymphoid, orbit, 272, **274–280**
Hyperplasia, nonpigmented ciliary epithelium, 145
Hyperplasia, pseudocarcinomatous (pseudoepitheliomatous)
conjunctiva, 53, **54**
eyelid, 13
Hyperplasia, pseudoadenomatous, retinal pigment
epithelium, 145
Hyperplasia, sebaceous, eyelid, 28
Hydrocystoma, eyelid, 22

Idiopathic orbital inflammation, **236**, 265
clinical features, 265, **266, 267**
differential diagnosis, 268, **269**
pathologic findings, 266, **266–268**
treatment, 269
Infantile hemangioma, orbit, 237
Inflammation, orbit, 263
Graves orbitopathy, 263, **263, 264**
idiopathic orbital inflammation (pseudotumor),
265, **266–269**
Inflammatory pseudotumor, orbit, 263
Intermediately differentiated diffuse lymphoma, orbit,
274, **274–280**
Intraepithelial neoplasia, conjunctiva
actinic keratosis, 55, **56–58**
carcinoma in situ, 59, **60–63**
dysplasia, 55, **59**
Inverted follicular keratosis, eyelid, **9**, 13, **13, 14**
Irritated seborrheic keratosis, eyelid, 13, **13, 14**

Juvenile fibromatosis, orbit, 249
Juvenile fibrosarcoma
eyelid, **11**
orbit, 249
Juvenile hemangioma
eyelid, 38
orbit, 237
Juvenile ossifying fibroma, orbit, **236**, 291, **292**
Juvenile pilocytic astrocytoma, optic nerve, 304, **305–308**
clinical features, 304, **305**
pathologic findings, 305, **306–308**
Juvenile xanthogranuloma, uveal tract, 202, **204–206**
Kaposi sarcoma, conjunctiva, **52**, 88, **89–91**
Keratoacanthoma

conjunctiva, 53
eyelid, **9**, 14, **15**
Keratosis, conjunctiva, actinic, 55, **56–58**
Keratosis, eyelid, **9**
actinic, 14, **16**
inverted follicular, 13, **13, 14**
seborrheic, 11, **12**
senile, 14, **16**
Keratotic plaque, conjunctiva, **51**, 53
Kimura disease, orbit, 268, **269**

Lacrimal gland and sac
anatomy and histology, 215, **215, 216**
classification and frequency of tumors, **2**, 216, **217**
Langerhans cell histiocytosis, orbit, 284, **285**
Leiomyoma, orbit, **235**, 249
Leiomyoma and mesectodermal leiomyoma, uveal tract,
159, 197, **199–202**
Leiomyosarcoma, orbit, **235**, 250
Lentigo simplex, eyelid, **10**
Lentigo maligna, conjunctiva, 78, **79–81**
Leukemia
conjunctiva, **51, 52**
eyelid, **11**
orbit, **236**, 283, **283**
retina, **101**, 138, **142**
uveal tract, 202, **203, 204**
Limbal dermoid, conjunctiva, 91, **92, 93**
Lipoma
eyelid, **11**
orbit, **235**, 257
Liposarcoma
eyelid, **11**
orbit, **235**, 257
Lymphangioma
conjunctiva, **52**
eyelid, **11**
orbit, **235**, 238
clinical features, 238, **240**
pathologic findings, 240, **241**
Lymphoepithelial lesion, lacrimal gland, **217**
Lymphoid hyperplasia, orbit, 272, **272, 273**
Lymphoid tumors, orbit, **235, 236**, 270
clinical correlations, 281
clinical features, 270, **271**
lymphoid hyperplasia, **236**, 272, **272, 273**
follicular lymphomas, 274
immunologic findings, **277**, 281
intermediately differentiated diffuse lymphomas,
274, **274–280**
malignant lymphomas, 274, **274–280**
pathologic findings, 271, **274–280**
poorly differentiated diffuse lymphomas, **278**, 280
treatment, 282
well-differentiated diffuse lymphomas, 274, **274–280**
Lymphoma
intermediately differentiated diffuse, orbit,
274, **276**
lacrimal gland, **217**
lacrimal sac, **228**
malignant
orbit, 274, **274–280**

retina, 100, **101**, 138, **139–142**
optic nerve, **300**
orbit, **236,** 271, **274–280**
poorly-differentiated diffuse, orbit, **278**, 280
secondary, uvea, 204, **274**
uveal tract, **159**
well-differentiated
    diffuse, orbit, 274, **274–277**
    uveal tract, 204, **274**

Magnocellular nevus, optic nerve, 301, **301–303**
Malignant astrocytoma of optic nerve and chiasm,
    309, **309**
Malignant lymphoma
    conjunctiva, **51**
    eyelid, **11**
    orbit, 274, **274–280**
    retina, 100, **101**, 138, **139–141**
    uveal tract, 204, **274**
Malignant melanoma, conjunctiva, **79**, 82, **83–87**
    clinical features, 84
    pathologic findings, **82**, 84, **83, 85, 86**
    prognosis, 86, **86–89**
Malignant melanoma, eyelid, **10**
Malignant melanoma in situ, conjunctiva, 78, **79–81**
Malignant melanoma, optic nerve, 304
Malignant melanoma, primary, orbit, **236,** 289, **290**
Malignant melanoma, uveal tract, **159**
    clinical features, 165
    cytology and histopathologic findings, 179, **185–189**
    differential diagnosis, 190
    etiology, 161
        age, 161
        associated tumors, 164, **165–167**
        genetic factors, 162
        geographic factors, 161
        predisposing lesions, 162, **162–164**
        racial pigmentation, 161
        sex, 161
    extraocular extension, 179, **183, 184**
    historical aspects and terminology, 161
    immunohistochemical findings, 190, **190, 191**
    pathologic findings, 167, **168–183**
    prognostic features, 191, **193**
    recurrence and metastasis, 193
    treatment, 194
Malignant mixed tumor, lacrimal gland, 220, **220, 221**
Malignant peripheral nerve sheath tumors, **235,** 262
Massive gliosis, retina, 136
Medulloepithelioma, ciliary epithelium, 143, **144–146**
Meibomian gland carcinoma, eyelid, 28, **30**
Melanocytic nevus
    conjunctiva, 72, **73-75**
    uveal tract, 159, **159, 160**
Melanocytoma
    optic nerve, **300,** 301, **301–303**
    uveal tract, 159, 301, **303**
Melanocytosis, ocular, 76
Melanocytosis, oculodermal, 77, **77**
Melanoma in situ, malignant, conjunctiva, 78, **79–81**
Melanoma, malignant

conjunctiva, **51**, 82, **83–89**
eyelid, **10**
optic nerve, **300,** 304
uveal tract, 161, **162–193, 207**
Melanoma, metastatic, orbit, **236**
Melanosis, benign acquired, conjunctiva, 78, **79–81**
Melanosis, congenital, orbit, 289, **290**
Melanosis, conjunctiva, 76
    dendritic-lentiginous, 78, **79–81**
    epithelial congenital, 76, **76**
    precancerous, 78, **79–81**
    primary acquired melanosis, 78, **79–81**
        clinical features, 78, **79**
        pathologic findings, 79, **80–82**
    secondary melanosis, 77, **78**
    subepithelial congenital melanosis, 76, **77**
Melanosis oculi, 76, 162, **162–164**
Meningioma, optic nerve, **300,** 309, **310–313**
    clinical features, 312
    pathologic findings, 314
Meningioma, secondary orbit, **236** 309, **312**
Merkel cell carcinoma, eyelid, **11,** 41, **42–44**
Mesectodermal leiomyoma, uveal tract, 197, **199–202**
Metastatic tumors
    eyelid, **11, 27,** 42
    orbit, 292, **293**
    optic nerve, **300,** 312
    retina, 149
    uveal tract, 207, **207–210**
Mixed tumor, lacrimal gland
    benign, 217, **217-219**
    malignant, 220, **220, 221**
Mixed tumor, sweat glands, eyelid, 24, **24**
Mucoepidermoid carcinoma
    conjunctiva, **51,** 65, **67–69**
    lacrimal gland, 227
Muir-Torre syndrome, 28
Multiple benign cystic epithelioma, eyelid, 35
Myelocytic sarcoma, orbit, 283, **283**
Myofibromatosis, orbit, 249
Myxoma, conjunctiva, **52**

Neoplasia, intraepithelial, conjunctiva, 55, **56–63**
Neuroblastoma, retina, **103**
Neuroendocrine carcinoma, conjunctiva, 41, **42–44**
Neuroepithelial tumors
    ciliary body, 142, **143–148**
    Fuchs adenoma, 145
    glioneuroma, 143, **143**
    medulloepithelioma, 143, **144–146**
    nonpigmented ciliary epithelium, 145, **147**
    pigmented ciliary epithelium, 148, **148**
    retinal pigmented epithelium, 148, **149–151**
Neurofibroma
    conjunctiva, **52**
    eyelid, **11**
    uveal tract, **159**
Neurofibromas, orbit, **235,** 258
    diffuse, 260
    isolated
        clinical features, 260
        pathologic findings, 260
    plexiform, 258

clinical features, 258, **259**
pathologic findings, 258, **259**
Nevus flammeus, 38, **195**
Nevus, melanocytic
conjunctiva, **51**, 72, **73–75**
eyelid, **10**, 38
uveal tract, 159, **160**
Nevus of Ota, 77, **77**
Nevus vasculosus, eyelid, 38

Ocular melanocytosis, 76, 162, **162–164**
Oculodermal melanocytosis, 77, **77**
Oncocytic adenoma, conjunctiva, 69, **70, 71**
Oncocytoma
conjunctiva, **51**, 69, **70, 71**
lacrimal sac, **228**
Optic nerve and optic nerve head
anatomy and histology, 299, **299, 300**
classification and frequency of tumors, **2**, 300, **300**
Orbit
anatomy and histology, 233, **233, 234**
classification and frequency of tumors, **2**, 235, **235, 236**
Ossifying fibroma, orbit, 291, **292**
Osteogenic sarcoma, orbit, 292
Osteoma, uveal tract, **159**
Oxyphilic adenoma, conjunctiva, 69, **70, 71**

Papillary syringoadenoma, eyelid, **10**
Papilloma
conjunctiva, 52, **53**
lacrimal sac, 228, **228, 229**
Persistent hyperplastic primary vitreous, **101**, 127, 129–132
Phakomatous choristoma, eyelid, **11**, 39, **39–41**
Pilar tumors, eyelid, **10**, 35, **36, 37**
Pilomatrixoma, eyelid, **10**, 36, **37**
Pineoblastoma
pineal gland, 101
Pinguecula, conjunctiva, 55
Plasma cell tumors, orbit, 282, **282**
Plasmacytoma
conjunctiva, **51**
lacrimal gland, **217**
Pleomorphic adenoma
conjunctiva, **51**
eyelid, 24, **24**
lacrimal gland, 217, **217–219**
Pleomorphic carcinoma, lacrimal gland, **217**, 220, **220, 221**
Pleomorphic, rhabdomyosarcoma, orbit, 254
Poorly differentiated diffuse lymphomas, orbit, **278**, 280
Porosyringoma, eyelid, 22
Port wine stain, eyelid, 38, **195**
Precancerous melanosis, conjunctiva, 78, **79–82**
Primary acquired melanosis, conjunctiva, **51**, 78, **79–82**
Primary malignant melanoma, orbit, 289, **290**
Primary small cell cutaneous carcinoma, eyelid, 41, **42–44**
Psammomatoid ossifying fibroma, orbit, 291, **192**
Pseudoadenomatous hyperplasia, retinal pigment
epithelium, 145
Pseudocarcinomatous (pseudoepitheliomatous) hyperplasia
conjunctiva, **51**, 53, **54**
eyelid, **9**, 13

Pseudogliomas, retina, 100, **101**, 127, **128–133**
Pseudoretinoblastomas, 100, **101**, 127, **128–133**
Pseudotumors, inflammatory, orbit, 261
Pterygium, conjunctiva, 55

Reactive lymphoid hyperplasia
conjunctiva, **51**
lacrimal gland, **217**
lacrimal sac, **228**
Retina
anatomy and histology, 97, **98–100**
classification and frequency of tumors, **2**, 100, **101**
Retinoblastoma, 100, **101, 103**
chromosomal deletion, 103, **104**
clinical features, 103, **104–107**
complete spontaneous regression, 111, **112–123**
differential diagnosis, 127
diffuse infiltrating retinoblastomas, 111
endophytic retinoblastomas, 108, **107–110**
epidemiology and genetics, 102, **103**
exophytic retinoblastomas, 108, **111, 112**
extraocular extension and metastasis, 123, **124–126**
familial, 103
mixed endophytic-exophytic tumors, 109
pathologic findings, 108
prognosis, 134, **134, 135**
second tumors in survivors, 102, **103**
treatment, 130
unsuspected retinoblastoma, 127
Retinocytoma, 101, 105, **107**, 122, **122, 123**
Retinoma, 101, 105, **107**, 122, **122, 123**
Rhabdomyosarcoma, conjunctiva, **52**
Rhabdomyosarcoma
eyelid, **11**
orbit, **235**
alveolar, 254, **255, 256**
clinical features, 250, **250, 251**
electron microscopic findings, 257
embryonal, 250, **252–254**
immunohistochemical findings, 254, **257**
pathologic findings, 250, **251**
pleomorphic (differentiated) rhabdomyosarcoma, 254
treatment and prognosis, 257

Sarcoma, granulocytic, orbit, 283, **283**
Sarcoma, osteogenic, orbit, 292
Sarcoma, uveal tract, **207**
Schwannoma, eyelid, **11**
Schwannoma (neurilemoma), orbit, **235**
clinical findings, 260
pathologic findings, 261, **261, 262**
Sebaceous adenocarcinoma, conjunctiva, **51**
Sebaceous adenoma
conjunctiva, **51**
eyelid, **10**, 28, **29**
Sebaceous gland tumors, eyelid, **10**
benign, 28, **29**
carcinoma, **10**
clinical features, 28, **29**
histologic findings, 30, **30, 31**
modes of spread, 31, **32–35**

sites of origin, 28
    treatment and prognosis, 34
Sebaceous hyperplasia, eyelid, **10,** 28
Seborrheic keratosis, eyelid, **10,** 11, **12**
Seborrheic wart, eyelid, 11, **12**
Second tumors, retinoblastoma survivors, 102, **103**
Secondary melanosis, conjunctiva, **51,** 77, **78**
Secondary lymphomas, uvea, 204, **274**
Secondary tumors
    optic nerve, 312
    orbit, 292, **293, 309,** 312
Seminoma, metastatic, orbit, **236**
Senile keratosis, **9**
    conjunctiva, 55, **56–58**
    eyelid, 14, **16**
Senile sebaceous nevus, eyelid, 28
Senile verruca, eyelid, 11, **12**
Sinus histiocytosis with massive lymphadenopathy, orbit,
    236, 285, **286**
Small cell neuroepithelial tumor, eyelid, 41, **42–44**
Soft tissue tumors
    conjunctiva, **51,** 88
    eyelid, **11,** 38
    orbit, 237, **238–262**
Solar keratosis
    conjunctiva, 55, **56–58**
    eyelid, 14, **16**
Squamous cell carcinoma
    conjunctiva, **51,** 60, **63–67**
    eyelid, 17, **17, 18**
Squamous cell papilloma
    conjunctiva, **51,** 52, **53**
    eyelid, **9,** 11
    lacrimal sac, 228, **230**

Strawberry nevus, eyelid, 38
Subepithelial congenital melanosis, conjunctiva, 76, **77**
Superficial spreading melanoma, conjunctiva, 78

Teratoma, orbit, **236,** 288, **288, 289**
Teratoneuroma, ciliary body, 143
Toxocara canis endophthalmitis, retina, **101,** 127, **128, 129**
Trabecular carcinoma of the skin, eyelid, 41, **42–44**
Trichilemmoma, eyelid, **10,** 36, **37**
Trichoepithelioma, eyelid, **10,** 35, **36**
Trichofolliculoma, eyelid, **10,** 35
Trilateral retinoblastoma, 102

Unsuspected retinoblastoma, 127
Uveal tract, **207**
    anatomy and histology, 155, **155, 158**
    classification and frequency of tumors, **2,** 159, **159**

Vascular tumors, retina
    angiomatosis retinae, 136, **137**
    cavernous hemangioma, 137
Von Hippel-Lindau syndrome, retina, 136, **137**

Well-differentiated diffuse lymphomas, orbit, 274,
    274–280
Well-differentiated lymphoplasmacytic lymphoma, orbit,
    279, **279, 280**
Well-differentiated small lymphocytic lymphoma,
    uveal tract, 204, **274**

Xanthogranuloma, juvenile, uveal tract, 202, **204–206**
Xanthomatous lesions, eyelid, **11**

Zeis gland carcinoma, eyelid, 28, **32**

✧ ✧ ✧